Borderline Personality Disorder

Editors

FRANK E. YEOMANS
KENNETH N. LEVY

PSYCHIATRIC CLINICS
OF NORTH AMERICA

www.psych.theclinics.com

Consulting Editor
HARSH K. TRIVEDI

December 2018 • Volume 41 • Number 4

ELSEVIER

1600 John F. Kennedy Boulevard • Suite 1800 • Philadelphia, Pennsylvania, 19103-2899

http://www.theclinics.com

PSYCHIATRIC CLINICS OF NORTH AMERICA Volume 41, Number 4
December 2018 ISSN 0193-953X, ISBN-13: 978-0-323-64213-2

Editor: Lauren Boyle
Developmental Editor: Kristen Helm

Psychiatric Clinics of North America (ISSN 0193-953X) is published quarterly by Elsevier Inc., 360 Park Avenue South, New York, NY 10010-1710. Months of issue are March, June, September, and December. Business and Editorial Offices: 1600 John F. Kennedy Blvd., Suite 1800, Philadelphia, PA 19103-2899. Periodicals postage paid at New York, NY and additional mailing offices. Subscription prices are $321.00 per year (US individuals), $666.00 per year (US institutions), $100.00 per year (US students/residents), $391.00 per year (Canadian individuals), $460.00 per year (international individuals), $838.00 per year (Canadian & international institutions), and $220.00 per year (Canadian & international students/residents). Foreign air speed delivery is included in all *Clinics*' subscription prices. All prices are subject to change without notice. **POSTMASTER:** Send address changes to *Psychiatric Clinics of North America*, Elsevier Health Sciences Division, Subscription Customer Service, 3251 Riverport Lane, Maryland Heights, MO 63043. **Customer Service: 1-800-654-2452 (US). From outside the United States, call 1-314-447-8871. Fax: 1-314-447-8029. E-mail: journalscustomerservice-usa@elsevier.com (for print support)** and **journalsonline support-usa@elsevier.com (for online support).**

Reprints. For copies of 100 or more, of articles in this publication, please contact the Commercial Reprints Department, Elsevier Inc., 360 Park Avenue South, New York, New York 10010-1710. Tel.: 212-633-3874, Fax: 212-633-3820, E-mail: reprints@elsevier.com.

Psychiatric Clinics of North America is covered in *MEDLINE/PubMed (Index Medicus)*, *Current Contents/Social and Behavioral Sciences*, *Social Science Citation Index*, *Embase/Excerpta Medica,* and PsycINFO.

Contributors

CONSULTING EDITOR

HARSH K. TRIVEDI, MD, MBA
President and CEO, Sheppard Pratt Health System, Baltimore, Maryland, USA

EDITORS

FRANK E. YEOMANS, MD, PhD
Clinical Associate Professor of Psychiatry, Director of Training, The Personality Disorders Institute, Weill Cornell Medical College, Adjunct Associate Professor, Columbia Center for Psychoanalysis, New York, New York, USA

KENNETH N. LEVY, PhD
Licensed Psychologist, Associate Professor, Department of Psychology, The Pennsylvania State University, University Park, Pennsylvania; Associate Director of Research, The Personality Disorders Institute, Weill Cornell Medical College, New York, New York, USA

AUTHORS

ANTHONY BATEMAN, MA, FRCPsych
Consultant to the Anna Freud National Centre for Children and Families and Visiting Professor, University College London, Mentalization Training Unit, Saint Ann's Hospital, North London, United Kingdom

JOSEPH BEENEY, PhD
Department of Psychiatry, University of Pittsburgh, Pittsburgh, Pennsylvania, USA

ANNA BUCHHEIM, PhD
Full Professor, Chair of Clinical Psychology, Institute of Psychology, University of Innsbruck, Innsbruck, Austria

ANDREA BULBENA-CABRÉ, MD, PhD
Department of Psychiatry, Icahn School of Medicine at Mount Sinai, New York, New York, USA; Mental Illness Research Education and Clinical Centers, VA Bronx Health Care System, Bronx, New York, USA; Department of Psychiatry and Forensic Medicine, Autonomous University of Barcelona (UAB), Barcelona, Cataluña, Spain

EVE CALIGOR, MD
Columbia University Center for Psychoanalytic Training and Research, Clinical Professor of Psychiatry, Columbia University College of Physicians and Surgeons, New York, New York, USA

JOHN F. CLARKIN, PhD
Clinical Professor of Psychology in Psychiatry, The Personality Disorders Institute, Weill Cornell Medical College, New York, New York, USA

TRACY CLOUTHIER, MS
Department of Psychology, The Pennsylvania State University, University Park, Pennsylvania, USA; Department of Psychiatry, Upstate Medical University, Syracuse, New York, USA

DIANA DIAMOND, PhD
Professor, City University of New York, Doctoral Program, Senior Fellow, The Personality Disorders Institute, Weill Cornell Medical Center, Adjunct Professor, New York University, New York, New York, USA

WILLIAM D. ELLISON, PhD
Assistant Professor, Department of Psychology, Trinity University, San Antonio, Texas, USA

KARIN ENSINK, PhD
Professor, School of Psychology, Laval University, Quebec, Quebec, Canada

ERIC A. FERTUCK, PhD
Department of Psychology, The City College of the City University of New York, New York, New York, USA

STEPHANIE FISCHER
Department of Psychology, The City College of the City University of New York, New York, New York, USA

MARIANNE GOODMAN, MD
Department of Psychiatry, Icahn School of Medicine at Mount Sinai, New York, New York, USA; Mental Illness Research Education and Clinical Centers, VA Bronx Health Care System, Bronx, New York, USA

SUSANNE HÖRZ-SAGSTETTER, PhD
Psychologische Hochschule Berlin, Berlin, Germany

OTTO F. KERNBERG, MD
Professor of Psychiatry, Weill Cornell Medical College, Director, The Personality Disorders Institute, NewYork-Presbyterian Hospital, USA Training and Supervision Analyst, Columbia University Center for Psychoanalytic Training and Research, New York, New York, USA

MARK F. LENZENWEGER
Adjunct Clinical Professor of Psychology in Psychiatry, Weill Cornell Medical College, New York, New York, USA; SUNY Distinguished Professor of Psychology, Binghamton University, The State University of New York, Binghamton, New York, USA

KENNETH N. LEVY, PhD
Licensed Psychologist, Associate Professor, Department of Psychology, The Pennsylvania State University, University Park, Pennsylvania, USA; Associate Director of Research, The Personality Disorders Institute, Weill Cornell Medical College, New York, New York, USA

SHELLEY McMAIN, PhD
Department of Psychiatry, Centre for Addiction and Mental Health, University of Toronto, Toronto, Ontario, Canada

KEVIN B. MEEHAN, PhD
Associate Professor of Psychology, Long Island University, Brooklyn, New York, USA; Adjunct Clinical Assistant Professor of Psychology in Psychiatry, Weill Cornell Medical College, New York, New York, USA

THERESA A. MORGAN, PhD
Clinical Assistant Professor, Department of Psychiatry and Human Behavior, The Warren Alpert Medical School of Brown University, Rhode Island Hospital, Providence, Rhode Island, USA

ANTONIA S. NEW, MD
Department of Psychiatry, Icahn School of Medicine at Mount Sinai, New York, New York, USA

ANAHITA BASSIR NIA, MD
Department of Psychiatry, Yale University School of Medicine, New Haven, Connecticut, USA

LINA NORMANDIN, PhD
Professor, School of Psychology, Laval University, Quebec, Québec, Canada

JOEL PARIS, MD
Professor of Psychiatry, McGill University, Research Associate, SMBD-Jewish General Hospital, Montreal, Quebec, Canada

MARIA MERCEDES PEREZ-RODRIGUEZ, MD, PhD
Department of Psychiatry, Icahn School of Medicine at Mount Sinai, New York, New York, USA

LIA K. ROSENSTEIN, MS
Department of Psychology, The Pennsylvania State University, University Park, Pennsylvania, USA

RAVI SHAH, MD
Research Fellow, Laboratory for the Study of Adult Development, McLean Hospital, Belmont, Massachusetts, USA; Department of Psychiatry, Harvard Medical School, Boston, Massachusetts, USA

CARLA SHARP, PhD
Department of Psychology, University of Houston, Houston, Texas, USA

BARRY L. STERN, PhD
Columbia University Center for Psychoanalytic Training and Research, Associate Clinical Professor of Medical Psychology (in Psychiatry), Columbia University College of Physicians and Surgeons, New York, New York, USA

CHRISTINA M. TEMES, PhD
Clinical and Research Fellow, Department of Psychiatry, McLean Hospital, Harvard Medical School, Belmont, Massachusetts, USA

PAULA TUSIANI-ENG, LMSW, MDiv
Executive Director, Emotions Matter, Inc, Garden City, New York, USA

SALOME VANWOERDEN, MA
Department of Psychology, University of Houston, Houston, Texas, USA

KIANA WALL, BA
Department of Psychology, University of Houston, Houston, Texas, USA

ALAN S. WEINER, PhD
Clinical Assistant Professor of Psychology in Psychiatry, The Personality Disorders Institute, Weill Cornell Medical College, White Plains, New York, USA

FRANK E. YEOMANS, MD, PhD
Clinical Associate Professor of Psychiatry, Director of Training, The Personality Disorders Institute, Weill Cornell Medical College, Adjunct Associate Professor, Columbia Center for Psychoanalysis, New York, New York, USA

MARY C. ZANARINI, EdD
Director, Laboratory for the Study of Adult Development, McLean Hospital, Belmont, Massachusetts, USA; Professor of Psychology, Department of Psychiatry, Harvard Medical School, Boston, Massachusetts, USA

MARK ZIMMERMAN, MD
Professor, Department of Psychiatry and Human Behavior, The Warren Alpert Medical School of Brown University, Rhode Island Hospital, Providence, Rhode Island, USA

GILLIAN ZIPURSKY
Department of Psychiatry, Icahn School of Medicine at Mount Sinai, New York, New York, USA

Contents

> This rich and comprehensive set of studies on the borderline personality disorder presents the reader with an up-to-date review of new findings and developments in our understanding of this serious and highly prevalent condition. It also outlines areas of controversies and open questions regarding conceptual models, psychopathology, genetic and environmental etiologic features, neurobiology, and treatment.

> The first of this two-part review evaluates the major approaches to conceptualizing Borderline Personality Disorder (BPD), from the traditional DSM diagnosis through the more recent Alternative Model in DSM-5, and the research domain criteria (RDoC) initiative responding to limitations of the DSM. While addressing the shortcomings of the DSM, the utilization of these alternative approaches has at times been reductive to specific (biological or trait) dimensions, in isolation from contextual interactions with one's sense of self affectively relating to an interpersonal environment. We highlight a number of emerging models that best conceptualize BPD as an emergent self in relational contexts.

> The second of this two-part review surveys social cognitive research findings to argue for a greater focus on a process approach to conceptualizing Borderline Personality Disorder (BPD). These studies highlight contextual aspects of the pathology, specifically the affective and relational conditions under which BPD features may become evident. Diffusely defined constructs that have been evaluated in BPD are teased apart, to identify at what level in a complex social cognitive process the pathology may emerge. Implications for future models are discussed, including the centrality of understanding BPD as an emergent phenomenon that cannot be reduced to single explanatory dimensions.

> Several studies of the prevalence of borderline personality disorder in community and clinical settings have been carried out to date. Although

results vary according to sampling method and assessment method, median point prevalence is roughly 1%, with higher or lower rates in certain community subpopulations. In clinical settings, the prevalence is around 10% to 12% in outpatient psychiatric clinics and 20% to 22% among inpatient clinics. Further research is needed to identify the prevalence and correlates of borderline personality disorder in other clinical settings (eg, primary care) and to investigate the impact of demographic variables on borderline personality disorder prevalence.

Differential Diagnosis of Borderline Personality Disorder

Joel Paris

Borderline personality disorder (BPD) has a wide range of symptoms and clinical features that overlap with other diagnostic categories. Diagnosis is important because different disorders respond to different forms of treatment. Differential diagnosis is particularly relevant for distinguishing BPD from bipolar spectrum disorders, requiring a careful evaluation of affective instability and hypomania. BPD may also be confused with major depression, schizophrenia, attention-deficit/hyperactivity disorder, and posttraumatic stress disorder.

Comorbidity of Borderline Personality Disorder: Current Status and Future Directions

Ravi Shah and Mary C. Zanarini

Patients with borderline personality disorder have high rates of comorbid mood, anxiety, substance use, and eating disorders. The longitudinal studies conducted on borderline patients over 10 years of prospective follow-up suggest that patients with borderline personality disorder experienced declining rates of Axis I disorders over time, but the rates of these disorders remained high compared with those with other personality disorders. In addition, patients whose borderline personality disorder remitted over time experienced a substantial decline in all comorbid Axis I disorders, but those whose borderline personality disorder did not remit over time, reported stable rates of comorbid disorders.

An Object-Relations Based Model for the Assessment of Borderline Psychopathology

Barry L. Stern, Eve Caligor, Susanne Hörz-Sagstetter, and John F. Clarkin

The authors describe an object-relations based model drawing on the work of Kernberg and colleagues for the assessment of borderline pathology. The substrate of internal object relations that constitutes borderline pathology internally or structurally is described and a model for assessing such pathology in a clinical interview format focusing on identity, defensive style, and quality of object relations is presented. Two clinical examples illustrate how these data can be compiled for purposes of psychodynamic case formulation and decisions about psychodynamic treatment.

The Borderline personality disorder (BPD) diagnosis has its origins in the concept of borderline personality organization (BPO). BPO is rooted in psychoanalytic object relations theory (ORT) which conceptualizes BPD and BPO to exhibit a propensity to view significant others as either idealized or persecutory (splitting) and a trait-like paranoid view of interpersonal relations. From the ORT model, those with BPD think that they will ultimately be betrayed, abandoned, or neglected by significant others, despite periodic idealizations. This article synthesizes the extant literature splitting and trust impairments in BPD, identifies avenues for further investigation, and discusses the relative promise of different methods to evaluate these clinical processes.

This article reviews the most salient neurobiological information available about borderline personality disorder (BPD) and presents a theoretic model for what lies at the heart of BPD that is grounded in those findings. It reviews the heritability, genetics, and the biological models of BPD, including the neurobiology of affective instability, impaired interoception, oxytocin and opiate models of poor attachment or interpersonal dysfunction, and structural brain imaging over the course of development in BPD; and posits that the core characteristic of BPD may be an impairment in emotional interoception or alexithymia.

Borderline personality disorder is associated with predominant insecure and unresolved attachment representations, linked history of trauma, impaired cognitive functioning and oxytocin levels, and higher limbic activations. Two randomized clinical trials on transference-focused psychotherapy assessed change of attachment representation and reflective functioning. The first showed that transference-focused psychotherapy was superior, demonstrating significant improvements toward attachment security and higher reflective functioning. The second randomized clinical trial study on transference-focused psychotherapy compared with therapy as usual replicated these results and additionally showed a significant shift from unresolved to organized attachment in the transference-focused psychotherapy group only, suggesting its effectiveness in traumatized patients.

Over the last 15 years, controversy over the construct of adolescent personality disorder has largely been laid to rest because of accumulating empirical evidence in support of its construct validity. In this article, four conclusions that can be drawn from recent literature on borderline disorder in adolescents are discussed, with the ultimate goal of building an argument to support the idea that adolescence is a sensitive period for the development of personality disorder.

Findings from decades of longitudinal research have challenged the long-held notion that borderline personality disorder (BPD) is a chronically disabling condition. Instead, several prospective, long-term follow-up studies have found that most patients with BPD experience a remission from the disorder, and many experience a full recovery over the course of their lives. These studies also indicate that symptoms of BPD wax and wane over time, although more acute, behavioral symptoms of the disorder tend to remit rapidly and recur rarely. Further, findings regarding predictors of good and poor outcomes in BPD could influence further developments in treatments for the disorder.

Patients experience difficulty in accessing the evidence-based treatments that exist for borderline personality disorder. This article identifies barriers to treatment within the US structural, economic, and political landscape and how families have created an advocacy movement to address this problem. It explores how the United States has addressed such barriers, in comparison to other countries. Finally, it offers recommendations for future advocacy to increase access to treatment for borderline personality disorder.

Findings from randomized controlled trials and meta-analyses suggest that there are several efficacious treatments for borderline personality disorder, including those based on cognitive behavior theories and psychodynamic theories. In addition, there are generalist and adjunctive approaches. These treatments and the corresponding evidence associated with each are described. It is concluded randomized controlled trials and meta-analyses suggest little to no difference between any active specialty treatments for borderline personality disorder; there are no differences between dialectical behavior therapy and non–dialectical behavior therapy treatments or between cognitive behavior–based and psychodynamic theory–based treatments. Thus, clinicians are justified in using any of these efficacious treatments.

Research on borderline personality disorder (BPD) in adolescence has helped to clarify the characteristics of BPD in young people. The

considerable emotional and economic cost associated with adolescent
BPD supports calls for early intervention and requires that the assessment
of personality functioning be an essential component in the psychological
evaluation of adolescents. Adult treatment models with demonstrated efficacy have been adapted for adolescents. This article describes the implementation of these treatment approaches, factors that frequently
complicate the recognition and diagnosis of BPD in young people, and
an overview of research on BPD in adolescents that delineates its clinically
relevant features.

PSYCHIATRIC CLINICS OF NORTH AMERICA

SERIES OF RELATED INTEREST

Child and Adolescent Psychiatric Clinics of North America
Neurologic Clinics

THE CLINICS ARE AVAILABLE ONLINE!
Access your subscription at:
www.theclinics.com

Preface

Borderline Personality Disorder

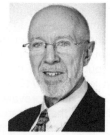
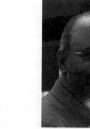

Frank E. Yeomans, MD, PhD   Kenneth N. Levy, PhD
Editors

This issue of the *Psychiatric Clinics of North America* on Borderline Personality Disorder (BPD) is very timely. Psychiatry has seen exponential growth in interest in this disorder since the 1970s and 1980s when the concept of the disorder, initially named by Adolph Stern[1] in 1938, was more fully elaborated, most particularly by Otto Kernberg[2] and Gunderson and Singer.[3] Those authors developed, respectively, a more psychoanalytic and a more descriptive understanding of the disorder. In the early 1990s, the research by Marsha Linehan and colleagues[4] on Dialectic Behavioral Theory inaugurated a phase of empirical investigation that now extends far beyond research on treatment modalities. As our understanding of BDP has advanced, it is more and more clear that it is a complex condition that can be a window into understanding many aspects of human psychopathology, and even the human condition itself.

The growth in interest in BPD is evident in the increase in the number of publications on this disorder over the last years. Based on data from the Library of Congress, Gunderson[5] showed that the number of books on BPD has more than doubled since 1990 and has increased almost 10 times since 1980. From 2013 to 2017, there has been an almost 20% increase in published articles (TARA4BPD). As recent research suggests,[6,7] BPD may represent the paradigm of severe personality disorders. Our appreciation of it has developed beyond seeing BPD as a constellation of symptoms to understanding it as a state of self in relation to others that involves all levels of psychiatric investigation. In this issue, we provide a view of the current understanding of BPD beginning with a commentary by Otto Kernberg, an author whose initial contributions to the field and whose thinking has never ceased to evolve as new information becomes available to us. We then launch into a comprehensive discussion of how the field views personality and personality pathology. The issue also provides a review of diagnostic and epidemiologic considerations, including a model of assessment, considerations of differential diagnosis,

Psychiatr Clin N Am 41 (2018) xiii–xv
https://doi.org/10.1016/j.psc.2018.09.001
0193-953X/18/© 2018 Published by Elsevier Inc.

and information on comorbidity and longitudinal course. When it comes to under-standing different levels of the disorder, there are articles on the genetics and biology of BPD and on what neuroscience and social cognition contribute to our un-derstanding of the disorder.

When it comes to clinical considerations, the reader will find articles on develop-mental perspective, attachment issues, and state-of-the-art treatments for adults and adolescents with BPD. The rest of the articles introduce the crucial area of re-sources, or the relative lack thereof, for patients with BPD and their families. In the context of vibrant research on BPD and great strides in our understanding of the condition, the medical, institutional, and governmental communities continue to fail in adequately acknowledging and addressing this major public health issue. Over the last 25 years, funding for BPD at the NIH has been less than 1/10th of that spent for bipolar disorder,[8] despite the fact that BPD is as or more prevalent than bipolar disorder and the completed suicide rate for BPD is more than six times that of bipolar disorder.[9] This is partly due to an unfortunate and enduring stigma associated with patients who have been considered "difficult" and partly due to the complexity of the disorder insofar as BPD is a condition requiring a bio-psychosocial approach at a time when psychiatry has been more focused on a bio-logical perspective.[10] One response to the lack of adequate understanding has been provided by the BPD Resource Center (BPDResourceCenter.org), and similar groups, such as TARA4BPD, NEA-BPD, and Emotions Matters, among others. These organizations provide support to those suffering from BPD and their families as well as resources. For example, the BPD Resource Center's mission is to provide information on the disorder to counter the lack of understanding. As part of its mission, the Resource Center gathered many specialists in the field to participate in a think tank in July 2018. Many of those who participated in that event are repre-sented in this issue in its effort to provide a state-of-the-art overview of how we currently understand BPD and try to help those afflicted by it. It is in this spirit of bringing together scientists, clinicians, and those directly affected by BPD that we offer this monograph.

Frank E. Yeomans, MD, PhD
Weill Cornell Medical College
Cornell University
Columbia Center for Psychoanalysis
122 East 42nd Street, Suite 3200
New York, NY 10065, USA

Kenneth N. Levy, PhD
Department of Psychology
Pennsylvania State University
362 Bruce V. Moore Building
University Park, PA 16802, USA

Personality Disorders Institute
Joan and Sanford I. Weill Cornell Medical College
Cornell University
New York, NY 10065, USA

E-mail addresses:
fyeomans@nyc.rr.com (F.E. Yeomans)
klevy@psu.edu (K.N. Levy)

REFERENCES

1. Stern A. Psychoanalytic investigation of and therapy in the borderline group of neuroses. Psychoanal Q 1938;7(4):467–89.
2. Kernberg OF. Borderline personality organization. J Am Psychoanal Assoc 1967; 15(3):641–85.
3. Gunderson JG, Singer MT. Defining borderline patients: an overview. Am J Psychiatry 1975;132:1–10.
4. Linehan MM, Armstrong HE, Suarez A, et al. Cognitive-behavioral treatment of chronically parasuicidal borderline patients. Arch Gen Psychiatry 1991;48: 1060–4.
5. Gunderson JG. Borderline personality disorder: ontogeny of a diagnosis. Am J Psychiatry 2009;166:530–9.
6. Sharp C, Wright AG, Fowler JC, et al. The structure of personality pathology: both general ('g') and specific ('s') factors? J Abnorm Psychol 2015;124(2):387–98.
7. Wright A, GC, Hopwood CJ, et al. Longitudinal validation of general and specific structural features of personality pathology. J Abnorm Psychol 2016;125(8): 1120–34.
8. Zimmerman M, Gazarian D. Is research on borderline personality disorder underfunded by the National Institute of Health? Psychiatry Res 2014;220(3):941–4.
9. Levy KN, Johnson BN. Personality disorders. In: Norcross J, VandenBos G, Friedheim D, editors. APA handbook of clinical psychology. Washington, DC: American Psychological Association; 2016.
10. Markowitz JC. There's such a thing as too much neuroscience. The New York Times 2016.

What's Next? A Clinical Overview

Otto F. Kernberg, MD[a,b],*

KEYWORDS

- Personality • Personality disorders • Psychological structure • Object relations
- Neurobiology • Attachment • Treatment • Advocacy

This rich and comprehensive set of studies on the borderline personality disorder (BPD) presents the reader with an up-to-date review of new findings and developments in our understanding of this serious and highly prevalent condition. It also outlines areas of controversies and open questions regarding conceptual models, psychopathology, genetic and environmental etiologic features, neurobiology, and treatment.

The controversial nature of the relevant conceptual models is well-illustrated in Kevin B. Meehan and colleagues' article, "Conceptual Models of Borderline Personality Disorder, Part 1: Overview of Prevailing and Emergent Models," in this issue. They rightly reject the reductionist descriptive-lexical 5 factor model, and the reductionist neurobiological research domain criteria, while stressing the criterion A of the alternative *Diagnostic and Statistical Manual of Mental Disorders*, 5th edition, section III model for personality disorders. This criterion stresses the function of the self (represented by identity and self-direction), and the interpersonal functions (represented by empathy and intimacy). Earlier work had described a 3-factor model for BPD: disturbed relatedness, behavioral dysregulation, and affective dysregulation, that Sharp's group condensed into one general "g" factor practically overlapping with the BPD diagnosis, and now considered representing the severity of the condition.

But here, I believe, we have to explore further what these concepts really mean, to be able to define more accurately the "g" factor. Disturbed relatedness clearly refers to the relationships with significant others, but so does affective dysregulation, which evinces in the instability of mood in relating to others, outbursts of rage, and sudden reversal of affective responses, and behavioral dysregulation again related to

---

Disclosure Statement: No relationships to disclose.
[a] Weill Cornell Medical College, The Columbia University Center for Psychoanalytic Center for Training and Research, New York, NY, USA; [b] New York Presbyterian Hospital, 21 Bloomingdale Road, White Plains, NY 10605, USA
* New York Presbyterian Hospital, 21 Bloomingdale Road, White Plains, NY 10605.
E-mail address: okernber@med.cornell.edu

Psychiatr Clin N Am 41 (2018) xvii–xxii
https://doi.org/10.1016/j.psc.2018.08.003
0193-953X/18/© 2018 Published by Elsevier Inc.

psych.theclinics.com

Abbreviation

BPD   Borderline personality disorder

interpersonal relations that trigger impulsive actions and suicidal and parasuicidal behaviors. At the bottom, an unstable self activates inappropriate reactions to ordinary and stressful interactions with others. Clinical observations demonstrate consistently that all affective activations represent, at the same time, the activation of a relationship, in reality or fantasy, with an important other. Abnormality of the internal world of relationship with significant others, and expression of this abnormality in actual interpersonal interactions, represent the core of BPD, and, we may add, of personality disorders in general.

Here comes another major issue, not really explored in this set of studies: What is personality? How do we conceptualize normal personality and differentiate it from personality disorders? I believe personality can be described as typical individual constancy throughout time and interaction with the surrounding interpersonal world, matched with a gratifying and effective expression of one's needs and desires in that surrounding world, and a capacity to relate, to depend, and to be autonomous. It shows in one's handling of major life tasks: work and profession, love and sex, and social life and creativity. Personality disorders can be defined as significant restrictions or limitations in any or all of these fields, and usually are expressed by rigidification of habitual behavior patterns, their exaggeration, inhibition, and/or chaotic alternation. Habitual behavior patterns coincide with individual character traits, and the diagnosis of functional and rigid character traits constitutes an important aspect of mental status examination, the really significant "traits" related to personality evaluation in contrast with the conventional "5-factor" ones. And habitual behavior patterns are determined and organized under the influences of a developing sense of consistent self and predictable relations to significant others.

The article on "An Object-Relations Based Model for the Assessment of Borderline Psychopathology" by Barry L. Stern and colleagues describes in depth the diagnostic process in the course of which a patient's personality disorder can be assessed in terms of his character structure, the integration or lack of integration of his self (identity) and the integrated or contradictory nature of his internal world of representation of significant others (object representation), and the nature of his interaction with significant others. In this context, the indissoluble combination of cognitive and affective experience of self and interactions illustrates the nature of cognitive and affective clarity or confusion, cognitive control over affective activation, and major conflicts between desired and feared interactions.

In their evaluation, patients with BPD show unrealistic, distorted representations of significant others, split idealized and persecutory images of parental and derived familial representations, and evince efforts to control, derive, or deny particularly aggressive impulses related to a predominance of the fight–flight affective system. Attribution of nonacknowledged negative affect to others may be related to the rejection–hypersensitive reaction of these patients, what clinically is seen as the combination of projective identification–denial–splitting defensive operation. Patients with BPD present these defensive operations very strongly. In the article on "Social Cognition and Borderline Personality Disorder: Splitting and Trust Impairment Findings," Eric A. Fertuck and colleagues summarize the empirical evidence of splitting and trust impairment mechanisms of BPD, and appropriately stress the crucial importance of faulty emotion recognition of others as well as faulty, self-devaluating reactions in that context.

The normal and abnormal development of self and internal object relations, cognitive affect control, flexible or rigid character patterns, and related, actual interpersonal relations depends, on the one hand, on the early psychosocial environment, and more fundamentally in terms of the development of these psychological structures on their neurobiological preconditions. The general reactivity of the organization already observable from birth on is a temperamental variable, genetically determined, as well as the predominately extraverted or introverted behavioral expressiveness. Maria Mercedes Perez-Rodriguez and associates overview the influence of functional alterations in the limbic system–neocortex equilibrium as a cause of affective hyperactivity of patients with BPD, the evidence for deficits in neuropeptides, hyperactivity of the amygdala, and dysregulation of oxytocin in their article, "The Neurobiology of Borderline Personality Disorder." In general, hyperactivity of the negative affect system, determining excessive activation of rage and fear responses may be a significant, genetic predisposition to the predominance of the negative affect determined construction of the representational world, combining with hyperreactive negativity originating in insecure attachment.

Anna Buchheim and Diana Diamond review the literature, empirical evidence, and psychotherapeutic implications of secure and insecure attachment in fostering, respectively, normal and pathologic development of self and internalized object relations in their article, "Attachment and Borderline Personality Disorder." We now know that normal mother–infant interaction fundamentally ensures secure attachment, and that BPD is associated with unresolved attachment, particularly fearful or preoccupied and angry/hostile attachment. This pathologic development is also associated with a lower oxytocin level and hyperactivity of the amygdala. By the same token, an increase in negative affective reactions related to insecure attachment is a significant contribution to the tendency to maintain splitting and related primitive mechanisms of defense in these patients, and transference focused psychotherapy, which centers on the resolution of splitting of self and object representations, normalizes insecure attachment.

It needs to be stressed that, although hypernegative affective development thus may derive from genetic determinants as well as early interpersonal (attachment) experiences, the impact of other affective systems in personality development has not been studied in detail. Thus, the influence of developments in the erotic affect system and play bonding (general affiliative) system are still open questions. Independent of the research on affects, the expanding knowledge of the neurobiology of cognition and cognitive control has provided crucial information about the formation of the self-concept and the construction of a realistic representation of the external world. The medial cerebral structures are largely involved with the development of the concept of the self, particularly the prefrontal cortex, the ventromedial prefrontal cortex, and the anterior cingulate cortex and insula. At the same time, the dorsolateral anterior cortex, the location of working memory functions, also is involved in cognitive construction of external reality, including the characteristics of significant others. Affective activation proceeding from deeper and superior limbic areas to the cortex in parallel to sensitive-cognitive information from the thalamic tract determine affective/cognitive structuring of self and other in interaction during affect activation, with the consequent setting up of affective memory structures (self–object–affect) in the hippocampus.

Adolescence is a particularly interesting life period during which an increase in borderline pathology seems to develop, to be followed by a decrease in early adulthood with only about 20% of the adolescent personality pathology remained with a BPD. In the article on "Adolescence as a Sensitive Period for the Development of

Personality Pathology," Carla Sharp and colleagues convincingly stress that the diagnosis of BPD can be made in adolescence. One may raise the gesture whether the diagnosis may be extended to childhood as well: until a few years ago, the literature denied strongly the possibility of the diagnosis before the age of 18. Paulina Kernberg had diagnosed narcissistic pathology and borderline pathology in children, and it may be that the lack of diagnostic instruments—related to bias—contributes to the lack of evidence available. I would raise the question, to what extent does the relative dominance of the growth of the limbic system predating later maturation of the prefrontal cortex determine affective hyperactivity and activation of borderline defense in adolescence, that then normalizes after adolescence. Another question is whether adolescent identity crises may be confused with chronic identity disturbance (identity diffusion) and appearance of adolescence BPD.

The article on "Comorbidity of Borderline Personality Disorder: Current Status and Future Directions" by Ravi Shah and Mary C. Zanarini documents the frequent comorbidity of mood disorders, particularly dysthymic disorder, anxiety disorders, eating disorders, and substance use, and their gradual remission, in parallel to the improvement of BPD over the years. As overviewed in great detail by Christina M. Temes and Mary C. Zanarini's article, "The Longitudinal Course of Borderline Personality Disorder," long-term follow-up studies indicate that most patients with BPD experience a remission of the disorder and many have a recovery. Drs Temes and Zanarini's overview summarizes lucidly the predictors for good and bad outcome in individual cases, and the prognosis for individual symptoms: self-mutilation and chronic depressed affect. Dr Zanarini and her group have been instrumental in shifting our prognostic criteria for BPD into a positive direction. At the same time, they also communicate that a significant (40%) subgroup of patients with BPD never recover, and this persistence is associated with vocational impairment and health problems.

From a clinical viewpoint, perhaps the most impressive article of this set of studies is Dr Paris' "Differential Diagnosis of Borderline Personality Disorder," He reviews systematically the most frequent problems in the diagnostic assessment of these patients. Their depressive symptoms differ from major depressive disorder, and do not respond to the same psychopharmacologic approaches. Bipolar illness tends to be overdiagnosed because their affective lability is misread as a hypomanic reaction. Attention deficit hyperactivity disorder tends to be overdiagnosed and stimulant treatment may become addictive. The overdiagnosis of PTSD "is another fact affecting critical health discussions."

William D. Ellison and colleagues' exploration of the "Community and Clinical Epidemiology of Borderline Personality Disorder" in this issue critically reviews an impressive number and variety of studies, and concludes that the prevalence of BPD is roughly 1% in community settings, 12% in outpatient psychiatric clinics, and 22% in inpatient psychiatric settings. Clinicians often miss the diagnosis and are resistant to diagnose it before the age of 18 years, except when participating in a specific diagnostic study. Many patients with BPD show up in medical settings for alcohol and substance use disorders, multiple somatic complaints, obesity, and sexual dissatisfaction. This study dovetails with Paula Tusiani-Eng and Frank Yeomans' moving article on "Borderline Personality Disorder: Barriers to Borderline Personality Disorder Treatment and Opportunities for Advocacy," in this issue They stress that, despite the severity of the illness, with 75% of patients with BPD attempting suicide during the course of the illness and 10% of those diagnosed ending their lives by suicide or drug overdose and although we now have effective treatments for this condition, a big gap exists between optimal care available and actual care delivered in health care activities.

Drs Tusiani-Eng and Yeomans point to the lack of clinical education and diagnostic training in BPD, insecurity of inadequately trained staff, a culture of stigma toward the patient with BPD, insufficient research and governmental funding support, the cost of long-term psychotherapy, and the reluctance of insurance agencies to support treatment of personality disorders. Federal and state policies do not list BPD as a serious mental illness, and access to treatment varies from state to state. The authors list efforts to overcome the treatment barriers—research and clinical advocacy as well as the role of nonprofit organizations—and these investigators mention specific efforts now under way, including in other countries. This article ends with a list of practical recommendations for further action, worth being studied by every reader of this overview of BPD.

BPD requires treatment with a long-term psychotherapeutic approach. All the effective treatments with empirical confirmation of their efficacy require 12 to 18 months of weekly or twice weekly sessions. Although psychopharmacologic treatment has no specific indication for this condition, it may have an auxiliary function for specific situations, symptoms or complications. The article on "Treatment of Borderline Personality Disorder" by Kenneth N. Levy and colleagues provides excellent overviews of the principal effective treatments, both cognitive–behavioral and psychodynamic. The description of these treatments, particularly dialectic behavioral therapy, mentalization-based therapy, and transference-focused psychotherapy, are clear and precise, and their outcomes, comparisons, and particular emphasis are beautifully highlighted. Dialectic behavioral therapy, mentalization-based therapy, and transference-focused psychotherapy, as well as general psychiatric management and schema-focused psychotherapy and others are referred to regarding their effectiveness and corresponding research interventions. A majority, but not all patients improve with all these treatments in comparison with treatment as usual approaches. However, there are patients who do not improve, and we do not yet have comparative studies that evaluate whether specific patients do better with one or another approach. This step is next in outcome research. How specific are the effects of these treatments? Are there common therapeutic factors in all or some of them? This question is another that is being explored presently. What impresses me is that all the treatments—cognitive–behavioral as well as psychodynamic—deal with patients' affective responses to their significant others, whether these reactions are evaluated in the patient–therapist relationship as well, or not. In fact, even in cognitive–behavioral approaches there probably is no possibility to avoid particular developments in that it is the relationship that is therapeutically relevant. All of this evidence points to the centrality of the vicissitudes of internalized object relations in the borderline pathology and its treatment.

The diagnosis of BPD in adolescence may be obscured by the prevalence of mood disorders, anxiety disorders, attention deficit hyperactivity disorder, and various conduct problems. As discussed elsewhere in this article, the differential diagnosis of identity crisis and identity diffusion require a sophisticated diagnostic evaluation that is not available in many places. Alan Weiner, Karin Ensink, and Lina Normandin examine the difficulties and methods to deal with the clarification of multiple symptoms that cloud the clinical picture of these patients, and point to the importance of differentiating specific treatment effects from general development and maturation in their article, "Psychotherapy for Borderline Personality Disorder in Adolescents," in this issue. They go on to outline dialectic behavioral therapy, mentalization-based therapy, and transference-focused psychotherapy and cognitive–analytic therapy for adolescents. In dialectic behavioral therapy, cognitive dysregulation and family conflict is treated with a special module to reduce all or nothing thinking ("walking the middle path"). Multifamily group and individual therapy may be combined. Mentalization-based therapy also combines family treatment and individual treatment components and mentalization-based treatment for families is a key modality of the approach. In transference-focused psychotherapy, the inclusion of families and the specific relationship of their participation in the structuring of the adolescent's interaction with them, is individually determined. Cognitive–analytic therapy provides up to a 24-session program in which psychotherapy, case management, and psychoeducation are combined. All these programs provide contracts with parents with teenagers and show coherence, consistency and continuity.

All the treatment approaches discussed center on the evaluation and modification of internal object relations as they affect interpersonal relations, affect control, and deepen understanding and reflections about the self and significant others. All these interventions deal with the vicissitudes, mutual influences, and organization of symbolic, subjective processes that directly influence behavior as well as experiencing transformations in the course of treatment. The underlying neurobiological predisposition also may affect behavior directly, or, more generally, determine the origin and development of those symbolic subjective structures and processes. Temperament, neurocognitive development, affective memory, working memory, and effortful control are biological structures influencing personality development directly, as do the major affect system and the underlying limbic structures and corresponding neurotransmitters.

My point is that we have here a complex interchange and integration of mental functioning at a genetic and neurobiological level, at a symbolic subjective level, and at a behavioral level. This situation is complex but not chaotic and can be classified and integrated conceptually. A major problem, in my view, has been the reluctance or unwillingness to consider these 3 levels directly, particularly ignoring the structuring effects of the intermediate, symbolic–subjective level of organization. This process has resulted in behavioral reductionism: the 5-factor system that ignores personality structure and development completely, and neurologic reductionism, the RDoC: (Research Domain Criteria) system, which ignores the complexity of the central nervous system in generating the affective–motivational structures of the mind, and the cognitive–evaluative system that is integrated with the affective–motivational one in the process of interpersonal interaction. And neurobiological centers, networks, and neurotransmitters directly and exclusively are supposed to result in behaviors.

To repeat and conclude: All affects imply object relations, conscious or unconscious; personality involves behavioral organization, intrapsychic organization, and neurobiological organization. It serves to tell us where we are, what we are, what we want, and how to put all of this together, in health or illness.

Conceptual Models of Borderline Personality Disorder, Part 1

Overview of Prevailing and Emergent Models

Kevin B. Meehan, PhD[a,b],*, John F. Clarkin, PhD[b],
Mark F. Lenzenweger, PhD[b,c]

KEYWORDS

- Borderline personality disorder • Neural systems model • Interpersonal model
- Cognitive-affective processing system model
- DSM-5 Alternative Model for Personality Disorders

KEY POINTS

- The first of this two-part review evaluates the major approaches to conceptualizing Borderline Personality Disorder (BPD), from the traditional DSM diagnosis through the more recent models responding to limitations of the DSM.
- While addressing the shortcomings of the DSM, alternative approaches have at times been reductive to specific (biological or trait) dimensions, in isolation from contextual interactions with one's sense of self affectively relating to an interpersonal environment.
- This review additional highlight a number of emerging models that best conceptualize BPD as an emergent self in relational contexts.

Borderline personality disorder (BPD) is a highly debilitating disorder that is prevalent in the general population (1.4% in a national sample[1]; see also Ref.[2]). Not only are there significant health care costs associated with the disorder, but also those with BPD have elevated rates of impairment in social and occupational functioning, such as unemployment[1] and foregone earnings. Thus, the costs of this disorder are multifaceted, including the personal, familial, economic, and societal.

Despite significant public health concern and research investment in BPD, conceptualizations of the disorder have remained controversial and continually evolving. On one level, difficulties with a clear conceptualization may in part be driven by the

[a] Long Island University, Brooklyn Campus, 1 University Plaza, Brooklyn, NY 11201, USA; [b] Weill Cornell Medical College, 21 Bloomingdale Road, White Plains, NY 10065, USA; [c] State University of New York at Binghamton, Science IV, Binghamton, NY 13902, USA
* Corresponding author. Long Island University, Brooklyn Campus, 1 University Plaza, Brooklyn, NY 11201.
E-mail address: kevin.meehan@liu.edu

Psychiatr Clin N Am 41 (2018) 535–548
https://doi.org/10.1016/j.psc.2018.08.001
0193-953X/18/© 2018 Elsevier Inc. All rights reserved.

polythetic nature of the disorder as well as the rampant comorbidity of BPD with other personality and symptom disorders, as articulated in the *Diagnostic and Statistical Manual for Mental Disorders (DSM-5)*.[3] Unfortunately, personality disorder comorbidity remains opaque, potentially reflecting an artifact of a system that encourages multiple diagnoses or genuine co-occurrence of 2 or more pathologic conditions. On another level, questions about how to conceptualize BPD intersect with broader questions of what constitutes a thorough and useful model of personality pathologic condition. In the authors' prior work,[4] they have delineated criteria for models of personality pathologic condition, including substantive foundations of the model, formal structure (core assumptions and major explanatory principles) of the model, the taxonomy that derives from the model, etiologic and developmental aspects, associated assessment and diagnostic approaches, and implications of the model for therapeutic intervention.

Conceptualizations of borderline personality pathologic condition must address multiple levels of analysis, including biological systems (genetic, neurobiological, neural circuitry), behavioral traits, and varying developmental outcomes, including relationship to one's sense of self and the interpersonal environment. All of these inputs interact to create the emergent outcome of BPD, which cannot be resolved to single underlying constituent components. Not only is it essential to understand the mechanisms underlying borderline personality pathologic condition at each of these levels but also models are needed for articulating the dynamic interactions between levels.[5] In short, one needs to understand how the underlying systems interact to allow BPD to emerge at the observable level[6] (cf. Refs.[7,8]).

Differing models of BPD can be useful in understanding the linkages between existing levels of knowledge and information. However, most importantly, models can be useful in making predictions for future research, which can either verify to some extent the model or bring it into question. With these elements in mind, one can as objectively as possible evaluate the current models and suggest advances for the future. In the first part of this review, the authors consider models of personality pathologic condition in general, and more specifically, models of BPD, because that disorder has attracted the most conceptual and empirical research among the categorical personality disorders.

HISTORY OF BORDERLINE PERSONALITY DISORDER IN THE *DIAGNOSTIC AND STATISTICAL MANUAL FOR MENTAL DISORDERS*
Evolution of Borderline Personality Disorder in the Diagnostic and Statistical Manual for Mental Disorders

Personality disorders (PDs) have been represented in the DSM since its inception.[9] At that time, PDs were represented by 3 major groupings: personality pattern disturbances representing "constitutional" causes (eg, schizoid, inadequate, cyclothymic, paranoid personalities), personality trait disturbances representing unstable/stress-reactive presentations (eg, emotionally unstable, passive-aggressive, compulsive personality), and sociopathic personality disturbance representing pathologic conditions related to societal nonconformity (antisocial, dissocial, sexual deviation, addiction, alcoholism). With the *DSM-III*[10] revolution came a significant reorganization of the PD categories, including for the first time the introduction of the diagnosis of BPD. A great deal of conceptual work laid the foundation for this shift, including Knight's[11] conceptualization of "borderline states," Grinker's[12] work on the "borderline syndrome," Kernberg's[13] articulation of a "borderline personality organization," and Gunderson and Singer's[14] synthesis of the emerging literature into a coherent categorical description. This work was influential to Spitzer and colleagues'[15] understanding of the fallacy of conceptualizing BPD patients as "on the border" of schizophrenia, and distinguishing it from schizotypal PD (see also Ref.[16]). The *DSM-III* articulated for the first time BPD as characterized by instability in 4 domains: affects, relationships, identity, and (impulsive) behaviors, with 5 of 8 (and later 9) symptoms needing to be present to meet criteria for the disorder; thereafter, the use of the BPD diagnosis soared.[17]

These BPD criteria have largely been retained in *DSM-IV*[18] and *DSM-5*[19] despite the growing awareness of the problems that its polythetic approach and excessive co-morbidity presented. Clarkin and colleagues[3,20] have argued that because of the poly-thetic nature of the criteria for BPD, patients may have distinct symptom profiles with pertinent prognostic implications (ie, suicidality), and yet each meets criteria for the disorder. There is considerable comorbidity in BPD, both among the PDs and between axis I and II disorders.[1] Notably, for those diagnosed with BPD, 84.5% met criteria for at least one axis I disorder (M = 3.2). Problems with differential diagnosis as well as concerns about stigma may lead clinicians to diagnose axis I but not PDs.[21]

Furthermore, factor analytical studies have not consistently identified BPD as a uni-tary construct (see Ref.[22]). Although Sanislow and colleagues[23] found in a large treatment-seeking sample a 3-factor model representing disturbed relatedness, behavioral dysregulation, and affective dysregulation, this did not substantially differ from the competing one-factor model. Sharp and colleagues,[24] in evaluating a bifactor model of PDs that allowed for both general and specific factors, found that BPD loaded almost entirely onto a large general factor of personality pathologic condition, suggesting that BPD is perhaps better conceptualized as a severity dimension rather than a specific diagnostic category. In hindsight, this may help explain why the most research on personality pathologic condition has been done with BPD patients.

Alternative Diagnostic and Statistical Manual for Mental Disorders-5, Section III Model for Personality Disorders

In anticipation of the revision for the 5th edition of the *DSM*,[19] a radical restructuring of PD criteria was suggested. The Personality and Personality Disorders Workgroup was acutely aware of the aforementioned problems and sought to address them in a novel diagnostic system.[25] Although ultimately not adopted, Section 3s "Alternative DSM-5 Model for Personality Disorders" offered an intriguing hybrid model that combined an assessment of personality *functioning* with personality *traits*.[19] Levels of personality functioning evaluate both self (identity, self-direction) and interpersonal (empathy, in-timacy) functioning (criterion A). For example, BPD functioning would be characterized by impairments in identity (diffuse, unstable, self-critical, empty), self-direction (un-clear goals, aspirations, plans), empathy (hypersensitive, difficulty recognizing others' emotions, negativity bias), and intimacy (intense, unstable, extreme perceptions). Di-mensions of personality traits (criterion B) evaluate the pathologic trait facets of antag-onism, disinhibition, detachment, negative affectivity, and psychoticism. For example, BPD trait pathologic condition would be characterized by negative affectivity (labile, anxious, depressive, separation insecurity), disinhibition (impulsive, risk taking), and antagonism (hostility).

Conceptually, this model includes 2 disparate literatures, namely an object relations/interpersonal focus on self-other functioning[13,26] combined with the descriptive approach of the 5 factor model (FFM) of personality traits.[27] However, in practice, levels of personality functioning (criterion A) has largely been operationalized as a measure of severity of personality pathologic condition,[28] although research suggests its constitu-ent domains may have descriptive value.[29] As a result, the alternative model has been used primarily in terms of describing PDs along 5 pathologic personality trait dimensions, plus a single severity dimension. Furthermore, a modified version of this model now being considered for the Personality Disorders and Related Traits section of the *International Classification of Diseases, Eleventh Revision*'s Mental and Behavioral Disorders removes the self (identity, self-direction) and interpersonal (empathy, intimacy) dimensions altogether in place of a unitary severity rating (mild/moderate/severe).[30,31]

Although Kernberg[13] and Yeomans and colleagues[32] have articulated a model emphasizing varying levels of personality organization along a severity dimension, that organization is not simply reducible to the number of symptoms/features present.[28] In fact, a lack of integration between functioning domains (eg, severe deficits in empathy in a highly self-directed narcissist) may be more reflective of a pathologic personality organization than higher mean features along many functioning domains (ie, modest deficits in both empathy and self-direction, with the latter example having a roughly similar "count" as the former). By simplifying the operationalization of self and interpersonal functioning, the complexity and nuance of personality types in these systems become entirely represented by trait dimensions.

Several critiques have been raised about organizing PD diagnosis around trait dimensions (see Ref.[33]). Trait dimensions have uncertain clinical utility, with disparate findings regarding how well clinicians can easily and accurately characterize their patients along these dimensions.[34–36] The precise nature of the underlying dimensional structure is neither defined nor known. That is, the dimension may not be entirely normal in shape, may reveal marked steps or thresholds, and/or may reflect only ordinal measurement at best. Furthermore, rather than relying on clinician-based assessment, the operationalization of these trait domains is primarily via patient self-report with the Personality Inventory for *DSM-5 (PID-5)*.[37] The broader problems with excessive reliance on self-report data in personality-disordered populations is well known.[38,39] Although there has been limited research evaluating how personality pathologic condition may bias self-reported trait-based ratings specifically, Morey[40] found that nonclinical participants with high BPD features overestimated their levels of trait agreeableness and conscientiousness, highlighting the importance of further evaluation in clinical PD samples. Unfortunately, to date research using the *PID-5* on clinical samples, as compared with nonclinical samples, is rather limited.[41]

Stepping back further, it is important to note that trait models do not necessarily represent psychological models of the mind. For example, in the BIG-5, the taxonomy of personality is represented by the latent structure of adjective descriptors naturally found in a natural language system (ie, dictionaries; lexical model) to represent the diversity of complex human attributes.[42] The so-called FFM is a close cousin of the BIG-5[27] and also provides a description of personality along 5 well-known trait dimensions. Although the interactions among these trait dimensions describe complex dispositions that are relatively stable across time and context, there is no assumption about the cause or processes that underlie these dispositions. As a result, the clinical application of the FFM, which posits that personality pathologic condition reflects extremes on these trait dimensions,[43,44] is fundamentally descriptive and lacking in causal force. As shall be discussed later, other systems have sought to map similar factors to underlying neurobehavioral systems, thus creating links between brain and personality.[6]

RESEARCH DOMAIN CRITERIA

Although the *DSM-III*[10] revolution was ostensibly a boon for psychiatric researchers, who benefitted from its reliably articulated criteria for categorical diagnoses, researchers from an experimental psychopathology tradition have long eschewed categories in favor of dimensions of psychopathology.[45] The nonetiologic approach of the DSM has been limited to many clinical and neurobiological researchers, who have favored a focus on underling systems from which manifest dysfunction arises. This culminated at the National Institute of Mental Health in an initiative to focus its research priorities on dimensions of neurobiological functioning that transcend a given categorical (*DSM*) disorder, called research domain criteria (RDoC).[46] The RDoC approach embraces the research foci and methodological preferences that have been long-standing in the fields of experimental and developmental psychopathology.

In theory, the RDoC framework is meant to evaluate psychopathology across levels of functioning, from brain to behavior (eg, genetics, neurotransmitters, neurocognitive functioning, psychological functioning). In practice, the focus has been overwhelmingly on biological systems of behavior: negative valence systems, positive valence systems, cognitive systems, social process systems, arousal/modulatory systems. The explicit goal of this framework is to allow for the identification of biomarkers of pathologic processes that would become the basis of a future diagnostic system.

With regard to BPD, this approach would move away from evaluation of this specific PD as diagnostic entity and shift the focus toward dimensions of psychopathology that may characterize an array of disorders (ie, fear responsivity). Biological systems of focus that are most relevant to BPD would likely include fear system reactivity, positive valence instability, reward system seeking, and deficits in constraint/effortful control. To be sure, the research to date on these systems has been fruitful in elucidating the pathologic processes underlying BPD (some of which is reviewed in the second part of this review, and in XXX this volume). However, as shall be discussed in subsequent sections, it is important to note that while underlying biological system dimensions (as well as their manifest trait dimensions) can be studied and understood, their interactive process gives rise to a more complex phenotype that is not merely the sum of its constituent parts.[6] The emergent properties of BPD, the level at which clinical assessment and intervention primarily occur, have not been operationally represented in the RDoC framework as of yet.

Furthermore, findings on the longitudinal course of BPD raise questions about the contributions of biological system dimensions (as well as their manifest trait dimensions) in accounting for both the stable and the unstable aspects of the pathologic condition. Four major longitudinal studies have now shown that BPD features decline with time; this includes symptom reductions in treatment (CLPS,[47] MSAD[48]) and even without the presence of treatment (CIC,[49] LSPD[50,51]). Thus, the natural history of BPD is one of decline in symptoms over time, whether treated or not treated. This research has resulted in speculation about what precisely is changing over time and what remains relatively stable (see Ref.[52]). For example, in BPD, the remission of acute symptoms such as suicidal behavior tend to change over time, in contrast to more stable temperamental features such as chronic anger.[48] This may suggest that basic temperamental dimensions are responsible for the more stable aspects of the PDs.[53] Thus, the specific focus of the RDoC framework on biological system dimensions may demonstrate the most utility in conceptualizing the relatively enduring aspects of BPD pathologic condition, but future models need to also account for the more unstable aspects of BPD pathologic condition (over time, in interaction with the social environment).

EMERGING MODELS
Neural Systems Model

Personality is argued to be the product of a complex interaction of underlying genetic, epigenetic, and trait dimensions that are contextualized by individuals' personal histories.[6] Depue and Lenzenweger[54,55] proposed a model that describes PDs as emergent products of the agentic approach, affiliation, anxiety, fear, and constraint systems, and they have recently expanded this model to include epigenetic influences.[6]

This model is based on a neurobiological understanding of neural systems that are reflected in phenotypically defined personality dimensions, thus seeking to link neurobehavioral systems and processes with their associated behavioral systems (ie, personality superfactors). This model is also compatible with the endophenotype approach[56] (see also Ref.[57] which focuses on genetically influenced indicators of psychopathology liability). Put differently, this approach eschews simplistic biological deterministic explanations (eg, all BPD features are due to abnormalities in one system, ie, serotonin) in favor of considering how multiple neurobehavioral systems interact and manifest themselves in discernible configurations at the observed level. This model also incorporates environmental inputs that impact the development and appearance of the phenotypic expressions of psychopathology, such as BPD.

A neural systems model would propose that deviations in basic processes may underlie the development of signs and symptoms of BPD. In an emergent view of BPD, the resulting configured PD phenotypes are not reducible in a straightforward manner to the underlying individual component systems or influences (not unlike how visual imagery cannot be understood solely in terms of individual brain systems). The contribution of stress and environmental conditions on the phenotypic BPD presentation will be magnified or mitigated by underlying neurobiological systems, which over time will tend to bias attention in perception in ways that will come to be reliable and recognizable behavioral expressions. However, manifestations of underlying systems are not stable over time, but rather vary greatly according to the affective and interpersonal context.

A neural systems model also departs from descriptive trait models in its conceptualization of the interaction of extreme trait dimensions. The same stressor may be differentially affecting underlying systems due to their differential thresholds, with perturbations in one system potentially cascading into others. For example, the high trait antagonism observed in BPD may differ greatly at conditions of high versus low trait negative affectivity not simply by type, but by virtue of the interaction of perturbations to anxiety, fear, and affiliative systems under varying conditions of arousal (see Ref.[6] for extensive detail).

Echoing the work of Depue and Lenzenweger,[54,55] a recent focus on what has been termed "personality neuroscience" has sought to integrate biological systems and trait models. In this approach, FFM traits are best understood in the context of their biological underpinnings (eg, neuroticism's link to the fear system), such that their motivational function is central (eg, threat assessment) (for example, see Ref.[58]). Turning their attention from normal personality to personality pathologic condition, Abram and DeYoung[59(p8)] note, "In effect, researchers can reconceptualize personality disorders as extreme variants of normal personality traits and formulate biological hypothesis regarding the sources of those traits." The advantage of this approach is that it provides a causal framework for what are otherwise descriptive trait features. However, as previously noted, both biological and trait-based models are likely to better capture the stable aspects of BPD pathologic condition. In fact, a personality neuroscience model of BPD posits that the instability that is the hallmark of the pathologic condition is best represented by low levels of trait domains associated with stability (that is, conscientiousness, agreeableness),[59] which fails to capture the contextual and sometimes even paradoxic responsiveness to situations of those with BPD.

Cognitive-Affective Processing System Model

Although trait-based models such as the FFM[27] have long dominated personality psychology, Mischel[60] emphasized the role of situational contexts in understanding how such dispositions may result in a complex array of behavioral outputs. As previously noted, whereas trait-based models may have utility in capturing the stable and enduring aspects of personality, they are less able to account for the unstable aspects of personality, or within-person differences in behavior that are driven by contextual factors.

The cognitive-affective processing system (CAPS)[61] provides a framework for understanding how situational contexts and individual differences in personality traits contribute simultaneously to both personality stability and behavioral variability. The CAPS model argues that personality manifests as a complex system of situational inputs ("*ifs*") and behavioral outputs ("*thens*") that are shaped by an individual's cognitive-affective units (CAUs). CAUs include an individual's unique values, motives, emotions, memories, and expectancies. Individual differences in the organization and accessibility of CAUs give rise to a stable pattern of situation-behavior contingencies, known as "*if-then*" behavioral signatures.[61] The chronic accessibility of maladaptive CAUs may result in individuals' distorting their perception of a given situation, leading to maladaptive responses.

Although the CAPS framework represents an established model in the field, recent work has sought to breathe new life into it by bringing it into contact with clinical phenomena. As with trait-based models, there are notable efforts underway in recent years to integrate "normal personality" and "personality disorder" domains in a meaningful way.[62,63] A CAPS model may help account for the situational nature of the expression of pathologic condition commonly observed in BPD. For example, a 40-year-old woman with BPD presents for treatment having achieved stability and even some degree of success in her profession, and yet her romantic relationships are characterized by instability and disappointment. A trait-based model might not easily account for the contrast between her collaborative nature at work and her antagonistic stance toward her romantic partner, nor the diminishment in disinhibited behaviors as her life circumstances have evolved in the last decade. Furthermore, there may be significant value in evaluating the same trait facet (ie, antagonism) at different levels of analysis (ie, self-reported attribution, behavioral manifestation), as discrepancies between levels often provide valuable information about the level of personality organization.[32,38,64] For example, disparities between her self-attributions (ie, "I am a victim") and interpersonal behaviors (ie, verbal aggression toward the partner) may suggest poor integration and thus greater pathologic severity. A CAPS-informed model might better account for the dynamic processes that give rise to such discrepancies in trait functioning.

The clearest application of a CAPS model to PDs research can be seen in longitudinal experience sampling designs (ie, ecological momentary assessment, daily diary) that evaluate unstable and context-specific expressions of personality pathologic condition.[62,65] Such intensive sampling methods, in which participants are asked to repeatedly provide brief ratings across a range of affective and interpersonal situations over time, are particularly well suited to evaluate *if-then* contingencies in daily functioning. Furthermore, these designs are often evaluated statistically with multilevel models that allow for both interindividual (between-person) and intraindividual (within-person) associations; although the former represents individuals' average behaviors across situations, the latter importantly captures moment-to-moment fluctuations around those averages.[66] This allows for the evaluation of dispositional characteristics (ie, personality traits, diagnostic categories) as moderators of event-level relationships between situational inputs (ifs) and behavioral outputs (thens).

Several experience sampling studies have evaluated the unstable and contextual nature of BPD pathologic condition (for a detailed review, see Ref.[67]). The variability of event-level affect ratings (within-person standard deviation) has been used as a measure of instability, with more extreme affects across a range of situations reflecting greater emotional lability in those with BPD as compared with controls,[68] and lag analyses have been used to demonstrate the greater persistence of negative affect over time and across events in those with BPD as compared with controls.[69] Research has identified several situational inputs that precede pathologic responsiveness unique to BPD. For example, Stiglmayr and colleagues[70] found that aversive tension/distress was preceded by situations of rejection, failure, and aloneness concerns in BPD patients but not controls; those with BPD also took longer to recover from their distress than controls. Coifman and colleagues[71] found that high-stress relational events were associated with greater extremes in affective ratings, and subsequent impulsive behaviors, in those with BPD but not controls. Berenson and colleagues[72] identified a relationship between momentary feelings of rejection (if) and rage (then) in those with BPD but not controls.

Although this research has been fruitful in evaluating the unstable and context-specific expressions of BPD pathologic condition, much of the focus has been limited to affective situations, rather than the larger relational configuration within which these events may be occurring. This may reflect a limitation of the CAPS model itself, because it provides no taxonomy of relevant situations or traits to guide the prediction of pathologic behaviors.[65,73] However, recent applications of interpersonal theory have provided a rich framework around which the CAPS framework has been operationalized.

Interpersonal Model

At its core, a wide swath of personality pathologic condition may be understood in terms of extremities in problem interpersonal behaviors, as reflected in criterion A of the DSM-5 Section III model.[19] Interpersonal theory, with roots in Sullivan[26] and Leary's[74] interpersonal approach and operationalized via the interpersonal circumplex[74,75] (see also Ref.[76]), provides a framework around which core themes of how interpersonal situations are perceived and how individuals respond in kind are clearly articulated. An interpersonal model also focuses on the rigidity of interpersonal styles; perhaps more important than manifest style is the ability to flexibly step out of characteristic ways of being in order to respond to the needs of others and situational demands. Furthermore, psychopathology is thought to powerfully interact with interpersonal dispositions in a "pathoplastic" relationship, with psychopathology and interpersonal signatures conceptualized as distinct but mutually influential.[77] This model shares the phenotypic emphasis of the neural systems model discussed earlier, in that interpersonal and personality dysfunction are understood to mutually shape each other's manifest expression, but importantly, one cannot be easily reduced to the other (ie, personality pathologic condition is not simply an outgrowth of interpersonal dysfunction; interpersonal dysfunction is not simply an outgrowth of personality pathologic condition).

Contemporary interpersonal theory offers a useful lens through which to further operationalize the CAPS framework, particularly interpersonal complementarity, which describes the patterning of agentic and communal interpersonal exchanges.[73,77] For example, perceiving high levels of dominance in the other person (if) invites the individual to respond with decreased dominance (then), thus forming the principle of *reciprocity.* Perceiving high or low levels of warmth in the other person (*if*) invites the individual to respond with similar levels of warmth (*then*), thus forming the principle of *correspondence.*[78,79] Longitudinal diary studies have generally confirmed this patterning of reciprocity and correspondence in naturally occurring social interactions,[73] whereas chronic deviations from these patterns are thought to lead to maladaptive cycles of relatedness.[78,79]

An interpersonally informed CAPS model differs from trait models in its emphasis on the stability of personality features within a given context that would not be expected between contexts (ie, within-person variability).[60] This distinction has significant implications for how pathologic aspects of personality are assessed. Rather than a conceptualization of BPD as extreme dispositional attributes, such as excessively high antagonism, an interpersonally informed CAPS model would emphasize the stability of the behavioral signature within which the attribute is observed. For example, from an interpersonal perspective, a behavioral signature might be observed in which the individual's antagonism is contextual; such an individual may be warm only when also in the dominant role (behavior covariation) or when experiencing the other person in the submissive role (perception covariation), whereas deviations from these covariant roles elicit an antagonistic (cold/dominant) response.[65] In this model, emergent phenotypes such as BPD may be understood as those with common organizing interconnections of CAUs in response to like contexts, thus sharing a characteristic set of *if-then* signatures.

In an experience sampling study using an interpersonally informed CAPS model, Sadikaj and colleagues[69] found in those with BPD had a greater tendency to respond with negative affect to perceptions of others' cold and assertive behaviors, but also importantly reported less benefit from warm, positive interpersonal exchanges. Furthermore, perceptions of others as cold, and the negative affect this elicits, were found to predict greater quarrelsome behaviors in those with BPD.[80] This suggests that the greater trait antagonism observed in those with BPD needs to be understood as contextual to the interpersonal situation.

Although many of these findings from an interpersonally informed CAPS model have thus far been mostly consistent with common conceptions of BPD, these methods have begun to produce findings that challenge us to expand our thinking about the nature of this pathologic condition. For example, Russell and colleagues[68] have found that although borderline patients were found to evidence higher overall mean levels of negative affect as compared with controls, greater affective variability was observed with regard to positive affect.[68] Furthermore, although on average BPD patients were more submissive and quarrelsome in their interpersonal behavior than were controls, significant variability was reported with regard to agreeableness. The aggregate findings are not surprising and consistent with past research, suggesting that borderline patients struggle with assertion and aggression. What is surprising and more powerful is the intraindividual variability within borderline pathologic condition; these data point to the inconsistency with which positive relatedness is experienced and subsequently elicited, and the potentially destabilizing ebb and flow of a good feeling for borderline patients.

Despite the rich potential of these data, an interpersonally informed CAPS model gives less attention to underlying neurobiological systems from which these *if-then* signatures arise. In this model, interpersonal dispositions are understood to interact with those neurobiological systems underlying psychopathology in a pathoplastic relationship, but to date, the focus on psychopathology has been on the manifest (diagnostic) level.[77] Ultimately a unified model of BPD should transcend any one level of analysis.

SUMMARY

In part 1 of this 2-part review, the authors sought to provide an overview of prevailing and emergent models for conceptualizing BPD. Although the need to refine their model of BPD stems from wide agreement about the limitations of the current DSM system, there is little agreement about what organizing framework should guide future articulations of BPD pathologic condition. The authors reviewed and critiqued models that seek to overwhelmingly define BPD along a single dimension (ie, pathologic traits, neurobiological functioning) and argue for models to incorporate multiple levels of analysis, including biological systems, behavioral traits, developmental process, in interaction with an emergent self affectively relating to an interpersonal environment under varying affective conditions. In part 2 of this review, the authors expand upon these ideas, arguing for the need to better capture the processes by which the "stable instability" of BPD emerges as central to future models of the disorder.[81]

REFERENCES

1. Lenzenweger MF, Lane MC, Loranger AW, et al. DSM–IV personality disorders in the National Comorbidity Study replication. Biol Psychiatry 2007;62(6):553–64.
2. Lenzenweger MF. Epidemiology of personality disorders. Psychiatr Clin 2008; 31(3):395–403.
3. Clarkin JF. Research findings on the personality disorders. In Session: Psychotherapy Pract 1998;4(4):91–102.
4. Lenzenweger MF, Clarkin JF, editors. Major theories of personality disorder. New York: Guilford Press; 2005.
5. Kosslyn SM, Cacioppo JT, Davidson RJ, et al. Bridging psychology and biology: the analysis of individuals in groups. Am Psychol 2002;57(5):341–51.
6. Lenzenweger MF, Depue RA. Toward a developmental psychopathology of personality disturbance: a neurobehavioral dimensional model incorporating genetic, environmental, and epigenetic factors. In: Cicchetti D, editor. Developmental psychopathology, volume 3, Maladaptation and psychopathology. 3rd edition. New York: Wiley; 2016. p. 1079–110.
7. Meehl PE, Sellars W. The concept of emergence. In: Feigl H, Scriven M, editors. Minnesota studies in the philosophy of science: vol. I: the foundations of science and the concepts of psychology and psychoanalysis. Minneapolis (MN): University of Minnesota Press; 1956. p. 239–52.
8. Rumelhart DE. The emergence of cognitive phenomena from the subsymbolic processes. In: Proceedings of the sixth annual conference of the cognitive science society. Erlbaum Hillsdale (NJ): The cognitive science society; 1984. p. 59–62.
9. American Psychiatric Association. Diagnostic and statistical manual of mental disorders. Washington, DC: Author; 1952.
10. American Psychiatric Association. Diagnostic and statistical manual of mental disorders. 3rd edition. Washington, DC: Author; 1980.
11. Knight RP. Borderline states. Bull Menninger Clinic 1953;17(1):1–12.
12. Grinker RR. The borderline syndrome: a behavioral study of Ego-functions. New York: Basic Books, Incorporated; 1968.
13. Kernberg OF. Borderline conditions and pathological narcissism. New Haven: Yale University Press; 1975.
14. Gunderson JG, Singer MT. Defining borderline patients: an overview. Am J Psychiatry 1975;132(1):1–10.

15. Spitzer RL, Endicott J, Gibbon M. Crossing the border into borderline personality and borderline schizophrenia: the development of criteria. Arch Gen Psychiatry 1979;36:17–24.
16. Loranger AW, Oldham JM, Tulis EH. Familial transmission of DSM-III borderline personality disorder. Arch Gen Psychiatry 1982;39(7):795–9.
17. Loranger AW. The impact of DSM-III on diagnostic practice in a university hospital: a comparison of DSM-II and DSM-III in 10 914 patients. Arch Gen Psychiatry 1990;47(7):672–5.
18. American Psychiatric Association. Diagnostic and statistical manual of mental disorders. 4th edition. Washington, DC: Author; 1994.
19. American Psychiatric Association. Diagnostic and statistical manual of mental disorders. 5th edition. Washington, DC: Author; 2013.
20. Clarkin JF, Levy KN, Lenzenweger MF, et al. The personality disorders institute/borderline personality disorder research foundation randomized control trial for borderline personality disorder. J Pers Disord 2004;18:52–72.
21. Paris J. Why psychiatrists are reluctant to diagnose: Borderline personality disorder. Psychiatry 2007;4:35–9.
22. Wright AGC, Zimmermann J. At the nexus of science and practice: answering basic clinical questions in personality disorder assessment and diagnosis with quantitative modeling techniques. In: Huprich S, editor. Personality disorders: assessment, diagnosis, and research. Washington, DC: American Psychological Association; 2015. p. 109–44.
23. Sanislow CA, Grilo CM, Morey LC, et al. Confirmatory factor analysis of the DSM-IV criteria for borderline personality disorder: findings from the collaborative longitudinal personality disorders study. Am J Psychiatry 2002;159:284–90.
24. Sharp C, Wright AG, Fowler JC, et al. The structure of personality pathology: both general ('g') and specific ('s') factors? J Abnorm Psychol 2015;124(2):387–98.
25. Krueger RF. Personality disorders are the vanguard of the post-DSM-5.0 era. Personal Disord 2013;4(4):355–62.
26. Sullivan HS. The interpersonal theory of psychiatry. New York: Norton; 1953.
27. McCrae RR, Costa PT Jr. Personality trait structure as a human universal. Am Psychol 1997;52(5):509.
28. Morey LC, Bender DS. Articulating a core dimension of personality pathology. In: Oldham JM, Skodol AE, Bender DS, editors. The American psychiatric publishing textbook of personality disorders. Washington, DC: American Psychiatric Association; 2014. p. 39–54.
29. Huprich SK, Nelson SM, Meehan KB, et al. Introduction of the DSM-5 levels of personality functioning questionnaire. Personal Disord 2017. [Epub ahead of print].
30. Herpertz SC, Huprich SK, Bohus M, et al. The challenge of transforming the diagnostic system of personality disorders. J Pers Disord 2017;31(5):577–89.
31. Hopwood CJ, Kotov R, Krueger RF, et al. The time has come for dimensional personality disorder diagnosis. Personal Ment Health 2017;12(1):82–6.
32. Yeomans FE, Clarkin JF, Kernberg OF. Transference-focused psychotherapy for borderline personality disorder: a clinical guide. Washington, DC: American Psychiatric Pub; 2015.
33. Meehan KB, Clarkin JF. A critical evaluation of moving toward a trait system for personality disorder assessment. In: Huprich SK, editor. Personality disorders: toward theoretical and empirical integration in diagnosis and assessment. Washington, DC: American Psychological Association; 2015. p. 85–106.

34. Huprich SK, Schmitt TA, Richard DCS, et al. Comparing factor analytic models of the DSM-IV personality disorders. Personal Disord 2010;1(1):22–37.
35. Paggeot A, Nelson S, Huprich S. The impact of theoretical orientation and training on preference for diagnostic models of personality pathology. Psychopathology 2017;50(5):304–20.
36. Shedler J, Westen D. Dimensions of personality pathology: an alternative to the five factor model. Am J Psychiatry 2004;161:1743–54.
37. Krueger RF, Derringer J, Markon KE, et al. Initial construction of a maladaptive personality trait model and inventory for DSM-5. Psychol Med 2012;42(9): 1879–90.
38. Bornstein RF. Behaviorally referenced experimentation and symptom validation: a paradigm for 21st-century personality disorder research. J Pers Disord 2003; 17(1):1–18.
39. Huprich SK, Bornstein RF, Schmitt TA. Self-report methodology is insufficient for improving the assessment and classification of Axis II personality disorders. J Pers Disord 2011;25(5):557–70.
40. Morey LC. Borderline features are associated with inaccurate trait self-estimations. Borderline Personal Disord Emot Dysregul 2014;1(4):1–6.
41. Al-Dajani N, Gralnick TM, Bagby RM. A psychometric review of the Personality Inventory for DSM–5 (PID–5): Current status and future directions. J Pers Assess 2016;98(1):62–81.
42. Goldberg LR. The structure of phenotypic personality traits. American psychologist 1993;48(1):26.
43. Trull TJ. The five-factor model of personality disorder and DSM-5. J Pers 2012; 80(6):1697–720.
44. Widiger TA, Mullins-Sweatt SN. Five-factor model of personality disorder: a proposal for DSM-V. Annu Rev Clin Psychol 2009;5:197–220.
45. Cicchetti D, Cohen DJ. Perspectives on developmental psychopathology. In: Cicchetti D, Cohen DJ, editors. Developmental psychopathology, vol. I. New York: Wiley; 1995. p. 3–22.
46. Cuthbert BN, Insel TR. Toward the future of psychiatric diagnosis: the seven pillars of RDoC. BMC Med 2013;11(1):126.
47. Skodol AE, Gunderson JG, Shea MT, et al. The collaborative longitudinal personality disorders study (CLPS): Overview and implications. J Pers Disord 2005; 19(5):487–504.
48. Zanarini MC, Frankenburg FR, Hennen J, et al. The McLean Study of Adult Development (MSAD): overview and implications of the first six years of prospective follow-up. J Pers Disord 2005;19(5):505–23.
49. Cohen P, Crawford TN, Johnson JG, et al. The children in the community study of developmental course of personality disorder. J Pers Disord 2005;19(5):466–86.
50. Lenzenweger MF, Hallquist MN, Wright AGC. Understanding stability and change in the personality disorders: methodological and substantive issues underpinning interpretive challenges and the road ahead. In: Livesley WJ, Larstone R, editors. Handbook of personality disorders. 2nd edition. New York: Guilford; 2018.
51. Lenzenweger MF. Stability and change in personality disorder features: the longitudinal study of personality disorders. Arch Gen Psychiatry 1999;56:1009–15.
52. Wright AGC, Hopwood CJ, Skodol AE, et al. Longitudinal variation of general and specific structural features of personality pathology. J Abnorm Psychol 2016;125: 1120–34.
53. Clark LA. Assessment and diagnosis of personality disorder: Perennial issues and an emerging reconceptualization. Annu Rev Psychol 2007;58:227–57.

54. Depue RA, Lenzenweger MF. A neurobehavioral dimensional model. In: Livesley WJ, editor. Handbook of personality disorders: theory, research, and treatment. New York: Guilford Press; 2001. p. 136–76.
55. Depue RA, Lenzenweger MF. A neurobehavioral model of personality disturbance. In: Lenzenweger MF, Clarkin JF, editors. Major theories of personality disorder. 2nd edition. New York: Guilford Press; 2005. p. 391–453.
56. Gottesman II, Gould TD. The endophenotype concept in psychiatry: etymology and strategic intentions. Am J Psychiatry 2003;160(4):636–45.
57. Lenzenweger MF. Thinking clearly about the endophenotype–intermediate phenotype–biomarker distinctions in developmental psychopathology research. Dev Psychopathol 2013;25(4 Pt 2):1347–57.
58. DeYoung CG. Personality neuroscience and the biology of traits. Soc Personal Psychol Compass 2010;4(12):1165–80.
59. Abram SV, DeYoung CG. Using personality neuroscience to study personality disorder. Personal Disord 2017;8(1):2–13.
60. Mischel W. Toward an integrative science of the person. Annu Rev Psychol 2004; 55:1–22.
61. Mischel W, Shoda Y. Toward a unified theory of personality. Handbook of Personality: Theory and Research 2008;208–41.
62. Eaton NR, South SC, Krueger RF. The Cognitive–Affective Processing System (CAPS) approach to personality and the concept of personality disorder: Integrating clinical and social-cognitive research. J Res Personal 2009;43(2):208–17.
63. Huprich SK, Nelson SM. Advancing the assessment of personality pathology with the cognitive-affective processing system. J Pers Assess 2015;97(5):467–77.
64. McWilliams N. Beyond traits: personality as intersubjective themes. J Pers Assess 2012;94(6):563–70.
65. Roche MJ, Pincus AL, Conroy DE, et al. Pathological narcissism and interpersonal behavior in daily life. Personal Disord 2013;4(4):315–23.
66. Bolger N, Laurenceau JP. Intensive longitudinal methods: an introduction to diary and experience sampling research. New York: Guilford; 2013.
67. Santangelo P, Bohus M, Ebner-Priemer UW. Ecological momentary assessment in borderline personality disorder: a review of recent findings and methodological challenges. J Pers Disord 2014;28(4):555–76.
68. Russell JJ, Moskowitz DS, Zuroff DC, et al. Stability and variability of affective experience and interpersonal behavior in borderline personality disorder. J Abnorm Psychol 2007;116(3):578.
69. Sadikaj G, Russell JJ, Moskowitz DS, et al. Affect dysregulation in individuals with borderline personality disorder: persistence and interpersonal triggers. J Pers Assess 2010;92(6):490–500.
70. Stiglmayr CE, Grathwol T, Linehan MM, et al. Aversive tension in patients with borderline personality disorder: a computer-based controlled field study. Acta Psychiatr Scand 2005;111(5):372–9.
71. Coifman KG, Berenson KR, Rafaeli E, et al. From negative to positive and back again: polarized affective and relational experience in borderline personality disorder. J Abnorm Psychol 2012;121(3):668–79.
72. Berenson KR, Downey G, Rafaeli E, et al. The rejection–rage contingency in borderline personality disorder. J Abnorm Psychol 2011;120(3):681–90.
73. Fournier MA, Moskowitz DS, Zuroff DC. Integrating dispositions, signatures, and the interpersonal domain. J Pers Soc Psychol 2008;94(3):531–45.
74. Leary T. Interpersonal diagnosis of personality: a functional theory and methodology for personality evaluation. New York: Ronald Press; 1957.

75. Wiggins J, Pincus A. Conceptions of personality disorders and dimensions of personality. Psychological Assessment: A Journal of Consulting and Clinical Psychology 1989;1:305–16.
76. Hopwood CJ, Wright AG, Ansell EB, et al. The interpersonal core of personality pathology. J Pers Disord 2013;27(3):270–95.
77. Pincus AL, Ansell EB. Interpersonal theory of personality. In: Suls J, Tennen H, editors. Handbook of psychology vol. 5: personality and social psychology. 2nd edition. Hoboken (NJ): Wiley; 2013. p. 141–59.
78. Carson RC. Self-fulfilling prophecy, maladaptive behavior, and psychotherapy. In: Anchin JC, Kiesler DJ, editors. Handbook of interpersonal psychotherapy. New York: Pergamon Press; 1982. p. 64–77.
79. Kiesler DJ. Interpersonal methods of assessment and diagnosis. In: Snyder CR, editor. Handbook of social and clinical psychology: the health perspective. New York: Pergamon Press; 1991. p. 438–68.
80. Sadikaj G, Moskowitz DS, Russell JJ, et al. Quarrelsome behavior in borderline personality disorder: influence of behavioral and affective reactivity to perceptions of others. J Abnorm Psychol 2013;122(1):195.
81. Schmideberg M. The borderline patient. In: Arieti S, editor. American handbook of psychiatry. New York: Basic Books; 1959. p. 398–416.

Conceptual Models of Borderline Personality Disorder, Part 2
A Process Approach and Its Implications

Kevin B. Meehan, PhD[a,b],*, John F. Clarkin, PhD[b],
Mark F. Lenzenweger, PhD[b,c]

KEYWORDS

- Borderline personality disorder • Social cognition • Emergence

KEY POINTS

- The second of this two-part review surveys social cognitive research findings to argue for a greater focus on a process approach to conceptualizing Borderline Personality Disorder (BPD).
- These studies highlight contextual aspects of the pathology, specifically the affective and relational conditions under which BPD features may become evident.
- Diffusely defined constructs that have been evaluated in BPD are teased apart, to identify at what level in a complex social cognitive process the pathology may emerge.
- Implications for future models are discussed, including the centrality of understanding BPD as an emergent phenomenon that cannot be reduced to single explanatory dimensions.

Borderline personality disorder (BPD) has both fascinated and frustrated clinicians and researchers since a label was first applied to the disorder, in part because the nature of the pathology features some apparent contradictions. For example, are interpersonal ruptures for those with BPD a product of underattending or overattending to social cues? Do those with BPD empathically relate too strongly to the feelings of others, or not strongly enough? Are those with BPD too guarded and suspicious of others, or too gullible and susceptible to the influence of others? Do those with BPD

[a] Long Island University, Brooklyn Campus, 1 University Plaza, Brooklyn, NY 11201, USA; [b] Weill Cornell Medical College, 21 Bloomingdale Road, White Plains, NY 10065, USA; [c] State University of New York at Binghamton, Science IV, Binghamton, NY 13902, USA
* Corresponding author. Long Island University, Brooklyn Campus, 1 University Plaza, Brooklyn, NY 11201.
E-mail address: kevin.meehan@liu.edu

Psychiatr Clin N Am 41 (2018) 549–559
https://doi.org/10.1016/j.psc.2018.08.002
0193-953X/18/© 2018 Elsevier Inc. All rights reserved.

underinterpret or overinterpret the mental states of others? Clinical observation suggests that for each the answer is "yes and yes," and research findings are riddled with contradictions suggesting both underperformance and overperformance in many of the aforementioned domains.

In the first part of this 2-part review, we promoted models of BPD that are not only taxonomically sound, but also that have causal force by virtue of incorporating etiologic and developmental considerations, and that can capture the unstable processes underlying (and not just content of) the psychopathology. In this second part of the review, we survey a number of exciting recent social cognitive research findings to highlight a greater need for a process approach in models of BPD that can account for these apparent contradictions. Although this review of recent social cognitive findings is by no means exhaustive (see Eric A. Fertuck and colleagues' article, "Social Cognition and Borderline Personality Disorder: Splitting and Trust Impairment Findings," in this issue), nor are any of the studies enthusiastically discussed as the last word on a given area, the work highlighted makes clear the importance of identifying at what level, in what context, and in interaction with what other capacities does the psychopathology become elicited. The literature on borderline pathology has been overreliant on studies demonstrating that patients with BPD look more pathologic on a given domain of functioning than nonpatients, or more pathologic than comparison anxious/depressed patients: we know that patients with BPD will look worse on a lot of things; such findings do not necessarily suggest an etiologic deficit central to the pathology. Research that more specifically aims to identify the level and context of the psychopathology's presence or absence may therefore be more useful in sharpening our models of BPD. We then discuss the implications of these findings for conceptualizing, researching, and treating BPD.

REJECTION AND SOCIAL OSTRACISM

The pain of rejection is not unique to BPD, and in fact may be understood as an adaptive response to the threat of loss of social connections.[1,2] Further, social rejection does in fact cause pain; research has clarified the significant overlap in neural systems that mediate both social and physical pain.[3] Those with BPD self-report heightened expectancies of rejection, and respond with strong negative affect to conditions of social exclusion.[4] Using Cyberball, a laboratory-based computer ball-toss game rigged to exclude the participant,[5] studies have demonstrated that those with BPD respond with heightened negative affect to social ostracism,[4,6] and these findings track closely with clinical observation. However, many of these laboratory-based studies of social exclusion have stopped short of clarifying the underlying processes that result in such affective expressions. Specifically, are those with BPD experiencing distortions at the level of their affective reactions to actual rejection events, or does the distortion lie at the level of biased perception of rejection events itself? Although not mutually exclusive, these are separate processes (social perception, affective reaction) that are best understood as distinct and in interaction.

De Panfilis and colleagues[7] turned this question on its head by evaluating overinclusion in BPD, with a modified version of Cyberball with conditions in which participants would be excluded (stop receiving the ball), included (ball received with the same frequency as others), or overincluded (disproportionally received as compared with others). Those with BPD indicated greater negative affect and felt less socially connected not only when excluded, but also when included. It was only when disproportionately overincluded that those with BPD had reduced levels of negative emotions, comparable with controls. This suggests those with BPD are not just overreacting to actual rejection events, but have a negative perception bias in conditions that may be objectively fair social conditions.

This study has important clinical implications, in that it suggests those with BPD may struggle to enjoy balanced and mutually rewarding social exchanges. Average expectable social rewards may not be enough; rather, dramatic displays of acceptance may be required to find comfort in the interaction. To date, our research on and models of BPD have focused overwhelmingly on negative affectivity in BPD; future research and conceptualizations should continue to evaluate the fraught relationship that those with BPD have to potentially rewarding, mutually enjoyable contexts within which positive affect might be most salient.[8]

EMOTION RECOGNITION

Although it has long been recognized that those with BPD may "misread" social situations, research that has specifically focused on recognition of emotion in the faces has produced results that are often quite contradictory, leaving ambiguity as to the exact nature of the dysfunction. Studies evaluating facial emotion recognition (FER) in BPD, in which still or morphing images of faces displaying a range of valenced emotions at various intensities, have collectively yielded inconsistent findings; including an underattention to emotional cues in faces, an "empathy paradox" in which those with BPD are hypersensitive to others' emotions, and a "negativity bias" toward interpreting neutral faces as emotional.[9]

The lack of clarity in this area of research may be related to a failure to distinguish among the many stages along which an emotion in a face comes to be detected, labeled, and subsequently interpreted. De Panfilis and colleagues[10] sought to address this by distinguishing between 2 separate processes: an earlier detection of emotion as it begins to subtly appear on a face (ie, "Is that an emotion?") versus a later appraisal of that emotion as it comes to be labeled (ie, "What emotion is that?"). Most FER tasks evaluate the latter, by asking to choose among a forced-choice set of emotions. Even tasks that slowly morph from neutral to a full expression of emotion require the participant to detect an emotion at the point at which they can subsequently label it. This may be too far "downstream" in the process of emotion recognition to capture the point at which a response bias is most evident in BPD.

Using an FER task that has 2 separate trials for detection versus identification of emotions, Meehan and colleagues[9] found that those with high BPD features evidenced a bias toward a very quick and reflexive detection of negative affect that is not there (mislabeling of neutral as negative emotion) or barely there (accurately detecting subtle negative emotion). For those with BPD, although a deliberative labeling of full emotional expressions may be relatively intact, a response bias may be more evident in reflexive decisions about subtle cues. Interpersonal ruptures may naturally follow from this; misperceiving a fleeting negative emotion in neutral face, or noticing a subtle cue of negative affect are each best not overattended to. Fertuck and colleagues[11] similarly found in evaluations of faces for trustworthiness in those with BPD that a bias toward "untrustworthy" appraisals are made in early stimulus processing, as indicated by electroencephalogram data, and are relatively stubborn to change through reappraisal. The larger implication of this research is that our studies and models need to be precise in articulating at what stage or level in these enormously complex mental processes amplifications/deficits arise that cascade into manifest pathologic behaviors. In BPD, it may be the case that biased appraisals are rapidly made during early detection, and not as amenable to change at later stages of reappraisal.

MENTAL STATE ATTRIBUTIONS

Clinical observation and research have each observed impairments in the capacity to reflect on mental states in oneself and others in those with BPD.[12,13] Sharp and colleagues[14] (see also Carla Sharp and colleagues' article, "Adolescence as a Sensitive Period for the Development of Personality Pathology," in this issue) have found a tendency to hypermentalize in those with BPD pathology; the tendency to overattribute mental states may lead to confusion among what is likely a mix of accurate and distorted observations. However, characterizing the exact nature of impairments in mental state attributions has produced mixed findings.

In social cognitive research, a preponderance of studies have used the Reading of the Mind in the Eyes (RMET[15]) task to evaluate accuracy in identifying the mental state isolated in the eye region. A meta-analysis by Richman and Unoka[16] found (despite significant heterogeneity between studies) that those diagnosed with BPD evidenced less accurate recognition of neutral (but not positive or negative) mental states than comparison samples, although this effect in neutral stimuli has not been borne out in studies using nonclinical samples with elevated BPD features.[17,18] Further complicating these findings, those diagnosed with major depressive disorder were found to have overall greater impairment in mental state recognition across valences than those diagnosed with BPD.[16] Further, Weinstein and colleagues[18] found that greater trauma exposure, not BP features, predicted enhanced accuracy for negative mental state identification. Taken together, these studies raise the question of whether those with BPD have distinctive impairments in their capacity to generally label mental states.

However, a recent study by Savage and Lenzenweger[19] suggests that impairments in mental state labeling may be contextually elicited by social threat. Participants were evaluated with the RMET, but randomized to be socially included versus excluded (via Cyberball) before labeling mental states. They found those with greater BP features to be less accurate in identifying neutral mental states after having been socially excluded, but this labeling impairment was not observed in the inclusion condition.

Thus, impairments in mental state recognition in those with BPD are likely best understood under conditions of social threat. This is consistent with the attachment literature, which has found a diminished capacity in those with BPD to maintain reflective functioning and narrative coherence during a very activating interview.[20] In probes about experiences of loss, rejection, and pain (during the Adult Attachment Interview), those with BPD struggle to reflect on experiences of self-affectively interacting with others, to a degree not seen when discussing less affect-laden topics. In terms of larger implications, research aiming to identify broad deficits, including those shared by other disorders, may have less utility than those seeking to articulate a more contextual understanding of the conditions under which BPD pathology is more or less likely to be observed.

EFFORTFUL CONTROL

Although disinhibition and low levels of constraint are often identified as core features of BPD, clinical observation suggests that those with BPD may simultaneously be planful, exercise caution, and persevere in given contexts. In our early work on the neurocognitive characteristics of patients with BPD,[20] we found that personality system impairments were associated with deficits in neurocognitive functioning requiring control, effort, and executive resources. More recently, we have continued to explore effortful control (EC), the neurocognitive process reflective of the control/constraint system,[21,22] as a useful construct for conceptualizing the contextual nature of impulse control, particularly as applied to BPD. EC is the aspect of temperament that is involved in the voluntary regulation of emotions, cognitions, and behaviors, and in successful conflict resolution between immediate desires and long-term goals.[23] Although EC underlies the development of the self-control component of the Big 5 trait "conscientiousness,"[24] it is a broader developmental construct that reflects the relative efficiency of executive attention, including the capacities to resist an inappropriate approach behavior, start a behavior when there is a strong tendency to avoid it, and shift attention when desired.[23] For those with low EC, when regulatory resources are taxed (such as under conditions of social threat or affective arousal), the capacity to be more planful may be diminished, with a greater reliance on automatic response tendencies.[25]

Those with BPD have been shown to rely on reflexive, automatically responding networks, whereas healthy controls make more use of networks with access to higher level conscious cortical processing[26]; further, those with BPD struggle to reduce negative affect by reappraisal.[27] Thus, for those with BPD, high EC may protect against reflexive responsiveness. High EC has been found to buffer the degree to which rejection sensitivity translates to increased BPD symptoms,[28,29] and to buffer against the automatic response tendency to detect negative affect in faces that is not or is barely there.[9] Thus, in the context of high EC, those with BPD may overcome their automatic tendencies toward amplifying minor signs of negative affect (or mistrust, or negative mental states) in others, resulting in better social adjustment.

The larger implication of this research is that traits such as impulse control are best not conceptualized as static capacities, in which more is simply better, but rather are contextual and best understood in interaction with other response tendencies. In fact, high constraint may not always be beneficial, as can be seen in the debate as to whether those who delayed on the classic "marshmallow task" grew to become more successful or more fearful later in life.[30,31] However, in the context of BPD specifically, it may be the case that EC provides a necessary buffer specifically in the context of otherwise automatic (negative, mistrustful, rejected) response tendencies.

EMPATHY

Mature empathic sensitivity depends on the integration of affective arousal, emotional understanding, and emotion regulation, all in the service of goal-directed, social behavior.[32] Although those with BPD are often described as exhibiting deficits in empathic relatedness, the exact nature of the dysfunction has been unclear, in part due to the nonspecificity of exactly what is meant by empathy. Empathy is generally defined as an affective response arising from the understanding of the other's emotional state or condition.[32,33] On one hand, under conditions of threat or distress, those with BPD may struggle to appreciate others' mental states.[19] On the other hand, those with BPD may powerfully resonate with the affect states of others.

The distinction between cognitive versus affective empathy has been used to conceptualize the deficits in empathic relatedness observed in BPD.[34,36] Affectively, those with BPD may strongly, even contagiously, identify with the feelings of others,[35] but cognitively may struggle to marshal the distance to experience others' emotion as separate from one's own, leading to affective contagion rather than an empathic resonance with the emotional states of others. Blair[36] further describes motor empathy, or the bodily mirroring of another's emotional expressions. Those with psychopathy features have been found to display less congruent affective expressions to emotions is other's faces[37]; no studies have evaluated motor empathy in BPD, although as a facet of affective empathy might anticipate amplified congruence in expressions.

As previously discussed, EC may protect against such automatic response tendencies. Affective empathy is understood to be a more automatic, reflexive process; whereas, the cognitive aspects of empathy are more reflective.[36] Those with low EC are more likely to be reactive to the emotional distress of others, as the affective overwhelm may lead to a turning inward in the service of self-focused regulation, at the expense of empathically attending to the feelings of others. By contrast, those with high EC, in the context of others' emotional distress, may be able to maintain an outward orientation that empathically focuses on others' needs, thus facilitating prosocial behavior.[38,39] The larger implication of this research is that affective-relational processes, such as empathic responsiveness, are the product of a complex interaction of capacities that can be understood only as an integrated whole.

IMPLICATIONS
Implications for Characterizing Borderline Personality Disorder Pathology

The biggest challenge in conceptualizing BPD pathology may also be its defining feature: stable instability.[40] From a longitudinal lens, although symptom severity may decrease over many years, the rank order stability of those symptoms is relatively enduring, and impairments in functioning remain generally consistent over time.[41,42] From a moment-to-moment lens, there can be enormous variability in function at the level of minutes, hours, and days. Therefore, BPD pathology is best understood in terms of unstable fluctuations, in response to situational demands, within a relatively stable longitudinal course. Pathologic processes that bias perception and attention are evidenced in situations that may not be elicited in other contexts, and may not be shared to the same extent by those without such pathology. Specifically, borderline symptoms are most evident in the context of social threat; interpersonal hypersensitivity contributes to affectivity, impulsivity, aggression, suicidality, and social dysfunction,[43] and the capacity for EC protects against automatic responsivity in such contexts.[28]

Neural systems, and their trait-based expressions, are centrally related to the more stable aspects of BPD pathology. However, poor effortful control/constraint also may be related to the momentary shifts (good vs bad; black vs white thinking) that are emblematic of BPD psychological experience.[22] As argued for by Depue and Lenzenweger,[21,22,44] we believe it is essential to conceptualize BPD pathology as an *emergent* phenotype that reflects a complex interaction among its underlying biological and behavioral trait systems. The internalization of affectively charged relational experiences result in unique and unstable self-other configurations, with the final result transcending deviation on any one component or process in the system. Longitudinally, it is important to note that the aforementioned process by which emergent phenotypes both arise from and influence the subsequent expression of underlying systems over time may lead to either a "hardening" or "softening" of the phenotypic features over time.[45]

Implications for researching borderline personality disorder pathology
The unstable aspects of BPD pathology are not adequately captured cross-sectionally. Research tools and techniques are needed that can model the contextual nature of dysfunctional processes in personality disordered individuals. Experience sampling methods are advances over self-report methods that are susceptible to memory bias,[19,46] in that participants are asked to provide brief but immediate ratings following specific events or random prompts at specified intervals. Such methods allow researchers to move away from aggregate ratings of a given behavioral or emotional experience to evaluate intraindividual variability. Future research should

seek to apply further methodologies that may track fluctuations over time and across contexts. For example, real-time coding of interpersonal patterns between 2 people has been fruitfully evaluated using the joystick method of Sadler and colleagues,[47,48] in which observers record real-time fluctuations in agency and communion among dyads (ie, patient and therapist, romantic couples).

Future research efforts also need to place emphasis on capturing borderline pathology in the contexts in which it is most evident, and the stage at which it most clearly emerges. Given the degree to which social threat taxes the regulatory resources of those with BPD, studies that evaluate the automatic response tendencies of those with BPD following a rejection experience are better positioned to delineate the nature of the pathology. Even then, such behavioral reactions are complex and cascading processes that unfold across multiple systems. Researchers need to be clearer, and seek to isolate, at what point and in interaction with what other capacities dysfunction processes emerge.

Implications for borderline personality disorder treatment
The negative response biases observed in BPD emerge very early in the process of emotion detection, based on subtle and fleeting cues of social threat that may or may not be present.[9] Subsequent interpretations of these social cues are often over-determined (or hypermentalized), and are stubborn to revision even when presented with additional information.[11,14] Clinically, revising these response biases will require enormous repetition, best accomplished in the context of the affectively charged relational experience with the therapist. For example, when sharing a painful loss, a 40-year-old woman with BPD tells her therapist, "I can tell you are sick of hearing this." Given that it is equally plausible the patient accurately perceived a flash of disgust across the therapist's face, or inaccurately attributed disgust to the therapists' neutrality, a focus on whether her perception was "correct" may be less fruitful than the question of selectivity; of all the social cues available, why were signs of the therapist's disgust sought and seized on, and why now? What mental states were then being attributed to the therapist, and why an overdetermined attribution when a simpler one would suffice? In response to clarifications, this patient acknowledged that the therapist's disgust might be easier to tolerate than his empathy for her painful story, which may make the loss "too real" and threaten to overwhelm them both. Disgust would signal, "I'm over this, you can get over this too": empathy would signal "this loss is real; we have a long road ahead to address it." Empathic relatedness is fraught for those with BPD, who want to feel validated but may also fear emotional contagion.

As with our conceptualizations of BPD, treatment has tended to focus on the impulsive and self-destructive aspects of the disorder. To be sure, these are the symptoms that interventions should focus on first, and in fact all of the major empirically supported treatments for BPD prioritize behaviors that threaten safety (to oneself, others, and the treatment itself[49–51]) Further, efficacy studies of these structured treatments suggest that the most unstable and emotion-driven behaviors, such as suicidal and self-destructive behavior, can be significantly reduced during the course of psychotherapy.

However, the work of Zanarini and colleagues[42] raises important questions about improving the level of social and work functioning to the point that work is gratifying and relationships are intimate. Although the negative affect storms may reduce, through psychotherapy or over time, positive affect often remains fraught for many with BPD; this has not been a major focus of our clinical and research efforts. The capacity for pleasure and intimacy is what allows for our relationships to be gratifying and meaningful, not just stable. Similarly, functioning can stabilize to the point of more structure in one's life, including the capacity to maintain employment. However, a sense of fulfillment through one's work, even enjoyment in one's occupational activities, often remains quite difficult for patients with BPD. Stability in relationships and in employment may still fall short of Freud's goal for our patients to have the capacity, "to love and to work."[52(p265)] A 35-year-old man diagnosed with BPD states, "I can never hold onto a good feeling; enjoyment is like gripping sand, I can feel it falling away through my fingers." Our clinical efforts should focus more on subjective experiences of pleasure and fulfillment in occupational and relational environments.

SUMMARY

Models of BPD will always be crude approximations of the enormous complexity evident in its psychopathology. Rather than seek to represent the totality of that complexity, in these reviews the investigators have aimed to identify leading edge questions that will push the refinement of our models forward. Specifically, the investigators have argued that models of BPD must address the following:

1. The organization of the emergent individual, reflecting a complex interaction of underlying neurobiological and behavioral trait features
2. The stable instability of the pathology, including the organizing principles that maintain aspects of borderline pathology in the long term but also allow for massive fluctuations in the short term
3. Both the idiopathic and nomothetic aspects of the pathology, highlighted by the intraindividual variability of each individual who manifests BPD

Recent empirical advances highlighted in this review are most useful in directing the headlight of research on the next question. Future refinement of models of BPD must also demonstrate their clinical utility; complex modeling of the pathology is of limited use unless helpful in the assessment and therapeutic intervention with borderline patients.

REFERENCES

1. Eisenberger NI, Lieberman MD. Why rejection hurts: a common neural alarm system for physical and social pain. Trends Cogn Sci 2004;8(7):294–300.
2. Kross E, Egner T, Ochsner K, et al. Neural dynamics of rejection sensitivity. J Cogn Neurosci 2007;19(6):945–56.
3. Eisenberger NI, Lieberman MD, Williams KD. Does rejection hurt? An fMRI study of social exclusion. Science 2003;302(5643):290–2.
4. Staebler K, Renneberg B, Stopsack M, et al. Facial emotional expression in reaction to social exclusion in borderline personality disorder. Psychol Med 2011; 41(9):1929–38.
5. Williams KD, Jarvis B. Cyberball: a program for use in research on interpersonal ostracism and acceptance. Behav Res Methods 2006;38(1):174–80.
6. Gratz KL, Dixon-Gordon KL, Breetz A, et al. A laboratory-based examination of responses to social rejection in borderline personality disorder: the mediating role of emotion dysregulation. J Personal Disord 2013;27(2):157–71.
7. De Panfilis C, Riva P, Preti E, et al. When social inclusion is not enough: implicit expectations of extreme inclusion in borderline personality disorder. Personal Disord 2015;6(4):301–9.
8. Russell JJ, Moskowitz DS, Zuroff DC, et al. Stability and variability of affective experience and interpersonal behavior in borderline personality disorder. J Abnorm Psychol 2007;116(3):578.

9. Meehan KB, De Panfilis C, Cain NM, et al. Facial emotion recognition and border-line personality pathology. Psychiatry Res 2017;255:347–54.
10. De Panfilis C, Antonucci C, Meehan KB, et al. Facial emotion recognition and social-cognitive correlates of narcissistic features. J Personal Disord 2018. [Epub ahead of print].
11. Fertuck EA, Grinband J, Stanley B. Facial trust appraisal negatively biased in borderline personality disorder. Psychiatry Res 2013;207(3):195–202.
12. Levy KN, Meehan KB, Kelly KM, et al. Change in attachment patterns and reflective function in a randomized control trial of transference-focused psychotherapy for borderline personality disorder. J Consult Clin Psychol 2006;74(6):1027–40.
13. Levy KN, Meehan KB, Temes CM. Attachment theory and personality disorders. In: Danquah A, Berry K, editors. Attachment theory in adult mental health. London: Routledge; 2013. p. 95–112.
14. Sharp C, Pane H, Ha C, et al. Theory of mind and emotion regulation difficulties in adolescents with borderline traits. J Am Acad Child Adolesc Psychiatry 2011; 50(6):563–73.
15. Baron-Cohen S, Jolliffe T, Mortimore C, et al. Another advanced test of theory of mind: evidence from very high functioning adults with autism or Asperger syndrome. J Child Psychol Psychiatry 1997;38(7):813–22.
16. Richman MJ, Unoka Z. Mental state decoding impairment in major depression and borderline personality disorder: meta-analysis. Br J Psychiatry 2015; 207(6):483–9.
17. Scott LN, Levy KN, Adams RB Jr, et al. Mental state decoding abilities in young adults with borderline personality disorder traits. Personal Disord 2011;2(2): 98–112.
18. Weinstein SR, Meehan KB, Cain NM, et al. Mental state identification, borderline pathology, and the neglected role of childhood trauma. Personal Disord 2016; 7(1):61–71.
19. Savage M, Lenzenweger MF. The impact of social exclusion on "Reading the Mind in the Eyes" performance in relation to borderline personality disorder features. J Personal Disord 2018;32(1):109–30.
20. Lenzenweger MF, Clarkin JF, Fertuck EA, et al. Executive neurocognitive functioning and neurobehavioral systems indicators in borderline personality disorder: a preliminary study. J Personal Disord 2004;18(5):421–38.
21. Depue RA, Lenzenweger MF. A neurobehavioral dimensional model. In: Livesley WJ, editor. Handbook of personality disorders: theory, research, and treatment. New York: Guilford Press; 2001. p. 136–76.
22. Depue RA, Lenzenweger MF. A neurobehavioral model of personality disturbance. In: Lenzenweger MF, Clarkin JF, editors. Major theories of personality disorder. 2nd edition. New York: Guilford Press; 2005. p. 391–453.
23. Evans DE, Rothbart MK. Developing a model for adult temperament. J Res Pers 2007;41(4):868–88.
24. Eisenberg N, Duckworth AL, Spinrad TL, et al. Conscientiousness: origins in childhood? Dev Psychol 2014;50(5):1331–49.
25. Vohs KD, Baumeister RF. Handbook of self-regulation: Research, theory, and applications. 2nd edition. Guilford Publications; 2011.
26. Koenigsberg HW, Siever LJ, Lee H, et al. Neural correlates of emotion processing in borderline personality disorder. Psychiatry Res Neuroimaging 2009;172(3): 192–9.
27. Koenigsberg HW, Fan J, Ochsner KN, et al. Neural correlates of the use of psychological distancing to regulate responses to negative social cues: a

study of patients with borderline personality disorder. Biol Psychiatry 2009; 66(9):854–63.

28. Ayduk Ö, Zayas V, Downey G, et al. Rejection sensitivity and executive control: joint predictors of borderline personality features. J Res Pers 2008;42(1):151–68.
29. De Panfilis C, Meehan KB, Cain NM, et al. Effortful control, rejection sensitivity, and borderline personality disorder features in adulthood. J Personal Disord 2016;30(5):595–612.
30. Bem DJ, Funder DC. Predicting more of the people more of the time: assessing the personality of situations. Psychol Rev 1978;85(6):485.
31. Mischel W. Toward an integrative science of the person. Annu Rev Psychol 2004; 55:1–22.
32. Decety J. The neurodevelopment of empathy in humans. Dev Neurosci 2010; 32(4):257–67.
33. Eisenberg N, Fabes RA. Prosocial behavior and empathy: a multimethod developmental perspective. In: Clark MS, editor. Review of personality and social psychology, vol. 12. Thousand Oaks (CA): Sage Publications, Inc; 1991. p. 34–61. Prosocial behavior.
34. Harari H, Shamay-Tsoory SG, Ravid M, et al. Double dissociation between cognitive and affective empathy in borderline personality disorder. Psychiatry Res 2010;175(3):277–9.
35. Niedtfeld I. Experimental investigation of cognitive and affective empathy in borderline personality disorder: effects of ambiguity in multimodal social information processing. Psychiatry Res 2017;253:58–63.
36. Blair RJ. Responding to the emotions of others: dissociating forms of empathy through the study of typical and psychiatric populations. Conscious Cogn 2005;14:698–718.
37. Khvatskaya Y, Lenzenweger MF. Motor empathy in individuals with psychopathic traits: a preliminary study. J Personal Disord 2016;30(5):613–32.
38. Taylor ZE, Eisenberg N, Spinrad TL. Respiratory sinus arrhythmia, effortful control, and parenting as predictors of children's sympathy across early childhood. Dev Psychol 2015;51(1):17–25.
39. Rueda MR. Effortful Control. In: Zentner M, Shiner RL (editors). Handbook of Temperament. New York: Guilford. p. 145–67.
40. Schmideberg M. The borderline patient. In: Arieti S, editor. American handbook of psychiatry. New York: Basic Books; 1959. p. 398–416.
41. Lenzenweger MF. Stability and change in personality disorder features: the longitudinal study of personality disorders. Arch Gen Psychiatry 1999;56:1009–15.
42. Zanarini MC, Frankenburg FR, Reich DB, et al. Attainment and stability of sustained symptomatic remission and recovery among patients with borderline personality disorder and axis II comparison subjects: a 16-year prospective follow-up study. Am J Psychiatry 2012;169(5):476–83.
43. Gunderson JG, Lyons-Ruth K. BPD's interpersonal hypersensitivity phenotype: a gene-environment-developmental model. J Personal Disord 2008;22(1):22–41.
44. Lenzenweger MF, Depue RA. Toward a developmental psychopathology of personality disturbance: a neurobehavioral dimensional model incorporating genetic, environmental, and epigenetic factors. In: Cicchetti D, editor. Developmental psychopathology, vol. 3, 3rd edition. New York: Wiley; 2016. p. 1079–110. Maladaptation and psychopathology.
45. Lenzenweger MF, Hallquist MN, Wright AGC. Understanding stability and change in the personality disorders: methodological and substantive issues underpinning interpretive challenges and the road ahead. In: Livesley WJ, Larstone R, editors.

Handbook of personality disorders. 2nd edition. New York: Guilford; 2018. p. 197–214.

46. Korfine L, Hooley JM. Directed forgetting of emotional stimuli in borderline personality disorder. J Abnorm Psychol 2000;109:214–21.

47. Sadler P, Ethier N, Gunn GR, et al. Are we on the same wavelength? Interpersonal complementarity as shared cyclical patterns during interactions. J Pers Soc Psychol 2009;97(6):1005–20.

48. Thomas KM, Hopwood CJ, Woody E, et al. Momentary assessment of interpersonal process in psychotherapy. J Couns Psychol 2014;61(1):1–14.

49. Bateman AW, Fonagy P. Mentalization-based treatment of BPD. J Personal Disord 2004;18(1):36–51.

50. Linehan M. Cognitive-behavioral treatment of borderline personality disorder. New York: Guilford Press; 1993.

51. Yeomans FE, Clarkin JF, Kernberg OF. Transference-focused psychotherapy for borderline personality disorder: a clinical guide. Washington, DC: American Psychiatric Pub; 2015.

52. Erikson EH. Childhood and society; 1950/1993 WW Norton & Company.

Community and Clinical Epidemiology of Borderline Personality Disorder

William D. Ellison, PhD[a],*, Lia K. Rosenstein, MS[b],
Theresa A. Morgan, PhD[c], Mark Zimmerman, MD[d]

KEYWORDS

- Borderline personality disorder • Prevalence • Epidemiology • Diagnosis

KEY POINTS

- The point prevalence of borderline personality disorder is roughly 1% in community settings.
- The point prevalence of borderline personality disorder in clinical settings is approximately 12% in outpatient psychiatric clinics and 22% in inpatient psychiatric clinics.
- Prevalence estimates of borderline personality disorder depend greatly on the use of standardized, validated methods for diagnosis; unstandardized or informal methods tend to underdiagnose borderline personality disorder.
- The prevalence of borderline personality disorder varies according to certain demographic factors, such as age; more research is needed into the demographic correlates of the disorder.

This article concerns the community and clinical epidemiology of borderline personality disorder (BPD)—its prevalence and characteristics in different community and treatment settings and among different populations of individuals. We focus on a categorically defined BPD entity, even if the exact definition varies across different diagnostic systems. Nevertheless, there is compelling evidence that BPD is not a discrete condition that pertains to a class of individuals (alongside another, complementary healthy class), but instead a dimensionally distributed construct. Taxometric studies using different operationalizations of BPD and conducted among different populations largely agree on this point,[1–4] as does a comparison of the fit of categorical and dimensional models of the latent structure of BPD.[5] However, the distribution

[a] Department of Psychology, Trinity University, One Trinity Place, San Antonio, TX 78212, USA;
[b] Department of Psychology, Pennsylvania State University, 140 Moore Building, University Park, PA 16801, USA; [c] Department of Psychiatry, Warren Alpert Medical School of Brown University, Rhode Island Hospital, 593 Eddy Street, Providence, RI 02903, USA; [d] Department of Psychiatry, Warren Alpert Medical School of Brown University, Rhode Island Hospital, 146 West River Street, Suite 11B, Providence, RI 02904, USA
* Corresponding author.
E-mail address: wellison@trinity.edu

Psychiatr Clin N Am 41 (2018) 561–573
https://doi.org/10.1016/j.psc.2018.07.008
0193-953X/18/© 2018 Elsevier Inc. All rights reserved.

Abbreviation	
BPD	Borderline personality disorder

of dimensionally defined borderline pathology is inadequately understood, and the extant large-scale research has generally assumed a categorical model for BPD. Therefore, the current review focuses on the epidemiology of the categorically defined BPD syndrome.

The authors also wish to highlight the importance of measurement for estimates of BPD prevalence, because studies suggest that clinicians who do not use a dedicated assessment tool to screen for or diagnose BPD tend to neglect the diagnosis. For example, Zimmerman and Mattia[6] found that clinicians left to their own judgments diagnosed BPD in only 0.4% of outpatients, compared with 14.4% by structured interview (a rate much more consistent with established outpatient prevalence rates of BPD). Simply providing results of positive BPD diagnoses to intake clinicians who had not used the interview themselves raised the diagnosis rate of BPD to 7%, suggesting the clinical usefulness of this information and the extent to which it can be neglected in routine practice. Likewise, Comtois and Carmel[7] compared BPD diagnoses produced by routine clinical records and diagnoses from semistructured research interviews among outpatients in a public mental health service. They found that the interviews identified BPD in 15.1% of patients, whereas this diagnosis appeared in records 6.9% of the time. Even when clinicians have the information necessary to make a BPD diagnosis, they often miss it. Hillman and associates[8] presented clinical vignettes describing individuals with major depression only or major depression with comorbid BPD to 186 experienced psychologists. Only 14% of respondents correctly made a BPD diagnosis when it was warranted.

Because of this discrepancy, when estimating community prevalence, we focus on epidemiologic studies using a well-validated instrument for diagnosing BPD, although there are some notable exceptions (described elsewhere in this article) in which a validated instrument was not used, but its prevalence was estimated systematically at a later date. However, for clinical prevalence, we review both BPD prevalence estimates derived from a BPD-specific diagnostic measure and those estimates derived from unstructured clinical assessment, and we highlight several additional studies that illustrate the importance of assessing for BPD in clinical settings.

MAJOR EPIDEMIOLOGIC STUDIES OF BORDERLINE PERSONALITY DISORDER IN THE COMMUNITY: UNITED STATES

In the United States, several large epidemiologic studies assessing BPD have been conducted since the introduction of the *Diagnostic and Statistical Manual of Mental Disorders* (DSM)-III criteria for the disorder. **Table 1** shows the prevalence rates obtained from each of these studies. The first of these was the National Institute of Mental Health's epidemiologic catchment area (ECA) studies.[9] The ECA studies collected interviews from more than 18,000 adult individuals across 5 catchment areas (New Haven, Baltimore, St. Louis, central North Carolina, and Los Angeles), oversampling elderly, Black, and Hispanic respondents. The NIMH Diagnostic Interview Schedule, a structured interview, provided information about DSM-III disorders. However, the only personality disorder directly assessed during this effort was antisocial PD. Although BPD was not directly assessed in the ECA studies themselves, 3 later studies attempted to derive BPD prevalence estimates from ECA respondents. Swartz and colleagues[10] used an empirically derived algorithm relating Diagnostic Interview Schedule symptoms to items from the Diagnostic Interview for Borderlines to estimate

Table 1
Epidemiologic studies of the prevalence of BPD in community samples

Study	N	Location	Criterion Set Used	BPD Measure	Prevalence (%)
Reich et al,[77] 1989	401	Iowa, USA	DSM-III	PDQ	1.3
Swartz et al,[10] 1990	1541	North Carolina, USA	DSM-III	DIS	1.8
Torgersen et al,[23] 2001	2053	Oslo, Norway	DSM-III-R	SIDP	0.7
Samuels et al,[12] 2002	742	Maryland, USA	DSM-IV	IPDE	0.5
Crawford et al,[15] 2005	716	New York, USA	DSM-IV	CIC-SR	2.2
Coid et al,[24] 2006	626	Great Britain	DSM-IV	SCID-II	0.7
Lenzenweger[20] 2007	5692	Continental United States	DSM-IV	IPDE	1.4
Trull et al,[22] 2010	34,653	United States	DSM-IV	AUDADIS-IV	2.7
Zanarini et al,[25] 2011	6330	Bristol, England	DSM-IV	UK-CI-BPD	3.2
ten Have et al,[26] 2016	5303	Netherlands	DSM-IV	IPDE	1.1

Abbreviations: AUDADIS-IV, Alcohol Use Disorder and Associated Disabilities Interview Schedule for DSM-IV; BPD, borderline personality disorder; CIC-SR, Children in the Community Self-report Scales; DIS, Diagnostic Interview Schedule; IPDE, International Personality Disorders Examination; PDQ, Personality Diagnostic Questionnaire; SCID-II, Structured Clinical Interview for DSM Personality Disorders; SIDP, Structured Interview for DSM Personality Disorders; UK-CI-BPD, UK Childhood Interview for DSM-IV Personality Disorder.

the prevalence of BPD in respondents from Wave II of the North Carolina site ECA study. Separately, Samuels and colleagues[11] followed 810 individuals from the Baltimore site who were selected for clinical reappraisal by psychiatrists. The reappraisals used a semistructured diagnostic instrument (the Standard Psychiatric Examination) that was not designed to diagnose DSM-III personality disorders, but rather general psychiatric symptoms, history, and functioning. Information about BPD was later coded from these interviews. Finally, Samuels and colleagues[12] reported on the prevalence of BPD among 742 individuals from the Baltimore ECA follow-up survey,[13] some of whom were among those examined by psychiatrists in the original ECA clinical reappraisal (other respondents in Samuels and colleagues' sample had a lifetime diagnosis of 1 of 6 Axis I disorders at follow-up or were drawn randomly from the remaining ECA respondents). These individuals were diagnosed via the International Personality Disorder Examination (IPDE).

The National Comorbidity Survey (NCS)[14] provided an update of the ECA findings using DSM-III-R criteria rather than those of DSM-III based on a stratified probability sample of individuals in the continental United States rather than a set of discrete catchment areas. Diagnoses were made using the World Health Organization's Composite International Diagnostic Interview, which was based on the Diagnostic Interview Schedule and, like its predecessor, was fully structured so that it could be used by lay interviewers. However, also like the ECA studies, the battery used in the NCS only included antisocial PD from among the DSM-III-R personality disorders, and no estimate of the prevalence of BPD in the NCS data has been made to date.

Crawford and colleagues[15] reported on the prevalence of personality disorders among 644 adult residents of 2 upstate New York counties who were screened as part of the longitudinal Children in the Community Study. Screening instruments were the Children in the Community-Self Report scales and the screener accompanying the Structured Clinical Interview for DSM-IV Axis II (SCID-II), the SCID-II-PQ. The SCID-II was then administered in an abbreviated fashion, omitting follow-up questions for those respondents who did not endorse enough screening questions to warrant further inquiry. The stability of BPD in the study cohort, as well as the cumulative prevalence for BPD from age 14 to age 33, are also available in separate reports.[16–18]

The NCS Replication[19] aimed to update the state of knowledge about the epidemiology of mental disorders in the United States, using DSM-IV criteria and an expanded list of assessed diagnoses. Importantly for BPD, the NCS Replication assessed personality disorders with the IPDE Screening Questionnaire and the IPDE itself for individuals screening positive. There were 9282 adults who participated in face-to-face interviews between 2001 and 2003. Lenzenweger and colleagues[20] reported on 12-month BPD prevalence in a probability subsample of 214 respondents who received a "clinical reappraisal" interview. This subsample oversampled those who screened positive for one of the core clinical disorders, but also included some individuals who did not screen positive.

The National Epidemiologic Survey on Alcohol and Related Conditions is a community-based survey of adults from all 50 US states and the District of Columbia. Face-to-face interviews were conducted with more than 40,000 respondents by census workers with minimal experience, who used an unvalidated Axis II diagnostic instrument, the Alcohol Use Disorder and Associated Disabilities Interview Schedule-DSM-IV. Lifetime BPD was assessed at wave 2 of the study,[21] which involved reinterviews of wave 1 respondents (34,653 of 43,093 wave 1 respondents gave reinterviews, or 86.7%). Importantly, Grant and colleagues[21] gave a lifetime BPD diagnosis if sufficient BPD symptoms were present and at least 1 symptom was associated with significant distress, impairment, or dysfunction. This method resulted in a lifetime prevalence estimate of 5.9%. However, some authors criticized this report as being overly inclusive, and resulting in exaggerated PD prevalence estimates. Trull and colleagues[22] revised the original National Epidemiologic Survey on Alcohol and Related Conditions scoring to require significant distress or impairment be present to count each PD criterion individually, rather than cumulatively. The authors then applied this revision to original National Epidemiologic Survey on Alcohol and Related Conditions algorithms, reporting a revised prevalence rate of 2.7%.

MAJOR EPIDEMIOLOGIC STUDIES OF BORDERLINE PERSONALITY DISORDER IN NON-US COMMUNITIES

Several studies of BPD prevalence in communities outside the United States have also been conducted. For example, Torgersen and coworkers[23] sampled individuals from the National Register of Oslo, Norway. Personality disorders were assessed with the SIDP-R, which was administered by nurses, medical students, and lay interviewers. Of the 3590 individuals selected for inclusion, 2053 (57%) were interviewed.

Coid and colleagues[24] reported the results of a national survey of adult community members in England, Wales, and Scotland. The initial screening for personality disorders was conducted under the British National Survey of Psychiatric Morbidity, which used computer-assisted interviews. Subsamples of the individuals screening positive in stage 1 for psychosis or a personality disorder, as well as a subsample screening negative for all disorders, were offered follow-up interviews. The stage 1 screening sample consisted of 8886 adults, of whom 628 individuals completed a follow-up interview with the SCID-II.

Zanarini and colleagues[25] reported on a survey of a cohort of 11-year-old community participants in Bristol, England, who were part of the Avon Longitudinal Study of Parents and Children. These children were interviewed with the UK Childhood

Interview for DSM-IV Borderline Personality Disorder, which was based on the Diagnostic Interview for DSM-IV Personality Disorders, but has modified language, content, and structure to accommodate juvenile respondents. Ther were 6330 children who gave complete interviews.

Finally, ten Have and colleagues[26] reported on the prevalence of BPD among adults in the Netherlands, using a sample from the Netherlands Mental Health Survey and Incidence Study-2. Like the British National Survey of Psychiatric Morbidity,[24] an initial stage of computer-assisted interviews was conducted on a probability sample of individuals (n = 6646). However, unlike that study, all respondents from this initial wave were approached for a follow-up, interview including the 8 BPD items from the IPDE, which were incorporated into the Composite International Diagnostic Interview. There were 5303 individuals who were included in the second wave sample.

COMMUNITY SUBPOPULATIONS: PREVALENCE OF BORDERLINE PERSONALITY DISORDER IN ADOLESCENTS AND OLDER ADULTS

Despite evidence that BPD emerges in adolescence, it has typically been thought of as an adult disorder. There has been resistance to diagnose it before the age of 18 on the basis that personality has yet to solidify and that instability in identity and relationships is part of normative development. However, owing to the seriousness of the disorder and marked burden on not only the individual but on the health care system, research efforts have shifted to focus on early detection and prevention.[27,28] These efforts parallel several recent findings that the BPD diagnosis can indeed be made in adolescents with adequate reliability, stability, and validity.[29,30]

A systematic review[31] found that rates of BPD in adolescent samples varied substantially depending on study design and sample characteristics, but overall tended to be higher than adult samples. For example, Levy and colleagues[32] found rates of BPD to be 43% in an adolescent inpatient unit (mean age, 15.5 years). Similar results were found by Grilo and colleagues,[33] with BPD prevalence rates of 49% in adolescent inpatients. Outside of inpatient settings, community and clinical prevalence rates of BPD in adolescents tend to look similar to adult cohorts,[20] with estimates ranging from 0.9%[34] to 3.0%[16] in community samples and 11% in outpatients.[35] Of note, although BPD tends to be more prevalent in adult women than adult men, this gender split is not apparent among adolescents.[31]

Although research shows that some personality pathology is exacerbated across the lifespan, BPD has been found to decrease and even remit as individuals age.[36,37] A review of personality disorder prevalence in younger and older age groups found rates of BPD to be significantly lower in older adults as compared with younger adults.[38] For example, 1 study found a prevalence rate of 22% in a sample of young adults and a rate of 7% in an elderly sample.[39] Another study found a BPD prevalence rate of 1% in a community sample of 200 adults over the age of 60.[40] Finally, a recent report of personality disorders in a community sample of individuals aged 55 to 64 found a BPD prevalence rate of 0.4%.[41] It has been hypothesized that this decrease in prevalence is secondary to burnout in symptoms such as impulsivity or lost social connections and therefore less interpersonal instability.[36] A majority of the research on prevalence rates is cross-sectional in design and more longitudinal studies extending into later life are needed with regard to aging and prevalence of BPD.

COMMUNITY SETTINGS: UNIVERSITY

An important community setting to consider when looking at diagnostic prevalence of any psychiatric disorder is universities. Given the high risk for suicide and comorbid disorders such as substance abuse, gaining estimates of BPD among university students is warranted. An early estimate of BPD prevalence among college students comes from Lenzenweger and colleagues,[42] who applied a 2-stage diagnostic procedure to a large sample of college students in Ithaca, New York, involving the IPDE-SQ and the IPDE. This study uncovered a point prevalence of 1.3%, although follow-up studies highlighted striking differences in the trajectories of PD symptoms in this cohort over a 4-year period.[43] This finding suggests that a BPD diagnosis may not be stable among undergraduates, perhaps owing to their relative youth or the fact that they are generally high functioning compared with other community populations. A recent metaanalysis found that reported rates of BPD among college samples ranged from as low as 0.5% to as high as 32.1%, likely reflecting the varying methodology among primary studies. Moreover, there was an average lifetime prevalence rate of 9.7% in this population, and BPD prevalence was significantly lower in Asian American college students than in other racial or ethnic groups.[44]

COMMUNITY SETTINGS: FORENSIC

Highly prevalent in community and clinical populations, research indicates that rates of BPD are higher still in forensic settings.[45–48] Black and colleagues[45] found a prevalence rate of 29.5% among a randomly selected sample of 220 individuals recently committed to prison. Within this sample, the prevalence of BPD in female offenders was more than twice the prevalence seen in male offenders (54.5% and 26.8%, respectively). In a female inmate sample, Jordan and colleagues[47] found a similar overall BPD prevalence rate of 28%. In a small male prison sample, Davison and associates[49] found a 45% rate of BPD using the SCID-II. Overall, research suggests that prevalence of BPD in a forensic setting falls between about 25% and 55%. Additional research is needed as to comorbidities and outcomes for individuals with BPD in prison settings.

CLINICAL EPIDEMIOLOGY OF BORDERLINE PERSONALITY DISORDER: PSYCHIATRIC CARE SETTINGS

In comparison with the general community population, BPD is highly prevalent in various types of psychiatric settings.[50] **Table 2** summarizes prevalence estimates of BPD in studies of psychiatric populations, focusing on samples that consist of consecutively admitted patients or other naturalistic groups. The mean prevalence rate of BPD among inpatient samples across these studies, weighted by sample size, is 22.4%, whereas the comparable mean for outpatient samples is 11.8%. As discussed elsewhere in this article, we wish to highlight the discrepancy in prevalence estimates derived from diagnostic practice as usual from those estimates derived through either a well-validated interview or a diagnostic process with deliberate attention to personality pathology. For example, Kantojärvi and colleagues'[51] inpatient prevalence estimate of 5.6%, derived through review of hospital records, is markedly lower than the inpatient average.

We also wish to highlight the Rhode Island Methods to Improve Diagnostic Assessment and Services (MIDAS) project, an ongoing study of diagnostic methods that has amassed a sample size of 3800 treatment-seeking outpatients.[52] To date, this is by far the largest outpatient sample to be diagnosed with semistructured diagnostic interviews and, as such, it provides perhaps the best single estimate of the outpatient prevalence of BPD. The most up-to-date estimate of BPD prevalence from the MIDAS project found 390 individuals with BPD among 3674 individuals completing the SIDP-IV (10.6%).[53]

Table 2
Epidemiologic studies of BPD prevalence in psychiatric samples

Study	N	Setting	Criterion Set Used	BPD Measure	Prevalence (%)
Stangl et al,[78] 1985	131	Inpatient and outpatient	DSM-III	SIDP	22.1
Kass et al,[79] 1985	609	Outpatient	DSM-III	Clinical	11.0
Koenigsberg et al,[80] 1985	2462	Mixed	DSM-III	Clinical	12.3
Dahl,[81] 1986	231	Inpatient	DSM-III	SIB	20.3
Fabrega et al,[82] 1993	18,179	Evaluation	DSM-III	Clinical	2.1
Herpertz et al,[83] 1994	231	Inpatient	DSM-III-R	AMPS	13.6
Molinari et al,[39] 1994	200	Inpatient	DSM-III-R	SIDP-R	6.5
Oldham et al,[84] 1995	100	Outpatient evaluation	DSM-III-R	PDE	18.0
Oldham et al,[84] 1995	100	Inpatient evaluation	DSM-III-R	PDE	64.0
Grilo et al,[33] 1998	138	Inpatient	DSM-III-R	PDE	49.3
Grilo et al,[33] 1998	117	Inpatient	DSM-III-R	PDE	42.7
Ottosson et al,[85] 1998	138	Mixed	DSM-IV	DIP-I	33.3
Marinangeli et al,[86] 2000	156	Inpatient	DSM-III-R	SCID-II	40.4
Fossati et al,[87] 2000	431	Inpatient and outpatient	DSM-IV	SCID-II	22.5
Chanen et al,[35] 2004	101	Outpatient	DSM-IV	SCID-II	10.9
Kantojärvi et al,[51] 2004	444	Inpatient	DSM-III-R	Clinical	5.6
Korzekwa et al,[88] 2008	360	Outpatient	DSM-IV	DIB-R	22.6
Kaess et al,[89] 2013	87	Inpatient and outpatient	DSM-IV	SCID-II	35.6
Ha et al,[90] 2014	418	Inpatient	DSM-IV	CI-BPD	32.8
Comtois & Carmel,[7] 2016	159	Outpatient	DSM-IV	PDE	15.1
Zimmerman et al,[53] 2017	3674	Outpatient	DSM-IV	SIDP	10.6

Abbreviations: AMPS, Aachen List of Items for the Registration of Personality Disorders; CI-BPD, Childhood Interview for DSM-IV Borderline Personality Disorder; DIB-R, Revised Diagnostic Interview for Borderlines; DIP-I, DSM-IV and ICD-10 Personality Interview; PDE, Personality Disorders Examination; SCID-II, Structured Clinical Interview for DSM Personality Disorders; SIB, Schedule for Interviewing Borderlines; SIDP, Structured Interview for DSM Personality Disorders.

CLINICAL SETTINGS: PRIMARY CARE

Whether an individual seeks consultation explicitly for their psychiatric symptoms or whether screened for psychopathology by their physician during routine medical practice, the gateway to psychiatric care for many individuals is through primary care providers. Although there is substantial information on the epidemiology of depression and anxiety in primary care settings, little is known about the prevalence of BPD in such facilities. One problem is that screening and assessment for BPD in primary care is lacking. For example, an examination of computerized databases of primary care records in the Catalan Health Institute in Spain[54] found a prevalence of recorded BPD of only 0.017%, which is much lower than the prevalence in the general population. This large discrepancy raises issues around screening for psychiatric disorders, particularly BPD, in primary care samples given the high rates of medical comorbidities in this population. Likewise, a study in an urban primary care practice found that 42.9% of cases later identified to have BPD had not been recognized as having psychiatric difficulties of any kind by their primary care physicians.[55] Given the increased risk of suicide and impaired psychosocial functioning, the authors of this study argued that properly assessing BPD is vital to better predicting and preventing potential ruptures in treatment and foreseeing issues in the patient–physician relationship. Further epidemiologic studies are needed with regards to BPD in primary care settings and behavioral medicine, with the ultimate goal of improving screening practice to help triage patients to appropriate treatment.

CLINICAL SETTINGS: NONPSYCHIATRIC SPECIALTY CARE

Reviews of the prevalence of BPD in medical settings suggest that individuals with BPD have been shown to be especially common among those presenting in medical settings with alcohol and substance use disorders, multiple somatic complains, chronic pain, obesity, sexual dysfunction (including sexual dissatisfaction and promiscuity), and trichotillomania.[56,57] This finding is essentially consistent with recent reviews documenting high levels of physical health problems among individuals with BPD.[58,59] It should be noted that the research basis for the connections between BPD and these physical complaints varies considerably in both quantity and quality; many primary studies used convenience samples rather than probability samples, self-report measures or chart review rather than well-validated diagnostic interviews, or had excessively small sample sizes.

Further reviews and primary studies have identified other specialty medical settings where individuals with BPD can be found in large numbers, such as aesthetic plastic surgery (especially to repair scars from deliberate self-injury)[60] and bariatric surgery.[61] Many of the large-scale epidemiologic studies reviewed herein have also provided their own evidence that BPD is associated with a wide array of physical health conditions.[62–65] In short, there is suggestive to strong evidence to indicate that BPD is prevalent among individuals seeking care for a wide variety of physical health complaints.

Given that personality pathology frequently cooccurs with alcohol and drug addiction, high rates of BPD are seen in substance abuse clinics and programs. One study[66] surveyed 320 patients enrolled in an outpatient addictions service targeting alcohol and opiate dependence and found the prevalence rate of personality disorders to be 62.2%. Although none of the sample met the criteria for schizotypal personality disorder and 13.8% qualified for an antisocial personality disorder diagnosis, BPD had the highest prevalence of any specific personality disorder at 15%. The authors also reviewed principal studies in the literature regarding the prevalence of personality pathology in substance abusing samples and found that the rates of BPD varied substantially between 3.2%[67] and 65.1%.[68]

SUMMARY AND AREAS IN NEED OF RESEARCH

BPD is relatively common in the general population, with a point prevalence of around 1%. There are also subpopulations in which the prevalence is higher (eg, incarcerated individuals) or lower (eg, elderly individuals) than this. The prevalence of BPD is substantially higher in clinical settings, around 12% in the outpatient psychiatric population and 22% among inpatients. Although there are no well-established prevalence rates in primary care, there is reason to believe that BPD is quite common among individuals seeking medical care for a variety of physical conditions.

There are some areas in which the epidemiology of BPD would particularly benefit from additional research. For example, although extant studies of racial and ethnic differences in the community prevalence of BPD do not show systematic differences,[21,69] a recent review identified racial differences in BPD prevalence in more specific settings.[70] Research also suggests that there may be differences among ethnic groups in the prevalence and extent of many indicators of BPD, such as suicidality[71,72] and deliberate self-harm.[73] In addition, the association between deliberate self-harm and borderline personality features differs among ethnic groups,[74] and African American individuals with BPD have been shown to report more affective instability and emotion dysregulation, but less suicidal behavior and deliberate self-harm, than white American individuals with the disorder.[75,76] Systematic studies of this topic are few, as are studies of the impact of other demographic variables (eg, socioeconomic status) on BPD presentation and prevalence. Our knowledge of BPD's epidemiology would be strengthened with greater attention to these important issues.

REFERENCES

1. Arntz A, Bernstein D, Gielen D, et al. Taxometric evidence for the dimensional structure of cluster-C, paranoid, and borderline personality disorders. J Pers Disord 2009;23:606–28.
2. Edens JF, Marcus DK, Ruiz MA. Taxometric analyses of borderline personality features in a large-scale male and female offender sample. J Abnorm Psychol 2008;117:705–11.
3. Rothschild L, Cleland C, Haslam N, et al. A taxometric study of borderline personality disorder. J Abnorm Psychol 2003;112:657–66.
4. Trull TJ, Widiger TA, Guthrie P. Categorical versus dimensional status of borderline personality disorder. J Abnorm Psychol 1990;99:40–8.
5. Conway C, Hammen C, Brennan PA. A comparison of latent class, latent trait, and factor mixture models of DSM-IV borderline personality disorder criteria in a community setting: implications for DSM-5. J Pers Disord 2012;26:793–803.
6. Zimmerman M, Mattia J. Psychiatric diagnosis in clinical practice: is comorbidity being missed? Compr Psychiatry 1999;40:182–91.
7. Comtois KA, Carmel A. Borderline personality disorder and high utilization of inpatient psychiatric hospitalization: concordance between research and clinical diagnosis. J Behav Health Serv Res 2016;43:272–80.
8. Hillman JL, Stricker G, Zweig RA. Clinical psychologists' judgments of older adult patients with character pathology: implications for practice. Prof Psychol Res Pr 1997;28:179–83.
9. Regier DA, Boyd JH, Burke JD, et al. One-month prevalence of mental disorders in the United States: based on five epidemiologic catchment area sites. Arch Gen Psychiatry 1988;45:977–86.
10. Swartz M, Blazer D, George L, et al. Estimating the prevalence of borderline personality disorder in the community. J Pers Disord 1990;4:257–72.
11. Samuels JF, Nestadt G, Romanoski AJ, et al. DSM-III personality disorders in the community. Am J Psychiatry 1994;151:1055–62.
12. Samuels J, Eaton WW, Bienvenu J, et al. Prevalence and correlates of personality disorders in a community sample. Br J Psychiatry 2002;180:536–42.
13. Eaton WW, Anthony JC, Gallo J, et al. Natural history of diagnostic interview schedule/DSM-IV major depression: the Baltimore epidemiologic catchment area follow-up. Arch Gen Psychiatry 1997;54:993–9.
14. Kessler RC, McGonagle KA, Zhao S, et al. Lifetime and 12-month prevalence of DSM-III-R psychiatric disorders in the United States: results from the National Comorbidity Survey. Arch Gen Psychiatry 1994;51:8–19.

15. Crawford TN, Cohen P, Johnson JG, et al. Self-reported personality disorder in the Children in the Community sample: convergent and prospective validity in late adolescence and adulthood. J Pers Disord 2005;19:30–52.

16. Bernstein DP, Cohen P, Velez N, et al. Prevalence and stability of the DSM-III-R personality disorders in a community-based sample of adolescents. Am J Psychiatry 1993;150:1237–43.

17. Johnson JG, Cohen P, Kasen S, et al. Age-related change in personality disorder trait levels between early adolescence and adulthood: a community-based longitudinal investigation. Acta Psychiatr Scand 2000;102:265–73.

18. Johnson JG, Cohen P, Kasen S, et al. Cumulative prevalence of personality disorders between adolescence and adulthood. Acta Psychiatr Scand 2008;118:410–3.

19. Kessler RC, Merikangas KR. The National Comorbidity Survey replication (NCS-R): background and aims. Int J Methods Psychiatr Res 2004;13:60–8.

20. Lenzenweger MF, Lane MC, Loranger AW, et al. DSM-IV personality disorders in the National Comorbidity Survey replication. Biol Psychiatry 2007;62:553–64.

21. Grant BF, Chou SP, Goldstein RB, et al. Prevalence, correlates, disability, and comorbidity of DSM-IV borderline personality disorder: results from the wave 2 national epidemiologic survey on alcohol and related conditions. J Clin Psychiatry 2008;69:533–45.

22. Trull TJ, Jahng S, Tomko RL, et al. Revised NESARC personality disorder diagnosis: gender, prevalence, and comorbidity with substance dependence disorders. J Pers Disord 2010;24:412–26.

23. Torgersen S, Kringlen E, Cramer V. The prevalence of personality disorders in a community sample. Arch Gen Psychiatry 2001;58:590–6.

24. Coid J, Yang M, Tyrer P, et al. Prevalence and correlates of personality disorder in Great Britain. Br J Psychiatry 2006;188:423–31.

25. Zanarini MC, Horwood J, Wolke D, et al. Prevalence of DSM-IV borderline personality disorder in two community samples: 6,330 English 11-year-olds and 34,653 American adults. J Pers Disord 2011;25:607–19.

26. ten Have M, Verheul R, Kaasenbrood A, et al. Prevalence rates of borderline personality disorder symptoms: a study based on the Netherlands Mental Health Survey and Incidence Study-2. BMC Psychiatry 2016;16:249.

27. Chanen AM, Thompson K. Preventive strategies for borderline personality disorder in adolescents. Curr Treat Options Psychiatry 2014;1:358–68.

28. Sharp C, Fonagy P. Practitioner review: borderline personality disorder in adolescence – recent conceptualization, intervention, and implications for clinical practice. J Child Psychol Psychiatry 2015;56:1266–88.

29. Kaess M, Brunner R, Chanen A. Borderline personality disorder in adolescence. Pediatrics 2014;134:782–93.

30. Miller AL, Muehlenkamp JJ, Jacobson CM. Fact or fiction: diagnosing borderline personality disorder in adolescents. Clin Psychol Rev 2008;28:969–81.

31. Sharp C, Romero C. Borderline personality disorder: a comparison between children and adults. Bull Menninger Clin 2007;71:85–114.

32. Levy KN, Becker DF, Grilo CM, et al. Concurrent and predictive validity of the personality disorder diagnosis in adolescent inpatients. Am J Psychiatry 1999;156:1522–8.

33. Grilo CM, McGlashan TH, Quinlan DM, et al. Frequency of personality disorders in two age cohorts of psychiatric inpatients. Am J Psychiatry 1998;155:140–2.

34. Lewinsohn PM, Rohde P, Seeley JR, et al. Axis II psychopathology as a function of axis I disorders in childhood and adolescence. J Am Acad Child Adolesc Psychiatry 1997;36:1752–9.
35. Chanen AM, Jackson HJ, McGorry PD, et al. Two-year stability of personality disorder in older adolescent outpatients. J Pers Disord 2004;18:526–41.
36. Oltmanns TF, Balsis S. Personality disorders in later life: questions about the measurement, course, and impact of disorders. Annu Rev Clin Psychol 2011;7: 321–49.
37. Paris J. Personality disorders over time: precursors, course and outcome. J Pers Disord 2003;17:479–88.
38. Balsis S, Zweig RA, Molinari V. Personality disorders in later life. In: Lichtenberg PA, Mast BT, Carpenter BD, et al, editors. APA handbook of clinical geropsychology, vol. 2. Washington, DC: American Psychological Association; 2015. p. 79–94.
39. Molinari V, Ames A, Essa M. Prevalence of personality disorders in two geropsychiatric inpatient units. J Geriatr Psychiatry Neurol 1994;7:209–15.
40. Ames A, Molinari V. Prevalence of personality disorders in community-living elderly. J Geriatr Psychiatry Neurol 1994;7:189–94.
41. Oltmanns TF, Rodrigues MM, Weinstein Y, et al. Prevalence of personality disorders at midlife in a community sample: disorders and symptoms reflected in interview, self, and informant reports. J Psychopathol Behav Assess 2014;36:177–88.
42. Lenzenweger MF, Loranger AW, Korfine L, et al. Detecting personality disorders in a nonclinical population: application of a 2-stage procedure for case identification. Arch Gen Psychiatry 1997;54:345–51.
43. Lenzenweger MF. The Longitudinal study of personality disorders: history, design considerations, and initial findings. J Pers Disord 2006;20:645–70.
44. Meaney R, Hasking P, Reupert A. Prevalence of borderline personality disorder in university samples: systematic review, meta-analysis and meta-regression. PLoS One 2016;11:e0155439.
45. Black DW, Gunter T, Allen J, et al. Borderline personality disorder in male and female offenders newly committed to prison. Compr Psychiatry 2007;48:400–5.
46. Blackburn R, Coid JW. Empirical clusters of DSM-III personality disorders in violent offenders. J Pers Disord 1999;13:18–34.
47. Jordan BK, Schlenger WE, Fairbank JA, et al. Prevalence of psychiatric disorders among incarcerated women: II. Convicted felons entering prison. Arch Gen Psychiatry 1996;53:513–9.
48. Mir J, Kastner S, Priebe S, et al. Treating substance abuse is not enough: comorbidities in consecutively admitted female prisoners. Addict Behav 2015;46: 25–30.
49. Davison S, Leese M, Taylor PJ. Examination of the screening properties of the personality diagnostic questionnaire 4+ (PDQ-4+) in a prison population. J Pers Disord 2001;15:180–94.
50. Zimmerman M, Chelminski I, Young D. The frequency of personality disorders in psychiatric patients. Psychiatr Clin North Am 2008;31:405–20.
51. Kantojärvi L, Veijola J, Läksy K, et al. Comparison of hospital-treated personality disorders and personality disorders in a general population sample. Nord J Psychiatry 2004;58:357–62.
52. Zimmerman M. A review of 20 years of research on overdiagnosis and underdiagnosis in the Rhode Island Methods to Improve Diagnostic Assessment and Services (MIDAS) project. Can J Psychiatry 2016;61:71–9.

53. Zimmerman M, Chelminski I, Dalrymple K, et al. Principal diagnoses in psychiatric outpatients with borderline personality disorder: implications for screening recommendations. Ann Clin Psychiatry 2017;29:54–60.
54. Aragonès E, Salvador-Carulla L, López-Muntaner J, et al. Registered prevalence of borderline personality disorder in primary care databases. Gac Sanit 2013;27: 171–4.
55. Gross R, Olfson M, Gameroff M, et al. Borderline personality disorder in primary care. Arch Intern Med 2002;162:53–60.
56. Sansone RA, Sansone LA. Borderline personality disorder in the medical setting. Prim Care Companion CNS Disord 2015;17(3). https://doi.org/10.4088/PCC. 14r01743.
57. Sansone RA, Sansone LA. Borderline personality disorder in the medical setting: suggestive behaviors, syndromes, and diagnoses. Innov Clin Neurosci 2015;12: 39–44.
58. Dixon-Gordon KL, Conkey LC, Whalen DJ. Recent advances in understanding physical health problems in personality disorders. Curr Opin Psychol 2018;21:1–5.
59. Dixon-Gordon KL, Whalen DJ, Layden BK, et al. A systematic review of personality disorders and health outcomes. Can Psychol 2015;56:168–90.
60. Morioka D, Ohkubo F. Borderline personality disorder and aesthetic plastic surgery. Aesthetic Plast Surg 2014;38:1169–76.
61. Kalarchian MA, Marcus MD, Levine MD, et al. Psychiatric disorders among bariatric surgery candidates: relationship to obesity and functional health status. Am J Psychiatry 2007;164:328–34.
62. El-Gabalawy R, Katz LY, Sareen J. Comorbidity and associated severity of borderline personality disorder and physical health conditions in a nationally representative sample. Psychosom Med 2010;72:641–7.
63. Lee HB, Bienvenu J, Cho S-J, et al. Personality disorders and traits as predictors of incident cardiovascular disease: findings from the 23-year follow-up of the Baltimore ECA study. Psychosomatics 2010;51:289–96.
64. McWilliams LA, Higgins KS. Associations between pain conditions and borderline personality disorder symptoms: findings from the National Comorbidity Survey Replication. Clin J Pain 2013;29:527–32.
65. Moran P, Stewart R, Brugha T, et al. Personality disorder and cardiovascular disease: results from a national household survey. J Clin Psychiatry 2007;68:69–74.
66. Casadio P, Olivoni D, Ferrari B, et al. Personality disorders in addiction outpatients: prevalence and effects on psychosocial functioning. Subst Abuse 2014; 8:17–24.
67. Driessen M, Veltrup C, Wetterling T, et al. Axis I and axis II comorbidity in alcohol dependence and the two types of alcoholism. Alcohol Clin Exp Res 1998;22: 77–86.
68. DeJong CAJ, van den Brink W, Harteveld FM, et al. Personality disorders in alcoholics and drug addicts. Compr Psychiatry 1993;34:87–94.
69. Chavira DA, Grilo CM, Shea MT, et al. Ethnicity and four personality disorders. Compr Psychiatry 2003;44:483–91.
70. McGilloway A, Hall RE, Lee T, et al. A systematic review of personality disorder, race, and ethnicity: prevalence, aetiology and treatment. BMC Psychiatry 2010; 10(33). https://doi.org/10.1186/1471-244X-10-33.
71. Borges G, Orozco R, Rafful C, et al. Suicidality, ethnicity and immigration in the USA. Psychol Med 2012;42:1175–84.
72. U.S. Department of Health and Human Services. Mental health: culture, race, and ethnicity—a supplement to mental health: a report of the surgeon general.

Rockville (MD): U.S. Department of Health and Human Services, Substance Abuse and Mental Health Services Administration, Center for Mental Health Services; 2001. Available at: http://www.surgeongeneral.gov/library/mentalhealth/cre/. Accessed April 29, 2011.

73. Gratz KL. Risk factors for deliberate self-harm among female college students: the role and interaction of childhood maltreatment, emotional inexpressivity and affect intensity/reactivity. Am J Orthopsychiatry 2006;76:238–50.

74. Gratz KL, Latzman RD, Young J, et al. Deliberate self-harm among underserved adolescents: the moderating roles of gender, race, and school-level and association with borderline personality features. Personal Disord 2012;3:39–54.

75. De Genna NM, Feske U. Phenomenology of borderline personality disorder: the role of race and socioeconomic status. J Nerv Ment Dis 2013;201:1027–34.

76. Newhill CE, Eack SM, Conner KO. Racial differences between African and White Americans in the presentation of borderline personality disorder. Race Soc Probl 2009;1:87–96.

77. Reich J, Yates W, Nduaguba M. Prevalence of DSM-III personality disorders in the community. Soc Psychiatry Psychiatr Epidemiol 1989;24:12–6.

78. Stangl D, Pfohl B, Zimmerman M. A structured interview for the DSM-III personality disorders: a preliminary report. Arch Gen Psychiatry 1985;42:591–6.

79. Kass F, Skodol AE, Charles E, et al. Scaled ratings of DSM-III personality disorders. Am J Psychiatry 1985;142:627–30.

80. Koenigsberg HW, Kaplan RD, Gilmore MM, et al. The relationship between syndrome and personality disorder in DSM-III: experience with 2,462 patients. Am J Psychiatry 1985;142:207–12.

81. Dahl AA. Some aspects of the DSM-III personality disorders illustrated by a consecutive sample of hospitalized patients. Acta Psychiatr Scand 1986; 1986(73):61–7.

82. Fabrega H, Ulrich R, Pilkonis P, et al. Personality disorders diagnosed at intake in a public psychiatric facility. Hosp Community Psychiatry 1993;44:159–62.

83. Herpertz S, Steinmeyer EM, Saß H. "Patterns of comorbidity" among DSM-III-R and ICD-10 personality disorders as observed with a new inventory for the assessment of personality disorders. Eur Arch Psychiatry Clin Neurosci 1994; 244:161–9.

84. Oldham JM, Skodol AE, Kellman HD, et al. Comorbidity of axis I and axis II disorders. Am J Psychiatry 1995;152:571–8.

85. Ottosson H, Bodlund O, Ekselius L, et al. DSM-IV and ICD-10 personality disorders: a comparison of a self-report questionnaire (DIP-Q) with a structured interview. Eur Psychiatry 1998;13:246–53.

86. Marinangeli MG, Butti G, Scinto A, et al. Patterns of comorbidity among DSM-III-R personality disorders. Psychopathology 2000;33:69–74.

87. Fossati A, Maffei C, Bagnato M, et al. Patterns of covariation of DSM-IV personality disorders in a mixed psychiatric sample. Compr Psychiatry 2000;41:206–15.

88. Korzekwa MI, Dell PF, Links PS, et al. Estimating the prevalence of borderline personality disorder in psychiatric outpatients using a two-phase procedure. Compr Psychiatry 2008;49:380–6.

89. Kaess M, von Ceumern-Lindenstjerna IA, Parzer P, et al. Axis I and II comorbidity and psychosocial functioning in female adolescents with borderline personality disorder. Psychopathology 2013;46:55–62.

90. Ha C, Balderas JC, Zanarini M, et al. Psychiatric comorbidity in hospitalized adolescents with borderline personality disorder. J Clin Psychiatry 2014;75: e457–64.

Differential Diagnosis of Borderline Personality Disorder

Joel Paris, MD

KEYWORDS

- Borderline personality disorder • Personality disorders • Bipolar disorders
- Major depression • Schizophrenia • Attention-deficit/hyperactivity disorder
- Posttraumatic stress disorder • Affective instability

KEY POINTS

- Borderline personality disorder (BPD) has a wide range of symptoms and clinical features that overlap with other diagnostic categories.
- Diagnosis is important because different disorders respond to different forms of treatment.
- Differential diagnosis is particularly relevant for distinguishing BPD from bipolar spectrum disorders, requiring a careful evaluation of affective instability and hypomania. BPD may also be confused with major depression, schizophrenia, attention-deficit/hyperactivity disorder, and posttraumatic stress disorder.

Classification in psychiatry is problematic because diagnoses of mental disorders are based on observable signs and symptoms, not etiologic and pathogenetic mechanisms. Almost no mental disorders are consistently correlated with biological markers.[1] Similar symptoms can derive from entirely different causes, and clustering of symptoms in a diagnostic category may only describe a syndrome, not a disease process. Diagnosis functions more as a way of communicating about patients than a guide to treatment. Yet diagnostic categories can become popular for reasons other than their validity. Clinicians may also prefer diagnoses that support the use of specific methods of treatment[2] and/or that are compatible with the insurance reimbursement system.

BPD is a complex multidimensional disorder characterized by unstable mood, impulsivity, and unstable relationships.[3] A diagnosis of BPD is, therefore, associated with a wide range of symptoms and extensive comorbidity, leading to problems in

Disclosure Statement: No disclosures.
McGill University, SMBD-Jewish General Hospital, 4333 Cote Ste Catherine, Montreal, Quebec H3A 1E4, Canada
E-mail address: joel.paris@mcgill.ca

Psychiatr Clin N Am 41 (2018) 575–582
https://doi.org/10.1016/j.psc.2018.07.001   psych.theclinics.com

differential diagnosis. Overlap between disorders, however, is built into the structure of the *Diagnostic and Statistical Manual of Mental Disorders* (Fifth Edition) (*DSM-5*) system and need not mean that patients have more than 1 diagnosis. For example, high levels of depression and anxiety are an intrinsic component of BPD but do not respond to the same treatments as in patients without BPD.[4] Making additional diagnoses is important if they point to treatment interventions that otherwise might not be offered. The best examples are substance use disorder and eating disorders, both of which are often comorbid with BPD but require a unique approach that may require separate treatments.[4]

DEPRESSION AND BORDERLINE PERSONALITY DISORDER

Major depression is common in BPD, and depressive symptoms are usually what bring patients to clinical attention.[5] Most patients with BPD meet criteria for depression sometime in the course of their illness.[6] Yet this is not surprising, given the low bar for diagnosis of major depressive episodes (2 weeks of 5 out of 9 symptoms). The question is whether depression in BPD is truly episodic or occurs in the context of mood instability, associated with problems in impulsivity, and interpersonal relationships.[6] The characteristic features of BPD are present for many years prior to the onset of depressive episodes. Moreover, the mood swings associated with BPD do not present with many of the vegetative symptoms seen in severe major depression.

Some mood disorder researchers have seen BPD as an atypical form of depression, either unipolar or bipolar.[7] But depressive symptoms not show the same pattern in BPD: they are chronic rather than episodic, associated with a mercurial and fluctuating mood that is highly responsive to interpersonal life events.[6] Moreover, BPD patients show higher levels of impulsivity than patients with depression alone, along with characteristic symptoms, such as self-harm and recurrent overdoses that are not common in major depression.[7] Depressive symptoms show only marginal improvement with antidepressants, and these agents never lead to remission of the disorder.[4] Finally, longitudinal studies show that depression in BPD usually declines when the personality disorder (PD) goes into remission.[8]

A crucial point is that the quality of depressive affect is different in BPD.[6] In classic depression, mood remains low independent of environmental input, and even the best news does not cheer up patients. In contrast, mood in BPD is both highly reactive and unstable and changes when the environment changes. That is why mood swings in BPD patients usually last for hours, not days.

For this reason, depressive symptoms do not show the same pattern in BPD: they are chronic rather than episodic, associated with a mercurial mood that is highly responsive to interpersonal life events.[6] BPD patients also show higher levels of impulsivity than patients with depression alone and have characteristic symptoms, such as self-harm and recurrent overdoses, that are uncommon in major depression.[3]

BORDERLINE PERSONALITY DISORDER AND THE BIPOLAR SPECTRUM

Proposals to extend the boundaries of bipolar disorder to a broader spectrum that includes BPD[7] are part of a radically expanded concept of bipolarity. The assumption is that mood swings of any duration, including cases marked more by irritability than euphoria, point to a bipolar diagnosis. This point of view proposes that patients can show soft bipolarity, that is a variant or subclinical form of classic bipolar disorder.[7] But this expanded spectrum has been defined entirely on the basis of phenomenological resemblances, not on a common etiology or pathogenesis.[8–10]

Manic-depressive illness (now renamed bipolar disorder) was defined by Kraepe-lin[11] as marked by a classic triad of symptoms: elevated affect, psychomotor excitement, and racing thoughts. The condition was also seen as episodic, with a relatively favorable long-term outcome. Classically, psychiatrists did not diagnose mania or hypomania in the absence of euphoria. But after the introduction of lithium, it was observed that some patients who respond to this drug have atypical features. This was interpreted to imply that states of excitement, irritability, and aggression in other categories of disorder could be viewed as symptoms of bipolarity.[12]

Overdiagnosis of bipolar disorders has been problematic, in that the wish to pre-scribe leads to the use of medications that are not effective in nonbipolar conditions that are also associated with mood instability. As a way of acknowledging this diffi-culty, DSM-5[13] changed the definition of a manic episode to require changes in energy as well as in mood.

The most generally accepted variant of the classical picture is bipolar II disorder.[14] This diagnosis describes mood swings from depression to hypomania rather than to full mania. But the bipolar II population is heterogeneous, and some of these patients meet criteria for personality disorders.[10]

The key issue is the assessment of hypomania. In DSM-5,[13] hypomanic episodes are defined as "a distinct period of persistently elevated, expansive, or irritable mood, lasting throughout at least 4 days, that is clearly different from the usual non-depressed mood." Patients must then have at least 3 of the following (4 if the mood is irritable and not euphoric): inflated self-esteem or grandiosity, decreased need for sleep, more talkativeness than usual or pressure to keep talking, flight of ideas or sub-jective experience that thoughts are racing, distractibility, increase in goal-directed activity (either socially, at work or school, or sexually) or psychomotor agitation, and excessive involvement in pleasurable activities that have a potential for painful conse-quences. Finally, and crucially, a hypomanic episode must be associated with an un-equivocal change in functioning that is uncharacteristic of the person when not symptomatic and should be observable by other people. In contrast to full mania, hy-pomania need not be severe enough to cause marked impairment in social or occu-pational functioning, rarely necessitates hospitalization, and is not associated with psychotic symptoms.

In short, hypomanic episodes have requirements defined by severity, time scale, and persistence. If following these criteria strictly, a bipolar II diagnosis should not be made in patients whose mood swings last less than 4 days or in whom mood does not remain abnormal over the entire period. Although it has been pointed out that the 4-day rule is not evidence based,[12] any other cutoff point would be equally arbitrary. To establish whether hypomanic episodes have occurred, it is not sufficient to take a brief history from patients, who can be vague about details; it can be helpful to interview family members to determine consistency of symptoms, time scale, whether mood changes lead to behavioral consequences, and whether they are noticeable to others.

Another variant of bipolar disorder in DSM-5[13] is a "mixed state," defined as at least a week in which a patient meets criteria for both major depression and mania. The research on mixed states is thin, and this category could be describing a heteroge-neous group of agitated patients.

Finally, DSM-5[13] allows for a diagnosis of bipolar disorder, unspecified. Like other unspecified diagnoses in the manual, this category describes patients with some but not all features of the disorder. In practice, this vague definition could be used to diagnose almost any patient with mood swings.

The proposal for a broader bipolar spectrum is not based on a gold standard for diagnosis or on biological markers derived from genetics or neurobiology.[10] Instead, epidemiologic and clinical studies estimate the prevalence of spectrum disorders using scales designed to assess subthreshold symptoms, leading to lack of precision.

In contrast to bipolar disorders, in BPD, important differences are seen in time scale and persistence in mood that can change by the hour, depending on vicissitudes in interpersonal relationships. Research using ecological momentary assessment confirms the view and suggests that BPD patients respond to interpersonal conflict with mood instability.[15] These changes usually last for hours rather than for days or weeks. Moreover, rapid shifts in mood are qualitatively different, with swings from depression to anger, whereas euphoria is rare.[16]

Several other lines of research point to important differences between BPD and bipolar disorders. The outcome of BPD is very different from (and much more favorable than) that of bipolar disorder: whereas classic bipolarity does not remit with age (and often gets worse), most BPD patients recover with time and no longer meet criteria for the disorder by middle age.[4] Moreover, family studies of patients with BPD find that diagnoses reflecting impulsivity (substance abuse and antisocial personality) are common in first-degree relatives, that unipolar depression is less common, and that bipolar disorders rare.[17] Finally, clinical trials fail to show that the drugs used to treat bipolar disorder are effective in putative spectrum disorders.[9] The few trials that have examined whether BPD responds to mood stabilizers in the same way as classic bipolar disorder show that the main impact of mood stabilizers in BPD is on impulsivity, not on mood.[4]

In summary, the fact that BPD and bipolarity both produce mood instability does not prove they are different forms of the same disorder. These differences can be conceptualized by viewing unstable mood as a nonspecific manifestation that could stem from either bipolarity or BPD.[16]

Mood swings that are responsive to the environment and that last only for a few hours can be described by the construct of affective instability (AI),[16] essentially equivalent to Linehan's[18] construct of emotion dysregulation. AI describes brief mood changes characterized by temporal instability, high intensity, and delayed recovery from dysphoric states. The construct emphasizes a distinction between environmentally driven, short-duration mood swings (AI) versus spontaneous, long-duration mood swings (bipolar and unipolar mood disorders). AI can be reliably measured and separated from mood intensity, is a heritable trait, and has been shown to be distinct from neuroticism.[16]

Because AI (or emotion dysregulation) is a key feature of BPD,[18] some investigators have suggested changing the name of the diagnosis to "emotional regulation disorder.[19] It is not clear, however, whether this affective domain accounts for all the psychopathology associated with BPD, which also includes a wide range of impulsivity, seriously disturbed interpersonal relationships, and micropsychotic phenomena.[20]

In summary, AI probably reflects a unique endophenotype. Although it is possible that some patients with BPD share neurobiological predispositions with bipolar patients, it cannot be assumed that all (or most) do.

Today one of the main obstacles to the diagnosis of BPD is the popularity of the bipolar diagnosis—what Zimmerman[21] has called the problem of diagnosing BPD in a bipolar world. Clinicians sometimes have a knee-jerk diagnostic response to mood swings. They may be unfamiliar with the concept of a PD but receive a continuous stream of claims for bipolar spectrum diagnoses, both from experts who believe in this idea and from pharmaceutical companies marketing their products. But as discussed, the consequences of misdiagnosis are bad for patients with BPD, who do not respond to the same treatment.

DIFFERENTIAL DIAGNOSIS WITH SCHIZOPHRENIA

It is not usually difficult to differentiate the hyperemotional pattern of BPD from schizophrenia, on which patients are consumed by delusions and/or emotionally unresponsive. Problems arise, however, when BPD patients have micropsychotic symptoms or brief psychotic episodes, as they often do.[22] These clinical features, in particular auditory hallucinations, are more common in BPD than is often recognized and are found in at least a quarter and up to half of cases.[23] Voices may tell BPD patients they are bad and should kill themselves. Initially, patients may consider such experiences, which are associated with severe dysregulation, as real. But because patients later realize that their imagination has been playing tricks on them, these symptoms can be called pseudohallucinations.

DIFFERENTIAL DIAGNOSIS WITH ATTENTION-DEFICIT/HYPERACTIVITY DISORDER

ADHD in adults, like bipolar disorder, is a category that is often overdiagnosed.[2] In most cases, the clinical picture of ADHD is not one of hyperactivity but of inattentiveness and a loss of mental focus, problems that can have many causes. But when practitioners are looking for something to medicate, it is tempting to consider stimulants for inattention.

What is sometimes forgotten is that ADHD begins in childhood and cannot be diagnosed in adults if it only appears in adolescence and young adulthood.[13] One longitudinal birth cohort study[24] found that almost all cases that have ADHD-like symptoms in adulthood had never had documented ADHD at any point in childhood. But because stimulants increase focus in almost everyone, the rate of their prescription has gone up dramatically.[25]

Studies of high-risk cohorts have found that childhood behavior disorders, such as ADHD and oppositional defiant disorder, can be precursors of BPD.[26] This does not mean that most cases of BPD begin as ADHD, however, or that both disorders are different manifestations of a common phenotype. Many types of temperamental variations can be associated with BPD, but the relationship between childhood risk factors and adult outcomes is complex, reflecting both equifinality (the same outcome arising from different risk factors) and multifinality (different outcomes arising from the same risk factor).[23]

DIFFERENTIAL DIAGNOSIS WITH POSTTRAUMATIC STRESS DISORDER

Several decades ago, data showing an unusually high rate of childhood trauma in BPD aroused excitement among clinicians and researchers. These reports were far from universal, however, and the types of childhood abuse most likely to lead to sequelae only occur in a minority of cases.[23,27] More severe adversities (eg, long-duration sexual abuse by family members) are associated with a greater risk, yet, even in these cases, most children do not develop BPD or other major mental disorders.[23] The association suggests that early adversity is a risk factor for many forms of psychopathology,[28] but that does not imply that BPD, a complex multidimensional disorder,[23] is a form of PTSD.

The tendency to overdiagnose PTSD, usually on the basis of trauma history alone, is another fad affecting mental health clinicians.[2] It is not justified to make this diagnosis in every patient who has experienced significant adversity: PTSD is defined by a specific set of symptoms that must be present.

Another concept that has gained some currency is *complex PTSD*,[29] in which a wider range of symptoms is assumed to be caused by multiple and repeated traumatic events. This diagnosis was not accepted by *DSM-5* but is expected to appear in the classification of the World Health Organization. The danger is that this category will encourage clinicians to focus on trauma in BPD rather on the broader picture.

BORDERLINE PERSONALITY DISORDER AND OTHER PERSONALITY DISORDERS

The classification of PD categories is unsatisfactory but was retained in *DSM-5* because alternatives, such as the dimensional system, found in Section III of the manual,[13] have not been widely researched. One result is that although some form of PD can be found in approximately half of all outpatients, the most common diagnosis is PD–not otherwise specified (now called PD unspecified).[30]

The most researched PDs are BPD and antisocial personality, and these are also probably the most valid categories.[31] Although some BPD patients, in particularly male patients, also meet criteria for antisocial, the presence of traits from other PD clusters need not be considered an example of comorbidity, given that the term describes overlaps between categories that are built into the *Diagnostic and Statistical Manual of Mental Disorders* system.[32] Thus, the presence of micropsychosis in BPD does not necessarily imply an overlap with cluster A disorders nor need the presence of avoidant or dependent patterns in relationship imply an overlap with cluster C disorders.

IMPLICATIONS FOR TREATMENT

Differential diagnosis is important when it leads to different treatment choices. Bipolar I and bipolar II disorder require pharmacologic management. Lithium is still the drug with the strongest support for both types in clinical trials,[33] and research also supports the use of anticonvulsant mood stabilizers and atypical neuroleptics.[34] But if the diagnosis is BPD, none of these drugs has more than marginal benefits.[35] The evidence strongly supports psychotherapy as the primary treatment of these patients.[36,37] Ironically, given lack of knowledge about or access to therapy, this is one of the reasons why BPD is missed.

Putting BPD patients on polypharmacy regimes derives partly from the misdiagnosis of BPD as bipolar disorder as well as the use of multiple pharmacologic agents to target specific BPD symptoms. But BPD is a diagnosis that informs clinicians that patients need to be referred for psychotherapies specifically tailored for their symptoms. The main obstacle to effective treatment of BPD lies in a lack of access to psychological services that are expensive and require well-trained therapists.[37] But this option may not be apparent if clinicians fail to take into account the disturbance of personality structure that precede and shape symptoms of mood instability and impulsivity.[38]

SUMMARY

BPD is a recognizable clinical syndrome but may be classified in other ways in the future when it is understood better.[39] Yet even within the limitations of a phenomenologically based system, some conclusions seem warranted. First, the AI that characterizes BPD can be distinguished from episodes of mood disorder, whether unipolar or bipolar. Second, the psychotic features of BPD can be distinguished from schizophrenia. Third, attentional difficulties in BPD can be differentiated from those seen in adult ADHD. Fourth, the effects of trauma in BPD do not usually resemble what is seen in PTSD.

None of these conditions, even when they are comorbid with BPD, can account for the complexity of the disorder. That is why differential diagnosis is crucial for choosing the best treatment.

REFERENCES

1. Hyman SE. The diagnosis of mental disorders: the problem of reification. Annu Rev Clin Psychol 2010;6:155–79.
2. Paris J. Overdiagnosis in psychiatry. New York: Oxford University Press; 2015.
3. Zanarini MC. Textbook of borderline personality disorder. Philadelphia: Taylor & Francis; 2005.
4. Paris J. Treatment of borderline personality disorder: a guide to evidence-based practice. New York: Guilford Press; 2008.
5. Zanarini MC, Frankenburg FR, Khera GS, et al. Treatment histories of borderline inpatients. Compr Psychiatry 2001;42:144–50.
6. Gunderson JG, Phillips KA. A current view of the interface between borderline personality disorder and depression. Am J Psychiatry 1991;148:967–75.
7. Akiskal H. Demystifying borderline personality: critique of the concept and unorthodox reflections on its natural kinship with the bipolar spectrum. Acta Psychiatr Scand 2003;110:401–7.
8. Gunderson JG, Morey LC, Stout RL, et al. Major depressive disorder and borderline personality disorder revisited: longitudinal interactions. J Clin Psychiatry 2004;65:1049–56.
9. Paris J, Gunderson JG, Weinberg I. The interface between borderline personality disorder and bipolar spectrum disorder. Compr Psychiatry 2007;48:145–54.
10. Paris J. The bipolar spectrum: diagnosis or fad? New York: Routledge; 2012.
11. Kraepelin E. Manic-depressive insanity and paranoia. Edinburgh (Scotland): E. and S. Livingstone; 1921.
12. Akiskal HS. The bipolar spectrum–the shaping of a new paradigm in psychiatry. Curr Psychiatry Rep 2002;4:1–3.
13. American Psychiatric Association. Diagnostic and statistical manual of mental disorders, text revision. 5th edition. Washington, DC: American Psychiatric Publishing; 2013.
14. Parker G, editor. Bipolar-II disorder: modelling, measuring, and managing. 2nd edition. Cambridge (England): Cambridge University Press; 2012.
15. Russell J, Moskowitz D, Sookman D, et al. Affective instability in patients with borderline personality disorder. J Abnorm Psychol 2007;116:578–88.
16. Koenigsberg H. Affective instability: toward an integration of neuroscience and psychological perspectives. J Personal Disord 2010;24:60–82.
17. White CN, Gunderson JG, Zanarini MC, et al. Family studies of borderline personality disorder: a review. Harv Rev Psychiatry 2003;12:118–9.
18. Linehan MM. Cognitive behavioral therapy for borderline personality disorder. New York: Guilford; 1993.
19. Livesley WJ. Integrated modular treatment for borderline personality disorder. Cambridge (England): Cambridge University Press; 2017.
20. Gunderson JG, Links PS. Borderline personality disorder: a clinical guide. 2nd edition. Washington, DC: American Psychiatric Press; 2008.
21. Zimmerman M. Improving the recognition of borderline personality disorder in a bipolar world. J Personal Disord 2016;30:320–3.

22. Zanarini MC, Gunderson JG, Frankenburg FR. Cognitive features of borderline personality disorder. Am J Psychiatry 1990;147:57–63.
23. Kelleher I, DeVylder JE. Hallucinations in borderline personality disorder and common mental disorders. Br J Psychiatry 2017;(210):230–1. https://doi.org/10.1192/bjp.bp.116.185249.
24. Zanarini MC. Childhood experiences associated with the development of borderline personality disorder. Psychiatr Clin North Am 2000;23:89–101.
25. Moffitt TE, Houts R, Asherson P, et al. Is adult ADHD a childhood-onset neurodevelopmental disorder? evidence from a four-decade longitudinal cohort study. Am J Psychiatry 2015;172:967–77.
26. Paris J. The development of impulsivity and suicidality in borderline personality disorder. Dev Psychopathol 2005;17:1091–104.
27. Olfson M, Blanco C, Wang S, et al. Trends in office-based treatment of adults with stimulants in the United States. J Clin Psychiatry 2013;74:43–50.
28. Courtois CA, Ford JD. Treating complex traumatic stress disorders. New York: Guilford Press; 2009.
29. Friedman MJ, Keane TM, Resnick PA. Handbook of PTSD, second edition: science and practice. New York: Guilford; 2014.
30. Zimmerman M, Rothschild L. The prevalence of DSM-IV personality disorders in psychiatric outpatients. Am J Psychiatry 2005;162:1911–8.
31. Paris J. A concise guide to personality disorders. Washington, DC: American Psychological Association Publishing; 2015.
32. Paris J. The intelligent clinician's guide to DSM-5 Oxford University Press, revised and expanded edition. New York: Oxford University Press; 2015.
33. Burgess S, Geddes J, Hawton K, et al. Lithium for maintenance treatment of mood disorders. Cochrane Database Syst Rev 2001;(3):CD003013.
34. Schatzberg AF, Nemeroff CB. The American psychiatric publishing textbook of psychopharmacology. 4th edition. Washington, DC: American Psychiatric Pubishing; 2004.
35. Stoffers J, Völlm BA, Rücker G, et al. Pharmacological interventions for borderline personality disorder. Cochrane Database Syst Rev 2010;(6):CD005653.
36. Stoffers JM, Völlm BA, Rücker G, et al. Psychological therapies for people with borderline personality disorder. Cochrane Database Syst Rev 2012;(8):CD005652.
37. Cristea I, Gentili C, Cotet C, et al. Efficacy of psychotherapies for borderline personality disorder: a systematic review and meta-analysis. JAMA Psychiatry 2017;74:319–28.
38. Kernberg OF, Yeomans F. Borderline personality disorder, bipolar disorder, depression, attention deficit/hyperactivity disorder, and narcissistic personality disorder: practical differential diagnosis. Bull Menninger Clin 2013;77:1–22.
39. Paris J. Stepped care for borderline personality disorder. Cambridge (MA): Academic Press; 2017.

Comorbidity of Borderline Personality Disorder
Current Status and Future Directions

Ravi Shah, MD[a,b], Mary C. Zanarini, EdD[a,b],*

KEYWORDS

- BPD • Comorbidity • Axis I disorders • Prevalence • Remission • Recurrence
- New onset

KEY POINTS

- All major types of disorders presenting at study entrance had a very high rate of remission over time (~90%).
- Recurrences were less common (~40%).
- New onsets were even less common (~25%).

INTRODUCTION

Borderline personality disorder (BPD) is a serious psychiatric illness associated with functional impairment, emotional instability, interpersonal problems, impulsivity, and suicidal behaviors. Studies over the past 2 decades have confirmed the coexistence of Axis I disorders in borderline patients and have documented high rates of comorbid Axis I disorders in these patients using cross-sectional and longitudinal study designs.

The borderline patients with comorbid Axis I disorders can be some of the most challenging patients for clinicians. Patients with BPD seem to have high rates of mood, anxiety, substance use, and eating disorders.[1–5] These studies were mostly conducted on borderline patients recruited from various clinical settings and had severe symptoms of BPD at the time of index admission or at the time of beginning outpatient treatment. It is quite possible that borderline patients residing in the community and other nonclinical settings may have less severe impairment and possibly fewer comorbid disorders. Furthermore, some of these studies have also documented the longitudinal associations between BPD and the commonly reported

Disclosure Statement: The authors report no relationship or financial interest with any entity that would pose conflict of interest with the subject matter of this article.
a Laboratory for the Study of Adult Development, McLean Hospital, 115 Mill Street, Belmont, MA 02478, USA; b Department of Psychiatry, Harvard Medical School, 401 Park Drive, Boston, MA 02215, USA
* Corresponding author. McLean Hospital, 115 Mill Street, Belmont, MA 02478.
E-mail address: zanarini@mclean.harvard.edu

Psychiatr Clin N Am 41 (2018) 583–593
https://doi.org/10.1016/j.psc.2018.07.009
0193-953X/18/© 2018 Elsevier Inc. All rights reserved.

Axis I disorders over the year of prospective follow-up. These findings were crucial to understanding the course of comorbid Axis I disorders in borderline patients over time. In particular, stability of Axis I disorders over time, rates of remission, recurrence, and new onset were revealed. For the purpose of this article, each comorbid Axis I disorder will be discussed separately under the following subheadings: baseline prevalence; prevalence over time; remission; recurrence; and new onset.

MOOD DISORDERS
Baseline Prevalence

Mood disorders are the most common comorbid conditions observed in patients with BPD. It has been estimated that 96% of patients with BPD have a mood disorder at some point during their life.[4,6] In particular, the prevalence of comorbid depression in borderline patients has been reported in the range of 32% to 83% by several cross-sectional studies.[1,3-5,7-9] Lower rates of comorbid depression in borderline patients were found in 2 out of 7 cross-sectional studies.[7,8] The lower rates observed in these 2 studies can be attributed to the differences in study population and sample size. The findings of Grant and colleagues[7] were based on a large-scale study conducted on an adult civilian population whereas that of Pope and colleagues[8] were from chart reviews of 39 former inpatients.

LONGITUDINAL COURSE OF MOOD DISORDERS IN BORDERLINE PATIENTS
Prevalence over Time

Three studies have assessed the prevalence of mood disorders in borderline patients longitudinally.[10-12] Links and colleagues[11] conducted a prospective follow-up study on former psychiatric in-patients 7 years after their discharge from one of the 4 general hospitals in Ontario, Canada. The prevalence rate of major depression in borderline patients was 37% 7 years after the index admission. The proportion of bipolar II and dysthymia in these borderline patients was 12% and 29.6%, respectively. The second study was conducted by Paris and Zweig-Frank[12] on former psychiatric in-patients at the Jewish General Hospital in Montreal, Canada. This follow-back study assessed the prevalence of major depression and dysthymia in borderline patients 27 years after their index admission. The overall prevalence of major depression and dysthymia in their sample was 3.1% and 22%, respectively. The third study was conducted by Zanarini and colleagues[10] on former psychiatric in-patients and was part of the McLean Study of Adult Development (MSAD). The participants were followed prospectively after their index admission, and 6-year follow-up data were collected through semistructured interviews. The prevalence of any mood disorders in borderline patients was found to be 75% whereas that of major depression, dysthymia, and bipolar II was 61.4%, 40.5%, and 6.7%, respectively. The lower rates of mood disorders observed in Paris's study can be attributed, in part, to the longer follow-up period.

The findings from these studies indicate that mood disorders are fairly common in borderline patients and remain stable over time. For example, the study conducted by Zanarini and colleagues[10] found that the rates of mood disorders in borderline patients at 6-year follow-up (75%) did not decrease much when compared with the baseline rates of 96.9%. These high rates of mood disorders in borderline patients could be attributed to the higher rates of relapse. This phenomenon was observed in the Collaborative Longitudinal Personality Disorders Study (CLPS) at 6-year follow-up. Their findings suggest that comorbid MDD relapsed more frequently in borderline patients compared with other personality disorders.[13]

Remission

Five naturalistic follow-along studies[13–17] from the CLPS examined the longitudinal interactions between BPD and mood disorders. A 2-year follow-up study from CLPS showed a bidirectional relationship in which improvement in either BPD or MDD predicted remission of the other disorder.[14] A 3-year follow-up study conducted by Gunderson and colleagues[15] indicated a unidirectional relationship; changes in BPD significantly predicted improvement in MDD but not vice-versa. Four-year follow-up data on comorbid bipolar disorder showed that neither bipolar I nor II had much effect on BPD's course.[16] Gunderson and colleagues[17] analyzed the interactions between BPD and mood disorders using the data collected over 10 years of prospective follow-up. Their findings suggest that BPD had no significant effect on bipolar disorder, but BPD and MDD had reciprocal negative effects on each other in terms of time to remission and time to relapse/onset. These findings are consistent with the 2-year follow-up study from CLPS. However, this bidirectional relationship was not evident in the 3-year follow-up study, wherein changes in the BPD predicted change in MDD but not vice-versa. This discrepancy may have resulted from using cross-lagged panel analyses (examining fine-tune changes in criteria) in the 3-year report as opposed to the proportional hazards regression analyses (examining remission/relapse events) used at 2- and 10-year follow-up.

Recurrence

The 6-year follow-up study conducted by Gunderson and colleagues[13] analyzed the rates of relapse of MDD in borderline patients. Their findings suggest that MDD relapsed more frequently in borderline patients compared with those with other personality disorders. In particular, the recurrence rate for MDD was 92% in borderline patients compared with 82% in other personality disorders by 6-year follow-up. Furthermore, in a 10-year follow-up study conducted by Gunderson and colleagues[17] reported that BPD significantly delayed MDD's time to remission and accelerated time to relapse ($P = .04$).

New Onset

The study conducted by Gunderson and colleagues[13] documented the new onset of major depression in the sample of borderline patients. Their findings suggest that 41% of BPD patients who did not meet the criteria for lifetime MDD at baseline had developed a new onset of MDD by 6-year follow-up. Another study conducted by the same group on borderline patients[16] reported the effects of BPD on bipolar disorders. Their findings suggest that BPD had a modest increased effect on new onsets of bipolar I and II disorders compared with those with other personality disorders.

ANXIETY DISORDERS
Baseline Prevalence

The prevalence of comorbid anxiety disorders in borderline patients has been documented by numerous cross-sectional studies, and it ranges from 0% to 35% for generalized anxiety disorder (GAD), 2% to 48% for panic disorder with or without agoraphobia, 3% to 46% for social phobia, 0% to 20% for obsessive compulsive disorder (OCD), and 25% to 56% for posttraumatic stress disorder (PTSD).[3,5,7,18,19] Furthermore, the co-occurrence of any anxiety disorder was found to be 88% in a study conducted on borderline patients recruited from psychiatric inpatient units.[4]

In addition, the lifetime prevalence of any anxiety disorder was found to be 74.2% in a large-scale community sample.[7]

LONGITUDINAL COURSE OF ANXIETY DISORDERS IN BORDERLINE PATIENTS
Prevalence over Time

Longitudinally, the prevalence of anxiety disorders in borderline patients was assessed in 3 studies[10,11,18] over 6, 7, and 10 years of prospective follow-up. At 6-year follow-up, the study conducted by Zanarini and colleagues[10] found that the co-occurrence of any anxiety disorder in borderline patients was 60.2% and that of panic disorder, social phobia, OCD, and GAD was 29.2%, 17.4%, 6.4%, and 7.2%, respectively. The study included PTSD as a part of anxiety disorders and its prevalence was found to be 34.9%. The study conducted by Links and colleagues[11] at 7-year follow-up reported the prevalence rates of 14.8%, 3.7%, and 7.4% for phobia, OCD, and GAD, respectively, in borderline patients. However, the overall prevalence of anxiety disorders was much lower in a 10-year follow-up. MSAD study conducted by Silverman and her colleagues[18] found that the prevalence of any anxiety disorder in borderline patients was 37.8% whereas that for panic, social phobia, OCD, and GAD were 22.9%, 7.2%, 10%, and 4.4%, respectively. It is important to note that Silverman's study excluded PTSD from data analyses when reporting the prevalence rates of anxiety disorders in borderline patients as the prevalence and course of this disorder was covered in another paper.[19] Overall, these studies indicate that anxiety disorder is relatively unstable over time, and the rates of anxiety disorders in borderline patients decreased significantly after 6 and 10 years of prospective follow-up. Although the rate of anxiety disorder was much lower at 10 years,[18] further exploration revealed a significant decrease in the rates of all anxiety disorders except for OCD and GAD over time.

Remission

The study conducted by Silverman and colleagues[18] reported that all anxiety disorders had high rates of remission by 10-year follow-up. Specifically, 77% of patients with OCD, 82% with panic disorder, 92% with simple phobia, 97% with social phobia, and 100% with GAD and agoraphobia who met the criteria for anxiety disorder at baseline experienced at least one 2-year remission by the time of 10-year follow-up. The remission rates of panic disorder reported in this study were consistent with the findings of the Harvard/Brown Anxiety Research Program (HARP) study at 8-year follow-up.[20] However, the rates of remission of social phobia, GAD, and OCD were substantially higher than the HARP study at 8- and 15-year follow-up.[21] These differences can be attributed to the fact that HARP study was following participants with primary anxiety disorders, whereas participants in the MSAD study primarily suffered from secondary anxiety disorders. Furthermore, the study conducted by Keuroghlian and colleagues[22] analyzed the interactions of BPD and anxiety disorders over 10 years of prospective follow-up. Their findings suggest that improvement in BPD significantly predicted remission from GAD and PTSD, but the course of anxiety disorders had no effects on BPD remission or relapse.

Recurrence

The 10-year follow-up study conducted by Silverman and colleagues[18] also reported the recurrence rates of panic disorder (65%), agoraphobia (30%), social phobia (40%), simple phobia (30%), OCD (37%), and GAD (32%) for borderline patients who met the criteria for these anxiety disorders at baseline and had remitted from anxiety disorders at an earlier follow-up period.

New Onset

This study has also demonstrated that new onsets of anxiety disorders are relatively uncommon in borderline patients who did not meet the criteria for an anxiety disorder at baseline. In a study conducted by Silverman and colleagues,[18] at 10-year follow-up, the rates of new onsets of anxiety disorders in borderline patients were 15% for agoraphobia, 17% for OCD, 23% for GAD, 24% for social phobia, 36% for simple phobia, and 47% for panic disorder.

POSTTRAUMATIC STRESS DISORDER
Baseline Prevalence

PTSD is common among patients with BPD and has been documented in several cross-sectional studies. The prevalence rates reported in these studies range from 25% to 56% (median = 46.9%).[3–5,7,23–25]

LONGITUDINAL COURSE OF POSTTRAUMATIC STRESS DISORDER IN BORDERLINE PATIENTS
Prevalence over Time

Two longitudinal studies have assessed the co-occurrence of PTSD in borderline patients.[10,19] Both studies were conducted by Zanarini and her colleagues at 6 and 10 years of prospective follow-up and provide substantial information about the course of comorbid PTSD in borderline patients. The 6-year follow-up study[10] demonstrated that 34.9% of the borderline patients had PTSD. In another study[19] at 10-year follow-up, the same group revealed a decline in the prevalence of PTSD in the borderline patients to 20.9%. Overall, these studies have indicated that the rate of PTSD in borderline patients tends to decrease over time.

Remission

It was estimated that 87% of borderline patients who met the criteria of PTSD at baseline experienced at least one 2-year remission by the time of 10-year follow-up.[19] The presence of childhood sexual abuse and the severity of abuse significantly predicted remission from PTSD. In other words, borderline patients with a history of childhood adversity were less likely to achieve a remission from PTSD compared with those without such history. The rate of remission reported at 10-year follow-up was in line with the rate of remission reported at 6-year follow-up.

Recurrence

This 10-year follow-up study[19] also reported the recurrence rate of PTSD in borderline patients who remitted from PTSD at an earlier follow-up period. It was estimated that 40% of these borderline patients had a PTSD recurrence by the 10-year follow-up.

New Onset

The 10-year follow-up study[19] also reported new onsets of PTSD in borderline patients who did not meet the criteria for PTSD at baseline. It was estimated that 27% of borderline patients who did not report having PTSD at baseline developed PTSD by 10-year follow-up. The rate of new onsets observed in this study was about 3 times higher than the longitudinal study of holocaust survivors followed for 10 years.[26] It is also about 5 times the rate of new onsets of PTSD found in Vietnam veterans followed for 14 years.[27] These differences in the rates of new onsets might be attributed to the nature of the trauma or severity of trauma experienced and/or the age at which these experiences occurred.

SUBSTANCE USE DISORDERS
Baseline Prevalence

Previous studies on borderline patients have frequently documented the presence of comorbid substance use disorders. Based on cross-sectional studies, the prevalence of comorbid substance use disorders in borderline patients ranges from 23% to 84% (median = 65.1%).[1,3,4,7,8,28] These studies have also reported that the co-occurrence of alcohol abuse or dependence in borderline patients ranges from 11.9% to 66% (median = 47%), whereas the prevalence of drug use or dependence ranges from 3.4% to 87% (median = 44.1%).[1,3–5,7,9,29,30]

LONGITUDINAL COURSE OF SUBSTANCE USE DISORDERS IN BORDERLINE PATIENTS
Prevalence over Time

Four longitudinal studies have assessed the prevalence of substance use disorders in samples of criteria-defined borderline patients.[10–12,31] The prospective follow-up study conducted by Links and colleagues[11] assessed the point prevalence of alcohol and drug use disorders in borderline patients 7 years after discharge from psychiatric in-patient units in Canada. The group found that 11.1% of the borderline patients met the criteria for alcoholism, whereas 7.7% met the criteria for drug use disorder at the time of interview. The second study was conducted by Paris and Zweig-Frank[12] on former psychiatric in-patients at the Jewish General Hospital in Montreal, Canada. The follow-up data collected after 27 years of postdischarge status found 4.7% of active substance use disorder in borderline patients. The other 2 prospective follow-up studies[10,31] were part of the MSAD. These 2 studies were conducted on former psychiatric in-patients who were enrolled in the study, and the data were collected prospectively 6 and 10 years after their index admissions. At 6-year follow-up, the prevalence of any substance use disorder in borderline patients was 18.9%, whereas that of alcohol and drug use disorders in borderline patients was 11.4% and 12.9%, respectively. As expected these rates continued to decline. At 10-year follow-up, the co-occurrence of any substance use disorders in borderline patients was 13.7%, whereas that of alcohol and drug use disorders was 8.8% and 7.2%, respectively. Overall, these findings suggest that substance use disorder is very common in borderline patients, but its prevalence tends to decrease substantially over time.

Remission

The study conducted by Zanarini and colleagues[31] reported that more than 90% of borderline patients who met the criteria for alcohol abuse/dependence or drug abuse/dependence at baseline experienced at least one 2-year remission by the time of 10-year follow-up. The rates of remission observed in this study were substantially higher than other studies conducted on primary substance use disorders.[32,33] It is quite possible that borderline patients with secondary substance use disorders may have less severe substance use disorder, which remitted significantly by 10 years of prospective follow-up.

Recurrence

The 10-year follow-up study conducted by Zanarini and colleagues[31] also reported the recurrence rates of alcohol abuse/dependence and drug abuse/dependence in borderline patients who remitted from these disorders. In particular, 35% of borderline patients who remitted from drug abuse or dependence also reported a recurrence of this disorder by the 10-year follow-up. Furthermore, 40% of borderline patients who remitted from alcohol abuse or dependence reported a recurrence of this disorder by the 10-year follow-up. The recurrence rate of alcohol abuse/dependence reported in this study was similar to the 45% found by Vaillant[34] in an 8-year follow-up study of patients initially hospitalized for alcohol withdrawal.

New Onset

The study conducted by Zanarini and colleagues[31] reported that the new onsets of drug abuse or dependence in borderline patients who did not meet the criteria for drug abuse/dependence at baseline were 21% by the time of 10-year follow-up. Furthermore, the new onsets of alcohol abuse or dependence in borderline patients who did not meet the criteria for these disorders at baseline were 20% by the time of 10-year follow-up. Similar but slightly lower rates of new onset of substance use disorders in borderline patients were found in a 7-year follow-up CLPS study conducted by Walter and colleagues.[35] Walter's study was conducted specifically to identify the new onset of substance use disorders, and their rates were 13% and 11% for new onset of alcohol and drug use disorder, respectively. Overall, these studies suggest that the new onset of substance use disorder is relatively uncommon in borderline patients who did not meet the criteria for alcohol abuse/dependence or drug abuse/dependence at baseline.

EATING DISORDERS
Baseline Prevalence

Eating disorders are common among patients with BPD, and its prevalence rates have been documented by several cross-sectional studies. These studies have reported that the co-occurrence of anorexia nervosa ranges from 0% to 21% (median = 6%), bulimia nervosa ranges from 3% to 26% (median = 10%), and eating disorder not otherwise specified (EDNOS) ranges from 14% to 26% (median = 22%).[1,3–5,8,9] These studies have also indicated that both anorexia nervosa and bulimia nervosa are relatively less common in borderline patients compared with EDNOS. Overall, the prevalence of any eating disorders was found to be in the range of 14% to 53% in these studies.[1,3,4]

LONGITUDINAL COURSE OF EATING DISORDERS IN BORDERLINE PATIENTS
Prevalence over Time

Two follow-up longitudinal studies on eating disorders[10,36] were conducted as a part of the MSAD. The prevalence of eating disorders in borderline patients was reported by 2 studies[10,36] at 6- and 10-year follow-up. At 6-year follow-up,[10] the prevalence of any eating disorders, anorexia, bulimia, and EDNOS in borderline patients was 33.7%, 2.7%, 5.3%, and 27.7%, respectively. As expected, at 10-year follow-up,[36] the prevalence of any eating disorders, anorexia, bulimia, and EDNOS in borderline patients was 19.7%, 1.6%, 1.6%, and 16.5%, respectively. Overall, these findings suggest that rates of eating disorders decreased significantly over time.

Remission

The study conducted by Zanarini and colleagues[36] reported that more than 90% of borderline patients who met the criteria for anorexia, bulimia, or EDNOS at baseline experienced at least one 2-year remission by the time of the 10-year follow-up. In particular, the rates of remission from anorexia, bulimia, and EDNOS at the 10-year follow-up were 100%, 97.4%, and 92%, respectively. These rates of remission were somewhat higher than the rates reported in other studies.[37–41] The higher rates of remission observed in Zanarini's study could be attributed to the differences in the study sample. The participants in those other studies were being treated for primary eating disorders, whereas those in Zanarini's study were suffering from secondary eating disorders. It is quite possible that borderline patients with secondary eating disorders may have a less severe eating disorder, which remitted significantly by 10 years of prospective follow-up.

Recurrence

The 10-year follow-up study conducted by Zanarini and colleagues[36] also reported the recurrence rates of anorexia, bulimia, and EDNOS in borderline patients who remitted from these disorders at an earlier follow-up. In particular, more than 50% of borderline patients who remitted from EDNOS reported a recurrence of this disorder by the time of 10-year follow-up. Furthermore, less than 30% of borderline patients who remitted from either anorexia or bulimia latter reported a recurrence of these disorders.

It is also important to note that diagnostic migrations were very common in borderline patients who met the criteria for anorexia and bulimia during their index admission. In particular, 87.5% of borderline patients who met the criteria for anorexia at baseline experienced change in their eating disorder diagnosis over time. Similarly, 70.7% of borderline patients reporting bulimia at baseline experienced change in their eating disorder diagnosis over time. Overall, the study indicated that the majorly of borderline patients with either anorexia or bulimia at baseline ultimately crossed over to EDNOS over time.

New Onset

Previous studies have also demonstrated that the new onset of eating disorders is relatively uncommon in borderline patients who did not meet the criteria for eating disorders at baseline. The study conducted by Zanarini and colleagues[36] at 10-year follow-up reported the new onsets of anorexia, bulimia, and EDNOS in borderline patients as 3.7%, 11.2%, and 42%, respectively.

COMPLEX COMORBIDITY

Clinical experience suggests that borderline patients often present with symptoms of comorbid axis I disorders. These initial symptoms may mask the underlying borderline psychopathology making it harder for early diagnosis. The study conducted by Zanarini and colleagues[4] analyzed a lifetime pattern of complex comorbidity as a predictor of BPD diagnosis. The concept of complex comorbidity was defined as meeting DSM-III-R criteria for both a disorder of affect (depression, bipolar disorder, and anxiety disorder) and a disorder of impulse (substance use or eating disorder) at the same time before the index admission. Their findings suggest that the pattern of complex comorbidity has a strong positive predictive power for the borderline diagnosis and can be used as a useful marker for it. It was also documented that a pattern of meeting lifetime criteria for both a disorder of affect and a disorder of impulse has strong sensitivity and specificity for the BPD diagnosis. Despite these promising findings, the complex model of comorbidity has not been widely used in clinical settings.

SUMMARY

Overall, this review suggests that Axis I disorders are very common in borderline patients and that prevalence rates tend to decrease gradually over time. The longitudinal studies conducted on borderline patients over 10 years of prospective follow-up suggest that patients with BPD experienced declining rates of Axis I disorders over time, and the rates of these disorders remained high compared with those with other personality disorders. Patients whose BPD remitted over time experienced a substantial decline in all comorbid Axis I disorders, but those whose BPD did not remit over time, reported stable rates of comorbid disorders.[10] These longitudinal studies have also assessed the stability of Axis I disorders over time in borderline patients. Borderline patients with mood disorders, OCD, and GAD tend to have stable rates of comorbidity over time compared with PTSD, substance use disorders, and eating disorders.

REFERENCES

1. Zanarini MC, Gunderson JG, Frankenburg FR. Axis I phenomenology of borderline personality disorder. Compr Psychiatry 1989;30(2):149–56.
2. Oldham JM, Skodol AE, Kellman HD, et al. Comorbidity of axis I and axis II disorders. Am J Psychiatry 1995;152(4):571–8.
3. Zimmerman M, Mattia JI. Axis I diagnostic comorbidity and borderline personality disorder. Compr Psychiatry 1999;40(4):245–52.
4. Zanarini MC, Frankenburg FR, Dubo ED, et al. Axis I comorbidity of borderline personality disorder. Am J Psychiatry 1998;155(12):1733–9.
5. McGlashan TH, Grilo CM, Skodol AE, et al. The Collaborative Longitudinal Personality Disorders Study: baseline Axis I/II and II/II diagnostic co-occurrence. Acta Psychiatr Scand 2000;102(4):256–64.
6. Biskin RS, Paris J. Comorbidities in borderline personality disorder. Psychiatric Times 2013. Available at: http://www.psychiatrictimes.com/borderline-personality/comorbidities-borderline-personality-disorder. Accessed March 20, 2018.
7. Grant BF, Chou SP, Goldstein RB, et al. Prevalence, correlates, disability, and comorbidity of DSM-IV borderline personality disorder: results from the Wave 2 National Epidemiologic Survey on Alcohol and Related Conditions. J Clin Psychiatry 2008;69(4):533–45.
8. Pope HG Jr, Jonas JM, Hudson JI, et al. The validity of DSM-III borderline personality disorder. A phenomenologic, family history, treatment response, and long-term follow-up study. Arch Gen Psychiatry 1983;40(1):23–30.
9. Coid JW. An affective syndrome in psychopaths with borderline personality disorder? Br J Psychiatry 1993;162:641–50.
10. Zanarini MC, Frankenburg FR, Hennen J, et al. Axis I comorbidity in patients with borderline personality disorder: 6-year follow-up and prediction of time to remission. Am J Psychiatry 2004;161(11):2108–14.
11. Links PS, Heslegrave RJ, Mitton JE, et al. Borderline psychopathology and recurrences of clinical disorders. J Nerv Ment Dis 1995;183(9):582–6.
12. Paris J, Zweig-Frank H. A 27-year follow-up of patients with borderline personality disorder. Compr Psychiatry 2001;42(6):482–7.
13. Gunderson JG, Stout RL, Sanislow CA, et al. New episodes and new onsets of major depression in borderline and other personality disorders. J Affect Disord 2008;111(1):40–5.
14. Shea MT, Stout RL, Yen S, et al. Associations in the course of personality disorders and axis I disorders over time. J Abnorm Psychol 2004;113(4):499–508.
15. Gunderson JG, Morey LC, Stout RL, et al. Major depressive disorder and borderline personality disorder revisited: longitudinal interactions. J Clin Psychiatry 2004;65(8):1049–56.
16. Gunderson JG, Weinberg I, Daversa MT, et al. Descriptive and longitudinal observations on the relationship of borderline personality disorder and bipolar disorder. Am J Psychiatry 2006;163(7):1173–8.

17. Gunderson JG, Stout RL, Shea MT, et al. Interactions of borderline personality disorder and mood disorders over 10 years. J Clin Psychiatry 2014;75(8):829–34.
18. Silverman MH, Frankenburg FR, Reich DB, et al. The course of anxiety disorders other than PTSD in patients with borderline personality disorder and axis II comparison subjects: a 10-year follow-up study. J Pers Disord 2012;26(5):804–14.
19. Zanarini MC, Horz S, Frankenburg FR, et al. The 10-year course of PTSD in borderline patients and axis II comparison subjects. Acta Psychiatr Scand 2011;124(5):349–56.
20. Yonkers KA, Bruce SE, Dyck IR, et al. Chronicity, relapse, and illness–course of panic disorder, social phobia, and generalized anxiety disorder: findings in men and women from 8 years of follow-up. Depress Anxiety 2003;17(3):173–9.
21. Marcks BA, Weisberg RB, Dyck I, et al. Longitudinal course of obsessive-compulsive disorder in patients with anxiety disorders: a 15-year prospective follow-up study. Compr Psychiatry 2011;52(6):670–7.
22. Keuroghlian AS, Gunderson JG, Pagano ME, et al. Interactions of borderline personality disorder and anxiety disorders over 10 years. J Clin Psychiatry 2015; 76(11):1529–34.
23. Mueser KT, Goodman LB, Trumbetta SL, et al. Trauma and posttraumatic stress disorder in severe mental illness. J Consult Clin Psychol 1998;66(3):493–9.
24. Yen S, Shea MT, Battle CL, et al. Traumatic exposure and posttraumatic stress disorder in borderline, schizotypal, avoidant, and obsessive-compulsive personality disorders: findings from the collaborative longitudinal personality disorders study. J Nerv Ment Dis 2002;190(8):510–8.
25. Golier JA, Yehuda R, Bierer LM, et al. The relationship of borderline personality disorder to posttraumatic stress disorder and traumatic events. Am J Psychiatry 2003;160(11):2018–24.
26. Yehuda R, Schmeidler J, Labinsky E, et al. Ten-year follow-up study of PTSD diagnosis, symptom severity and psychosocial indices in aging holocaust survivors. Acta Psychiatr Scand 2009;119:25–34.
27. Koenen KC, Stellman JM, Stellman SD, et al. Risk factors for course of posttraumatic stress disorder among Vietnam veterans: a 14-year follow-up of American Legionnaires. J Consult Clin Psychol 2003;71(6):980–6.
28. Frances A, Clarkin JF, Gilmore M, et al. Reliability of criteria for borderline personality disorder: a comparison of DSM-III and the diagnostic interview for borderline patients. Am J Psychiatry 1984;141(9):1080–4.
29. Swartz MS, Blazer DG, George LK, et al. Identification of borderline personality disorder with the NIMH Diagnostic Interview Schedule. Am J Psychiatry 1989; 146(2):200–5.
30. Shearer SL. Dissociative phenomena in women with borderline personality disorder. Am J Psychiatry 1994;151(9):1324–8.
31. Zanarini MC, Frankenburg FR, Weingeroff JL, et al. The course of substance use disorders in patients with borderline personality disorder and Axis II comparison subjects: a 10-year follow-up study. Addiction 2011;106(2):342–8.
32. Hser YI, Hoffman V, Grella CE, et al. A 33-year follow-up of narcotics addicts. Arch Gen Psychiatry 2001;58(5):503–8.
33. Vaillant GE, Clark W, Cyrus C, et al. Prospective study of alcoholism treatment. Eight-year follow-up. Am J Med 1983;75(3):455–63.
34. Vaillant GE. A long-term follow-up of male alcohol abuse. Arch Gen Psychiatry 1996;53(3):243–9.
35. Walter M, Gunderson JG, Zanarini MC, et al. New onsets of substance use disorders in borderline personality disorder over 7 years of follow-ups: findings from

the Collaborative Longitudinal Personality Disorders Study. Addiction 2009; 104(1):97–103.

36. Zanarini MC, Reichman CA, Frankenburg FR, et al. The course of eating disorders in patients with borderline personality disorder: a 10-year follow-up study. Int J Eat Disord 2010;43(3):226–32.

37. Grilo CM, Pagano ME, Skodol AE, et al. Natural course of bulimia nervosa and of eating disorder not otherwise specified: 5-year prospective study of remissions, relapses, and the effects of personality disorder psychopathology. J Clin Psychiatry 2007;68(5):738–46.

38. Deter HC, Herzog W. Anorexia nervosa in a long-term perspective: results of the Heidelberg-Mannheim Study. Psychosom Med 1994;56(1):20–7.

39. Herzog DB, Dorer DJ, Keel PK, et al. Recovery and relapse in anorexia and bulimia nervosa: a 7.5-year follow-up study. J Am Acad Child Adolesc Psychiatry 1999;38(7):829–37.

40. Eddy KT, Dorer DJ, Franko DL, et al. Diagnostic crossover in anorexia nervosa and bulimia nervosa: implications for DSM-V. Am J Psychiatry 2008;165(2): 245–50.

41. Fichter MM, Quadflieg N. Long-term stability of eating disorder diagnoses. Int J Eat Disord 2007;40(Suppl):S61–6.

An Object-Relations Based Model for the Assessment of Borderline Psychopathology

Barry L. Stern, PhD[a],*, Eve Caligor, MD[a],
Susanne Hörz-Sagstetter, PhD[b], John F. Clarkin, PhD[a]

KEYWORDS

- Psychoanalytic psychotherapy • Borderline • Borderline personality disorder
- Personality organization • Assessment

KEY POINTS

- The authors describe an object-relations based model drawing on the work of Kernberg and colleagues for the assessment of borderline pathology.
- The substrate of internal object relations that constitutes borderline pathology internally or structurally is described and a model for assessing such pathology in a clinical interview format focusing on identity, defensive style, and quality of object relations is presented.
- Two clinical examples illustrate how these data can be compiled for purposes of psychodynamic case formulation and decisions about psychodynamic treatment.

Psychodynamic clinicians have long been troubled by the disconnect between the official psychiatric diagnostic classification codified in the *Diagnostic and Statistical Manual of Mental Disorders* (DSM),[1,2] and the underlying, internal characteristics of disordered personality, our understanding of what is pathologic in personality disorders, and how personality disorders are treated therapeutically. This disconnect has diminished somewhat in the past several years, with the development of both the *Psychodynamic Diagnostic Manual* (PDM)[3,4] and the Alternate Model for Personality Disorders in Section III of the DSM-5 (AMPD),[2] both of which move beyond assessment of symptoms to the acknowledgment of core psychological features of a patient's personality, specifically, the patient's experience of the self and the relation of that experience to others, that lies at the heart of personality disorders.

Disclosure statement: Work on the STIPO-R, which is a significant focus on this paper, has been provided by the American Psychoanalytic Association, and the International Psychoanalytic Association.

[a] Columbia University Medical Center, 122 East 42nd Street, Suite 3200, New York, NY 10168, USA; [b] Psychologische Hochschule Berlin, Clinical Psychology and Psychotherapy, Am Köllnischen Park 2, 10179 Berlin, Germany
* Corresponding author. Columbia University Medical Center, 122 East 42nd Street, Suite 3200, New York, NY 10168.
E-mail address: bs2137@cumc.columbia.edu

Psychiatr Clin N Am 41 (2018) 595–611
https://doi.org/10.1016/j.psc.2018.07.007
0193-953X/18/© 2018 Elsevier Inc. All rights reserved.

Abbreviations

BPO   Borderline personality organization
STIPO   Structured Interview of Personality Organization

The psychodynamic assessment of borderline pathology unfolds in the initial meetings with a patient according to the particular therapist's frame of reference as well as the level of acuity with which the patient presents. Along with providing appropriate containment of affect and assessments of risk and safety, the therapist's questions in the initial sessions allow the therapist to develop a map of the patient's internal world and how this internal experience in turn fits with the therapist's model of health and pathology. Part of this assessment involves the patient's capacities, for example, for reflection, interpersonal relatedness, reality testing, coherence of self, impulse control, and anxiety tolerance, all features related to borderline symptoms as well as dynamic conceptions of personality disorder.[5,6] The patient's primary defensive style can also be ascertained in these initial meetings; is there flexibility and openness, or clear "no-go" areas of inquiry that would suggest the patient's need for control and the operation of splitting-based defenses. An assessment process that conveys at the outset an interest in the person through which maladaptive behaviors and symptoms are expressed, in his or her capacities, proclivities, and defenses, frames a treatment focused on this broader conception of personality, proposing that a better understanding of this person is intimately related to the success and durability of the treatment.

Before elaborating further our particular psychodynamic model of personality disorder assessment, we need to frame this discussion in the context of a major shift in the empirical, theoretic, and clinical classification of personality disorders. Criticism of the DSM's categorical classification system, for the lack of any empirical support for distinct personality disorders, for the significant criterion overlap and the associated, clinically meaningless comorbidity of diagnosis, and for the lack of reliability for individual personality disorder diagnoses, has been long and well-documented.[7–10] Furthermore, the current present or absent, 10-category diagnostic system provides no information about severity of illness, prognosis, or likely course of treatment. The broad chorus echoing these complaints, along with scores of empirical studies, has led to a groundswell of support for a reconceptualization of personality disorder diagnosis based on a dimensional approach,[11–15] a shift that has been expressed to varying degrees in the revisions of each of several major diagnostic systems, including the PDM 2,[4] the Alternative Model for Personality Disorders in the DSM-5,[2] and the still in-process *International Classification of Diseases*, 11the edition.[11]

Despite clear consensus that a shift to dimensional thinking better fits the empirical data and is more clinically useful, 2 questions remain somewhat less clear: what definition of personality are we considering when we say "a dimensional approach to personality assessment" and, then, what specific variables or domains related to personality health and pathology ought we assess in this dimensional manner? One definition or conceptual model for personality with a long tradition of empirical research across cultures involves dispositional traits (ie, The Big Five).[16–20] An approach to personality assessment based on dispositional traits has been lobbied effectively for inclusion in personality disorder diagnostic systems, in part owing to their recognizability, replicated links to personality disorders, and biological and evolutionary underpinnings. For many dynamic clinicians, however, an individual's trait signature (eg, extraverted, antagonistic, open to experience, self-conscious, vulnerable) provides little information about the person's "characteristic adaptations,"[21] the psychosocial and interpersonal context of the person over time, and his or her motivations, interests, characteristic tendencies, conflicts, and overall adaptation. Although the assessment model we elaborate is a specific psychodynamic model of personality within this latter category of "characteristic adaptations," and with specific domains of functioning, surveyed dimensionally, it is notable that both the DSM-5, the AMPD, and to some extent the PDM 2 are hybrid models in which both dispositional traits and styles of characteristic adaptation are assessed.

The remainder of this article addresses the question of which specific domains of adaptation or functioning related to personality we assess, why these particular domains, and how they are assessed. It is notable that we are speaking of several domains, each sampled dimensionally, and that, taken together, form a full picture of the individual's personality functioning, one into which the individual's symptoms and clinical problems can be contextualized, for example, one's sense of self over time, stability versus instability in experience of others, coping and defensive style, aggression and hostility, and moral functioning. They provide the clinician with both an index of severity of illness, as well as a sense of the patient's competence and resiliencies, all of which help to contextualize the patient's difficulties in the language of the therapist's theory of technique, clinical experience, and his or her own personality.

The assessment model that follows is born of the belief that the symptoms of borderline personality disorder, as well as most of the other personality disorders cataloged in the DSM IV and 5, share certain core or "structural" features forming a syndrome called borderline personality organization (BPO). Derived from modern object relations theory,[5,6] we conceptualize a personality disorder as a pathology of "internal object relations," in which the integration of positively and negatively charged representations of self and others, required for a realistic and stable sense of self across time and situations, is not attained. This lack of integration of positive and negative aspects of the self is referred to as identity diffusion. It is from this internal structure that the various symptomatic expressions of personality disorder in the borderline range (eg, borderline proper, schizoid, narcissistic, paranoid) derive and that the experience of borderline symptomatology, at various levels of severity follows.

BORDERLINE PERSONALITY ORGANIZATION AS A PATHOLOGY OF INTERNAL OBJECT RELATIONS

Of the several features that come to a clinician's mind when thinking of borderline personality, problems with identity and splitting as a defensive posture are among the more prominent and defining. Almost indistinguishable empirically,[22–24] identity pathology and splitting-based defenses also work hand-in-glove psychically and together constitute the core of the internal world of the borderline patient. Splitting-based defenses such as primitive denial, omnipotent control, idealization/devaluation, and black-and-white thinking, operate intrapsychically and interpersonally to divide the full experience of the self, splitting off experiences and representations that are undesirable, disturbing, or incongruent with a desired self-image and assigning, or projecting them, onto others. The result of this process is the internally segmented world that we term "identity diffused," meaning that the self is experienced as discontinuous over time and across situation as different aspects of the self, dissociated from one another, are experienced in a back-and-forth and abruptly shifting manner. When representations of self and other fail to consolidate to form an integrated sense of self and others, and the good and desirable qualities never touch and thus modulate the bad or undesirable qualities and vice versa, and the result is a brittle, rigid caricature of a self, and a correspondingly brittle caricature of others, one lacking in the depth, nuance, and realistic feel of an integrated, healthier personality. This internal split leaves the individual vulnerable to typical borderline symptoms such as mood lability, idealization/devaluation, instability, and a lack of coherence in the sense of self, with corresponding difficulties in the steady, realistic experience of others.

ASSESSMENT OF BORDERLINE PERSONALITY ORGANIZATION

Our evaluation approach begins with a discussion of presenting symptomatology and allows for the determination of both phenomenological (DSM) and structural diagnoses. Our approach follows the form and content of Kernberg's Structural Interview,[5] a free-form clinical interview that typically might take 60 to 90 minutes over 1 or 2 evaluation sessions, and that queries all aspects of the patient's difficulties—cognitive, emotional, physical, and interpersonal, both their history and current manifestation. The Structural Interview is typically conceived in 3 phases: an initial phase focusing on the specific presenting complaint and symptom inquiry, a middle phase explicitly oriented to the assessment of personality disorder features and structural diagnosis, and a concluding phase seeking information on the patient's family history and current life situation, sharing with the patient a diagnostic formulation, and outlining a framework for treatment if psychotherapy is indeed recommended.

The interview begins with an initial probe to the effect of, "Please tell me what problem or problems bring you here today, any other difficulties—emotional, cognitive, or physical—that you may have, how you understand your problems, and what you hope to gain from therapy?" The initial phase focuses in turn on each of the presenting difficulties identified by the patient, querying their history and the extent of associated impairment. This initial phase of symptom inquiry constitutes a concurrent mini mental status examination and initial test of the patient's personality organization and overall mental and emotional functioning: Can the patient hold the questions in mind? Are the responses coherent and logical? Are they realistic, suggesting an appropriate matching of verbal content to emotional valence? And what is the patient's reflective capacity? Throughout its various stages, the method of the interview itself constitutes an in vivo test of the patient's defensive system and reality testing through a focus on how the patient is functioning in the here-and-now interaction with the interviewer. Are the patient's responses open or guarded or evasive, agreeable or defensive or argumentative, realistic or superficial or caricature-like? The operation of splitting-based defenses can be discerned in various ways: when we sit with a patient whose hostility is palpable and by whom we feel controlled during the interview; when, after an hour of examination we feel confused, as though we have learned nothing of the patient, where information seems to have no substance or cannot attach to anything in the clinician's model of health and pathology. In such cases, it is not the content but rather interview process itself, our experience and feeling about the same, which suggests the influence of splitting-based defensive operations and the presence of borderline pathology.

The middle phase of the structural interview serves 2 functions:

1. To elicit information related to the structural diagnosis and the assessment of acuity within the borderline range, ie, as described, is the patient's sense of identity unintegrated, supported by splitting-based or "primitive" defenses, or is the internal structure integrated, and coherent, supported by more adaptive, higher-level defenses; and
2. To inquire more directly around the symptoms of DSM-5 borderline personality disorder.

In this middle phase of the interview, we further assess the patient's defensive system by gauging his or her response to gentle inquiries into contradictions in his or her responses, contradictions within the verbal report, between the patient's verbal report and his or her behavior, and between the patient's report and collateral information. Does this "confrontation" of discrepant information lead to an increase in hostility, paranoia, and control, or is the patient relaxed in response, openly providing information that clarifies what had seemed to be contradictory? Whereas the former suggests the operation of splitting-based defenses leaning toward a borderline diagnosis, the latter suggests some initial guardedness or anxiety that dissipates, and the associated flexibility and trust associated with greater openness in the interview.

As we proceed to discuss this middle section of the Structural Interview, the domains of functioning to assess and the specific questions one might ask to clarify a structural diagnosis, we must note several problems with the Structural Interview method. First, the ability to conduct the Structural Interview requires significant clinical tact and skill, coupled with a deep understanding of the structural features of personality disorder. Further, the method suffers from a lack of clinical "reliability"; two theoretic interviewers assessing the same theoretic patient would conduct the interview in the exact same way, and thus might not arrive at the same diagnosis. Further, each interviewer is subject to biases and blind spots within any given interview (a positive or negative halo effect, for example) that might lead the interviewer to omit content essential to determining a BPO diagnosis.

It was with the goal of developing a reliable and valid research tool, as well as the desire to provide language for clinicians assessing personality disorders in patients, that we developed the Structured Interview of Personality Organization (STIPO, Clakin, Caligor, Stern, & Kernberg, 2004, unpublished manuscript, Personality Disorders Institute, Weill Cornell Medical College, New York), an interview that provides coverage of the content domains sampled in the Structural Interview in a semistructured interview format familiar to personality disorder researchers. The STIPO has proved instrumental in our training of medical residents, psychology interns, analytical candidates, and transference-focused therapy trainees alike, providing language that operationalizes the structural features of personality disorder. In addition to items that tap identity and defenses (a spectrum including adaptive and primitive defenses), the domains central to making a structural diagnosis, the STIPO also assesses quality of object relations, aggression, and moral values, domains essential for determining the level of severity within the borderline range.

The items for the original STIPO and its recent revision were drawn from the experience of clinicians who for years practiced and studied psychodynamic psychotherapy with borderline patients. The original STIPO was tested in 2 separate clinical samples with empirical results supporting the reliability and validity of the various domains,[22,24] and the more focused, revised interview (Clarkin JF, Caligor E, Stern B, et al. Structured interview of personality organization-revised [STIPO-R]. Unpublished manuscript, Personality Disorders Institute, Weill Cornell Medical College, New York, 2016) which can be found in English online at www.istfp.org/measures/stipo-r, is also available in German, Italian, Spanish, French, and Turkish translations. This discussion weaves some of the language of the STIPO-R and its content domains into our discussion of the middle phase of the more free-form Structural Interview, during which our task as clinicians is to form a map in our clinical minds of the patient's sense of self, defensive and relational capacities, and overall life situation.

IDENTITY

Healthy identity is marked by a sense of coherence and continuity in the sense of self across time and situation, and in a correspondingly stable and coherent representation of significant others. To allow for a sense of the feel of the STIPO-R interview items, several sample items that reflect coherence and continuity of the identity domain are listed.

- Consistent sense of self in present
  - Would you say that you come across like a different person to different people in your life so that each of them get a different sense of who you are as a person?
  - Do you act in ways that appear to others as unpredictable and erratic (…or do people generally know what to expect from you)?
- Sense of self: Intimate relationships
  - In the course of an intimate relationship (your marriage), or as one begins to develop, are you afraid of losing a sense of yourself, of what's important to you?
- Self-esteem: Stability
  - Would you say that your self-esteem alternates, with you seeing yourself at times as special or unique, and at other times as small, boring, or defective?
  - If yes, would you say that the shifts in your self-esteem are quite severe, that they happen frequently, or that they are upsetting you?

For each item queried in the STIPO-R we typically ask follow-up probes designed to determine, for affirmative responses, the severity, frequency, and pervasiveness of the problem across various relationships and/or situations.

Open-ended self-descriptions are also elicited, assessing the patient's capacity to provide a coherent, ambivalent (freely accessing and tolerating positive and negative attributes), realistic, and on balance, positive, description of self that is a hallmark of consolidated, integrated, identity: "Tell me about yourself, what are you like as a person? Let's say that you wanted me to get to know you as quickly as possible, in just a few minutes—how would you describe yourself to me so that I get a live and full of picture of the kind of person you are?" Our objective in this exercise is to determine whether the description is realistic and nuanced versus superficial, and integrated and balanced realistically between positive and negative qualities, or whether the description tends toward split idealization or devaluation. In assessing the capacity to form stable, integrated representations of others, we ask the patient to describe a significant person in his or her life, following this same open-ended format, as well as specific questions related to the patient's confidence and stability in his or her experience of significant others. One can also develop impressions related to narcissistic pathology to the extent that the descriptions of others tends toward excessive idealization or devaluation, lacks depth and differentiation, and/or is largely self-referential.

One primary manifestation of a consolidated identity is the ability to direct oneself effectively, with purpose and pleasure, toward one's primary role, whether that be academic or occupational, and similarly, the capacity to "invest" the self in recreational pursuits. We ask how effective the patient is in his or her primary role, probing for grade reports, the ability to meet deadlines, promotions/raises/performance reviews, and the patient's subjective sense of effectiveness. We ask about the consistency of their engagement over time (significant absences, periods when not working), whether their goals have been consistent or shifting, and whether they experience a sense of pleasure in doing the work, rather than a mere sense of obligation. We similarly ask about the presence of significant recreational pursuits with a demonstrated "invest-ment" in learning or growing their involvement in the activity, probing the consistency of involvement over time and the sense of pleasure/satisfaction derived from the activity.

DEFENSES

If we conceive of identity as an ego function that reflects the organization of disparate internal object relations into either a coherent, integrated stable whole, or a chaotic, unintegrated and unstable internal world, it is the patient's defensive style that deter-mines this quality of identity. During our interview, and in the STIPO-R, we assess healthy defenses such as suppression, proactive coping, and flexibility to determine whether they work effectively or in an overly rigid and less adaptive manner. We also assess the use of splitting-based defenses because these strategies, operating largely outside conscious awareness, serve to maintain splits in the experience of the self and others that, were they to break down, would lead to intense anxiety. Externalization helps patients to maintain largely favorable representations of self by deflecting responsibility for any adverse experience onto others. Projective identifica-tion involves the assignment of that which is undesirable in the self to others, while the patient him or herself is concurrently expressing, either in thought or behavior and at varying levels of awareness, that very same quality—that is, he or she remains identi-fied with that undesirable quality, even if only in behavior—while also projecting it. Om-nipotent control, whether it be through the subtle threat of hostility or otherwise, operates to shut off areas of uncomfortable dialogue or interaction with others, including the therapist, whereas idealization/devaluation works to split up the fullness of the self, dividing good from bad, positive from negative, and splitting these valences between self and other.

The identification of identity diffusion as described elsewhere in this article, and the experience or manifestation of primitive defensive operations during the interview con-firms the diagnosis of BPO. Several factors help to determine the severity and prognosis for patients in the borderline range. The first of these involves the quality of the patient's object relations[a]: How isolated is the patient, socially and romantically? What is the quality of his or her relationships? The second involves aggression, the severity of aggression or hostility, how frequently expressed or well-controlled it is, and whether it is directed primarily at the self, others, or both. Last, we assess the patient's capacity for concern over his or her actions, the capacity for guilt and remorse, and the extent to which such feelings provide a check on the patient's impulsive aggression. The greater the extent of the aggression, as described, the less concern and remorse related to that aggression, and the poorer the state of the patient's interpersonal relationships, the lower in the BPO spectrum the patient falls, and the poorer the patient's prognosis in psychodynamic treatment. Each of these 3 areas is elaborated further.

QUALITY OF OBJECT RELATIONS

This section of the structural interview and STIPO-R involves an assessment of the pa-tient's social connectedness, socially and romantically, and the quality of those

---

[a] Object relations refers to both the relation between internal representations of self and other within the mind, and also to the person's interpersonal relations, both of which are assessed in the Quality of Object Relations section of the STIPO-R and the Structural Interview.

connections. We ask who the patient's friends are, assessing both the breadth and depth of his or her social network. We ask about the duration of close friendships, the frequency and mode of contact, and the extent of tension and volatility in the friendship as well as the level of reciprocity, support, and mutual dependency. In terms of romantic and sexual relationships, we inquire as to the presence of romantic and sexual partners at the current time and in the recent past, and the duration, depth, and quality of those relationships: Are they brief, superficial, and volatile or chaotic? or, are they deep, mutually dependent, reciprocal, loving relationships? We ask about the patient's sexual functioning: Do they have sex? With whom? How frequently? and is the sex in the context of an ongoing relationship or not? Are they satisfied with the sexual aspect of their relationships? and What do they mean by "satisfied?"

The final section of the Quality of Object Relations domain is termed Investment in Others, a set of questions that essentially assesses narcissistic object relations. Among the aspects we assess in this section are the capacity for empathy, the patient's attitude toward lending support and nurturance to others, the extent of the patient's preoccupation with fairness or equality in relationships, and the tendency toward boredom in friendships and romantic relationships.

AGGRESSION

The extent of a patient's aggression, against the self in the form of severe neglect, self-injury, and suicidality, as well as aggression felt and/or enacted against others, is central to the determination of the acuity and treatability of patients in the borderline range. In the Structural Interview, we inquire as to the number of suicide attempts, their mode, state of intent, and lethality. We also ask about various modes of self-injury, their frequency, and severity, because these behaviors need to be contained in some stable manner for the effective conduct of any dynamic treatment (see, eg, our writings on treatment contracting in transference-focused therapy).[25,26] The assessment of hostility, resentment, and enacted aggression against others is also a crucial prognostic factor. In the Structural Interview and STIPO-R, we ask about the frequency and extent of rage manifest through tantrums and verbal dyscontrol, as well as tendencies toward physical altercations and assault.

MORAL VALUES

Closely related to the assessment of aggression is the patient's moral functioning. In addition to asking about any frank antisocial behaviors, criminal history, and legal involvement, we also attempt to assess the patient's capacity for remorse and guilt, as well as the patient's capacity for genuine concern for another, and how that concern might influence his or her aggressive inclinations. When focusing during the Structural Interview on acts of interpersonal aggression in a patient's presentation and history, the interviewer attempts to determine whether that aggression is ego syntonic or dystonic: Does the patient feel entitled to or justified in his or her expressions of hostility, that the injury to the target is deserved and just, or does the patient express any regret for such behavior based on a sense that it has violated some internal moral code or out of concern for the hurt or damage done to another? In the STIPO-R, we are interested in examples in which the patient behaved in ways that either hurt others, were patently immoral, or that violated his or her internal moral code. We ask how the patient felt about his or her behavior, probing for feelings of guilt and/or remorse, and we ask what the patient did in response to his or her behavior? Did he attempt to avoid getting caught, avoid the target person, or seek that person out for purposes of apology and repair?

NARCISSISM

Throughout the structural interview, we pay attention to manifestations of narcissistic pathology, which often co-occur with a diagnosis of borderline personality disorder,[27] including features such as grandiosity, the signature feature of narcissistic personality disorder, and a corresponding devaluation of others, including the interviewer and/or treatment team; feelings of entitlement; an excessive need for admiration; expressions of envy; and statements reflecting a preoccupation with one's social standing (looks, job status and finances, sexual exploits, etc) and self-esteem. In addition to items in the content domains described that address features of narcissism (eg, boredom in, and an economic or quid pro quo view of interpersonal relationships, idealization/devaluation), the STIPO-R also includes several items specifically related to the assessment of narcissistic features, including the patient's need for admiration and reaction to a withdrawal of attention/admiration, and his or her experience of envy.

THE STRUCTURAL INTERVIEW: CONCLUDING PHASE

Having covered the patient's presenting problems and conducted a thorough assessment of symptomatology (phase I), and evaluating (by testing, challenging) the patient's defensive system while assessing the extent of personality symptoms and structural features (phase II), the concluding phase of the interview involves a discussion of the patient's motivation for treatment, of factors that may interfere with the safe and effective conduct of psychodynamic treatment (assessment of acute danger to self, and the presence of treatment-interfering behavior), and as well as a discussion of the patient's family and personal history as related to current difficulties, recognizing that these are subject to distortions of memory and motivation, but are yet useful as an expression of the patient's representations of significant others. At the conclusion of the interview, diagnostic formulations, both structural and phenomenological, are shared with the patient, along with the outline of a proposed treatment.

STRUCTURAL ASSESSMENT: CLINICAL VIGNETTES

The evaluation of a patient's character pathology in clinical settings does not generally follow a structured protocol such as the STIPO-R. Rather, the therapist's idiosyncratic adaptation of the more free form Structural Interview, covering the content domains outlined herein and perhaps using or informed by the language of the STIPO-R, allows for the collection of relevant clinical information but in a manner that allows for clinical flexibility and the building of rapport.[28] A thorough evaluation typically requires a minimum of 90 minutes; more extended evaluation sessions in some cases are warranted, allowing for the collection of information from collateral sources (past treaters, family members) that can then be fed back into the ongoing consultation process when that information conflicts with the patient's direct report. Information obtained in this manner, particularly related to the nature of the patient's expressed aggression, moral functioning, and secondary gain, are, again, crucial for determining acuity within the borderline range, and helping the therapist to ascertain whether a viable treatment can be established.

These clinical vignettes summarize the results of structural interviews of patients with 2 different levels of borderline pathology.

Case 1. Shelly

Shelly, a 45-year-old married woman, mother of 2 teenage children, was referred by a colleague, a cognitive–behavioral therapist whom she had seen for 3 years owing to "anxiety." The colleague stated that she had "exhausted her bag of tricks," that is, strategies to help Shelly calm herself under stress, regulate her emotions, and manage interpersonal challenges, and that she felt a more dynamic approach might help the patient to grow further.[b] The colleague acknowledged that the patient, rather than becoming more independent and stable as a result of their work, had become increasingly unstable, acute, and unmanageable in recent months, related in part to her use of the therapist for emotional support outside the treatment sessions, throwing verbal tantrums and threatening her when she was not sufficiently available or helpful to her via phone or text.

Shelly was intolerant of the new clinician's evaluation process, rolling her eyes, angry and impatient—she wanted to get going already, why did she have to talk about herself again to someone new??!! She agreed with his impression that her sense of omnipotence gets activated when her immediate needs are not met, and that others' needs, including the new clinician's needs with regard to starting a treatment, should not matter when the issue of her discomfort or desire is at play. Further, despite her eagerness, Shelly repeatedly pushed back the clinician's lines of questioning, his sense of what was important, and the overall interventional stance of the treatment, that is, exploratory rather than overtly supportive, protesting that such a treatment felt like an abandonment, leaving her to "suck it up" on her own. At the end of each evaluation session, Shelly underscored that she felt unhelped and was reluctant to leave. Further, upon return to the next session she stressed how difficult the session had been and how emotionally draining she experienced the days in between our meetings. Upon inquiry, it was quite difficult for Shelly to articulate the nature of her upset; instead, she would describe her focus on one thing the clinician had said, or had not said in the prior session, and how angry the perceived lack of tact or callous omission made her feel.

In terms of her identity, Shelly demonstrated the capacity to invest herself quite fully and with pleasure in multiple areas of functioning, including her job as an attorney at her own boutique law firm, her role as a mother, and 2 serious recreational pursuits (tennis and choral singing), both of which were activities that she deeply enjoyed, studied, and had engaged in at a very high level (the latter semiprofessionally), consistently, for many years. Her sense of self in the present was stable, although her description of self was highly superficial, as was her ability to think in depth about her emotional states and motivations and those of others. She described herself largely through the lens of her neediness, and the sense of being the victim of an unjust world that did not understand or support her. Shelly's self-esteem was labile, up and down depending on interpersonal setbacks and disappointments in her recreational and professional pursuits; she alternated between thinking extremely highly of herself, and also feeling as though there were things deeply wrong with and lacking in herself.

Shelly displayed the capacity for significant healthy defenses, including her ability to plan effectively and proactively, and to work to a high standard in many areas of her life without the tyranny of rigid perfectionism. At the same time, when emotionally stressed, her capacity for suppression and flexibility were compromised, and splitting-based defenses became activated. Shelly had a tendency to be rejecting of support and help when it could not magically solve her problems or discomforts, while

---

[b] The authors frequently have the experience of receiving referrals of this nature, wherein the patient, consistent with the current climate in psychiatry and mental health treatment, was evaluated for symptoms and Axis I diagnoses, but not for features of personality disorder. This unfortunate and all too common experience often leads unnecessarily to years of symptom-chasing treatments that provide little relief.

concurrently feeling rejected and abandoned by others who failed to meet such an unrealistic, idealized standard. This tendency toward projective identification was profound, causing considerable tension in her close interpersonal relationships, including the one with her previous therapist. Externalization was evidenced through a brittle, unrealistic idealization of the new clinician and the treatment, along with a superficial sense of hopefulness—"I really hope this will work"—a sense devoid of any personal responsibility or agency for change.

Shelly had a largely good relationship with a quiet, emotionally reserved husband, whom she experienced as dedicated and loving, but also devalued as ineffectual. Her description of her best friend was highly idealized and superficial—"She's the best... I don't know....I mean I just love her, our kids grew up together, we've shared so much. I don't know what to say, she's always there for me, whatever I need, whenever....you know what I mean.... I don't know what you want." When asked to elaborate further on her friend, she could describe her beauty and intelligence, but little in terms of an example or story between the 2 of them that could bring any quality of her friend's to life. Other friendships were long-standing and durable, with some ups and downs, but few ruptures. The clinician's sense was that Shelly was able to maintain relational stability, but only to a minimal depth and at the price of true intimacy and dependency. The lack of depth and openness with others resulted in a predominance of superficial relationships, wherein the lack of true intimacy protected her from exposing her poor self-esteem and tendency to break down under emotional stress, whereupon she would withdraw into extended periods of angry depression.

Shelly's hostility was well-controlled. She did not injure herself and took good care of herself physically. Although she did not lose verbal or physical control with others, she harbored considerable feelings of resentment toward others whom she felt did not accord her the respect, attention, or support she deserved. Last, Shelly, had good moral functioning; there was no evidence of antisocial or exploitive behaviors, and a clear capacity for guilt and remorse over her actions, an awareness when pressed that her behaviors and emotional immaturity hurt others, and a tendency to make reparation to others, particularly her husband and children, after having behaved poorly.

These were the data the clinician gathered from Shelly over a 90-minute initial session, one 45-minute follow-up session, and a brief discussion with the referring therapist. Shelly met the DSM diagnostic criteria for borderline personality disorder, characterized by difficulties with her sense of identity, mood lability, feelings of abandonment, difficulties with intense anger, tendencies toward idealization or devaluation, and difficulties in her interpersonal relationships. Structurally, Shelly falls within the range of BPO with prominent narcissistic features, including identification with both a grandiose and vulnerable self, feelings of entitlement and a tendency toward devaluing others who do not meet her expectations, and significant difficulties in her interpersonal relationships characterized by a lack of depth and mutual dependency. The ability to largely control the expression of her hostility and aggression, and her concern over the same, place Shelly in the high borderline range, and her motivation for treatment and historical dedication to the same, despite her difficulty using a more supportive treatment to develop emotionally, suggested that she would be a good candidate for an exploratory psychodynamic treatment.

Case 2: Mark

At the first meeting, Mark, a 23-year-old college dropout, described the circumstances of his referral, namely, his dismissal from a therapeutic residential community for repeated violations of its rules of sexual conduct. His disregard and disdain for the rules, lack of any guilt or remorse, and retributive attacks on the community's staff and therapists, including his well-organized attempts to rally other residents against the staff, resulted in Mark and his hostility coming to be seen as too toxic and destructive to the community to sustain his residence therein.

Mark detailed his sense of mistreatment by the staff, stating that they were "just all over me," for infractions that he felt ridiculous and unhealthy for people whose problems involve difficulties in relationships: "How ridiculous is that??!! To ban being in a relationship while being in treatment for difficulties in relationships?" This statement condenses Mark's intelligence with his oppositionality and expresses a disingenuousness with highly perverse and destructive elements that left no room to "submitting" himself to others for his own potential benefit.

Mark described a repeated pattern since his high school years of doing well for brief periods of time in school before becoming engaged in some dramatic acting out in which administrators and fellow students were aligned against him. His self-righteousness and clever arguments left no room for an alternate view of the circumstances. When, in the first session, the evaluating clinician confronted him with the fact that his repeated attempts to "just find a place to learn and share the good I have inside with others" had not worked out for him, following a familiar pattern of subversion, sowing conflict, and eventual dismissal, the clinician was breezily dismissed without a shred of reflection or remorse. Mark had held several jobs, obtained for him through connections with his influential family, each of which he had left after brief periods of time, citing either a lack of interest, a change in life plan, or a good opportunity to travel that had arisen and to which he "could not say no." In fact, Mark had demonstrated no ability to invest in school, work, or recreation, no consistent sense of what appealed to him, and no track record of consistent engagement or achievement anywhere.

Mark's open-ended self-description focused solely on how misunderstood and mistreated he was. Said differently, he used the probe of asking him to describe himself as an opportunity to demonstrate the defense of projective identification, that is, how others have treated him with a dismissive, uncaring attitude, while demonstrating that very same dismissive, uncaring attitude toward himself and toward the clinician during the interview. When prompted to describe further his personality, he provided positive, idealized adjectives with superficial elaboration, and when confronted with the ways in which those adjectives contradicted data from collateral sources (the referring therapist), these were again met with no evidence of reflection but only with angry disbelief that the clinician would challenge his narrative, and that a view other than his own might actually have any merit.

Mark described no relationships of any significant duration, and none that were free of conflict. He described his closest friend as someone he had met at the hospital several months earlier and with whom he had partied on several occasions since, meaning, binged for several days on cocaine and alcohol. Many of his male friends from high school had, for reasons difficult to discern in the interview, dropped out of touch with him in the ensuing years. Similarly, Mark had never been in a serious romantic relationship of any duration, or one that was free of chronic conflict and involved any mutuality or dependency.

Mark's defensive style was characterized significantly by splitting-based, primitive defenses, including denial, projective identification, idealization (of self) and devaluation (of others), and omnipotent control. There was no demonstration of adaptive, higher level defenses, perhaps because Mark had never committed to any circumstance wherein such defenses would have been required for success (proactive coping, flexibility, suppression), or perhaps because he avoided any deeper professional or academic commitments owing to some awareness that he was not equipped for the associated challenges to his coping capacities.

The varied expressions of Mark's aggression was impressive: binge drug and alcohol use; illegal procurement of sedative medication; impulsive sex with strangers without protection; gleeful, deliberate revenge against staff who had confronted and set limits on his behavior and against friends who, in his view, had "betrayed him"; repeated self-injury; and, finally, his blithe and highly provocative affirmation of his plan to kill himself by his 26th birthday if he had not completed college and found a girlfriend. Mark's discussion of the foregoing was triumphant; he beamed when discussing it, while completely denying his pleasure in the same when it was pointed out to him. His lack of concern for himself was demonstrated by the grandiose triumph of his destructiveness, his proof that it was stronger than anyone's "therapeutic" or helpful influence, even stronger than the weakened part of himself that might want a better life, which he too had vanquished.

In terms of structural diagnosis, Mark would fall in the low borderline range, with a severe narcissistic personality disorder, demonstrated by his substantial grandiosity, his complete inability to consider others for their own sake, independent of his needs, and his thorough use of splitting-based defenses to assign all the negative, weak qualities in himself to others. The severity and pervasiveness of Mark's perverse aggression, as well as his complete lack of remorse, accounts for his placement in the low range of BPO. Mark's poor prognosis was signaled through his proudly stated commitment to self-destructiveness and by the sense of pleasure and triumph that accompanied that.

ALTERNATIVE MODELS

Having outlined in detail our approach to the psychodynamic assessment of personality disorders, it is worthwhile to comment briefly on 2 alternative models to the assessment of borderline pathology that clinicians will likely encounter.

The Diagnostic and Statistical Manual of Mental Disorders

Although the narrative portions of the personality disorders section of the last 2 versions of the DSM have discussed difficulties in the sense of self or identity, and difficulties in the realm of self-regulation and interpersonal relationships, these features have not been systematically included in the diagnostic system proper. Although the most recent revision of the DSM (the DSM-5)[2] did not include major changes to the official 10-disorder classification system for personality disorders, the AMPD brings these core features into the actual diagnostic system. Whereas one aspect of the AMPD involves the assessment of specific maladaptive traits that vary or combine according to specific personality disorder styles, the criteria also elaborate "impairment in self and interpersonal functioning," defined further as difficulties in the areas of identity and self-direction (self) and empathy and intimacy (interpersonal relations). Scales have been developed to operationalize both aspects of the AMPD: The Levels of Personality Functioning Scale for the self and interpersonal functioning criteria,[29–32] for which there has also been developed a diagnostic interview to specifically provide the clinical data to inform a Levels of Personality Functioning Scale rating[33,34]; and, for the maladaptive personality traits, the Personality Inventory for DSM-5,[35] for which there is also a significant and growing body of empirical support (see Refs.[36,37] for a recent review). The authors are of the view that these aspects captured in the AMPD are indeed the domains central to the diagnosis of BPO, the group of personality disorders characterized structurally, internally, by a pathology of internal object relations described elsewhere in this article in our model of borderline pathology and assessment.

The Psychiatric Diagnostic Manual

The PDM[3] was developed to provide a more clinically meaningful and useful diagnostic alternative to the DSM and *International Classification of Diseases*, 10th edition. The PDM and its recent revision, the PDM-2, reflect a psychodynamic tradition that conceptualizes personality disorder in terms of personality traits and styles and also the psychological functions that underlie healthy/normal and pathologic personality. The PDM-2 is integrative, with aspects related to personality reflected in all 3 axes of its diagnostic system for adults, which in combination constitute a multidimensional approach that describes the patient's overall functioning, symptoms, psychological capacities, and modes in which he or she is likely to engage the therapeutic process. Said differently, the manual attempts to provide a comprehensive and clinically useful taxonomy of the person, rather than a taxonomy of disorders.

Personality disorder features are folded into 3 axes of the PDM-2. The P axis, of personality patterns and disorders, is explicitly grounded in the object-relations model elaborated elsewhere in this article. The focus is on identifying both a level of personality organization (neurotic, borderline, psychotic as elaborated in the work of Kernberg),[5,6] as well as a determination of which personality style best fits the person. The personality styles are drawn largely from the personality disorders listed in the DSM 5, but considered less as disorders than prototypic themes or organizing principles that characterize the person and his or her conflicts, and without a resulting cutoff for disorder status but rather an impression of the patient's rigidity, dysfunction, impairment, and subjective suffering.

The M axis yields a profile of mental functioning that also integrates much of our thinking as to the structural factors related to the diagnosis of BPO. The M profile assesses psychological capacities in 4 areas:

1. Cognitive and affective processes (eg, ability to communicate and understand, mentalization, and attentional capacities);
2. Identity and relationships (capacities for differentiation and integration, for relationships and intimacy, and for self-esteem regulation);
3. Defensive style and coping (including impulse control and regulation, primary defensive style [splitting based vs higher level], and overall adaptation and resiliency); and
4. Self-awareness and self-direction (including the capacity for self-observation and to develop and use an internal moral code).

Finally, the S axis incorporates much of DSM Axis I, with a focus on present symptomatology, with a recognition that individual with similar symptoms patters may present in different ways and with differing degrees of subjective distress and impairment owing to the nature of their person (Axes P and M). Although integrative and clinically rich, the PDM-2 does not provide a categorical diagnosis of any personality disorder. Methods for organizing the PDM-2 data are currently under development and investigation (see the Psychodiagnostic Chart[38]), and these will in time speak to the usefulness of PDM-2 formulations in clinical settings and discussions of subtypes of patients on dimensions of personality.

SUMMARY

The landscape of personality disorder assessment is experiencing a generational shift. The move from a categorical diagnostic system to one combining a trait focus with a concurrent focus on capacities and tendencies related to the experience of the self, and the self in relation to others, is monumental. This shift promises to lend greater validity to personality disorder diagnostics and to yield a diagnostic language that is of greater usefulness to clinicians, who must determine the nature and severity of an individual's pathology, as well as that individual's suitability for treatment.

REFERENCES

1. American Psychiatric Association. Diagnostic and statistical manual of mental disorders. 4th edition. Washington, DC: Author; 2000. text rev.
2. American Psychiatric Association. Diagnostic and statistical manual of mental disorders. 5th edition. Washington, DC: Author; 2013.
3. PDM Task Force. Psychodynamic diagnostic manual. Silver Spring (MD): Alliance of Psychoanalytic Organizations; 2006.
4. Lingiardi V, McWilliams N. Psychodynamic diagnostic manual, version 2 (PDM-2). New York: Guilford Press; 2017.
5. Kernberg OF. Severe personality disorders. New Haven (CT): Yale; 1984.
6. Kernberg OF, Caligor E. A psychoanalytic theory of personality disorders. In: Lenzenweger M, Clarkin J, editors. Major theories of personality disorder. New York: Guilford; 2005.
7. Trull T, Durrett C. Categorical and dimensional models of personality disorder. Annu Rev Clin Psychol 2005;1:355–80.
8. Verheul R. Clinical utility of dimensional models for personality pathology. In: Widiger TA, Simonsen E, Sirovatka PJ, et al, editors. Dimensional models of personality disorders: refining the research agenda for DSM-V, 203-218. Washington, DC: American Psychiatric Association; 2006.
9. Westen D, Arkowitz-Westen L. Limitations of Axis II in diagnosing personality pathology in clinical practice. Am J Psychiatry 1998;155:1767–71.
10. Widiger T, Samuel DB. Evidence-based assessment of personality disorders. Psychol Assess 2005;17(3):278–87.
11. Hopwood CJ, Kotov R, Krueger RF, et al. The time has come for dimensional personality disorder diagnosis. Personal Ment Health 2018;12:82–6.
12. Krueger RF, Markon KE. The role of the DSM-5 personality trait model in moving toward a quantitative and empirically based approach to classifying personality and psychopathology. Annu Rev Clin Psychol 2014;10:477–501.
13. Markon K, Kreuger RF, Watson D. Delineating the structure of normal and abnormal personality: an integrative hierarchical approach. J Pers Soc Psychol 2005;88(1):139–57.
14. Morey LC, Hopwood CJ, Gunderson JG, et al. Comparison of alternative models for personality disorders. Psych Medicine 2007;37(3):983–94.
15. Widiger TA, Livesley WJ, Clark LA. An integrative dimensional classification of personality disorder, Psychological assessment 2009;21(3):243–55.
16. Costa PT, Widiger TA, editors. Personality disorders and the five factor model of personality. Washington, DC: American Psychological Association; 1994.
17. Digman JM. Higher-order factors of the big five. J Pers Soc Psychol 1997;73: 1246–56.
18. John OP. The "Big Five" factor taxonomy: dimensions of personality in the natural language and in questionnaires. In: Pervin LA, editor. Handbook of personality: theory and research. New York: Guilford; 1990. p. 66–100.

19. McCrae RR, Costa PT Jr. Toward a new generation of personality theories: theoretical contexts for the five-factor model. In: Wiggins JS, editor. The five-factor model of personality: theoretical perspectives. New York: Guilford; 1996. p. 51–87.

20. Widiger TA, Trull TJ. Plate tectonics in the classification of personality disorder: shifting to a dimensional model. Am Psychol 2007;62:71–83.

21. McAdams DP, Pals JL. A new Big Five: Fundamental principles for an integrative science of personality. American Psychologist 2006;61(3):204–17.

22. Doering S, Burgmer M, Heuft G, et al. Reliability and validity of the German version of the Structured Interview of Personality Organization (STIPO). BMC Psychiatry 2013;13:210.

23. Lenzenweger MF, Clarkin JF, Kernberg OF, et al. The Inventory of Personality Organization: psychometric properties, factorial composition, and criterion relations with affect, aggressive dyscontrol, psychosis proneness, and self-domains in a nonclinical sample. Psychol Assess 2001;13:577–91.

24. Stern B, Caligor E, Clarkin JF, et al. The Structured Interview of Personality Organization (STIPO): preliminary psychometrics in a clinical sample. J Pers Assess 2010;91:35–44.

25. Yeomans FE, Clarkin JF, Kernberg OF. Transference-focused psychotherapy for borderline personality disorder: a clinical guide. Washington, DC: American Psychiatric Publishing; 2015.

26. Yeomans FE, Delaney J, Levy K. Behavior action in TFP: the role of the treatment contract in transference-focused psychotherapy. Psychotherapy 2017;54(3): 260–6.

27. Diamond D, Levy K, Clarkin J, et al. Attachment and mentalization in female patients with comorbid narcissistic and borderline personality disorder. Personal Disord 2014;5:428–33.

28. Hörz-Sagstetter S, Caligor E, Preti E, et al. Clinician-guided assessment of personality using the structural interview and the Structured Interview of Personality Organization (STIPO). J Pers Assess 2018;100:30–42.

29. Bender DS, Morey LC, Skodol A. Towards a model for assessing level of personality functioning in DSM-5, Part I: a review of theory and methods. J Pers Assess 2011;93(4):332–46.

30. Hutsebaut J, Feenstra DJ, Kamphuis JH. Development and preliminary psychometric evaluation of a brief self-report questionnaire for the assessment of the DSM-5 level of personality functioning scale: the LPFS Brief Form (LPFS-BF). Personal Disord 2016;7(2):192–7.

31. Morey LC, Berghuis H, Bender DS, et al. Towards a model for assessing level of personality functioning in DSM-5, Part II: empirical articulation of a core dimension of personality pathology. J Pers Assess 2011;93(4):347–53.

32. Rockland LH. Supportive therapy for borderline patients: a psychodynamic approach. New York: Guilford; 1992.

33. Bender DS, Skodol AE, First MB, et al. Module I: structured clinical interview for the level of personality functioning scale. In: First MB, Skodol AE, Bender DS, et al, editors. Structured clinical interview for the DSM-5 alternative model for personality disorders (SCID-AMPD). New York: New York State Psychiatric Institute; 2016.

34. Hutsebaut J, Kamphuis JH, Feenstra DJ, et al. Assessing DSM–5-oriented level of personality functioning: development and psychometric evaluation of the Semi-Structured Interview for Personality Functioning DSM–5 (STiP-5.1). Personal Disord 2017;8(1):94–101.

35. Krueger RF, Derringer J, Markon KE, et al. Initial construction of a maladaptive personality trait model and inventory for DSM-5. Psychol Med 2012;42:1879–90.

36. Al-Dajani N, Gralnick TM, Bagby RM. A psychometric review of the Personality Inventory for DSM-5 (PID-5): current status and future directions. J Pers Assess 2016;98(1):62–81.
37. Bagby, 2016.
38. Gordon RM, Bornstein RF. Construct validity of the psychodiagnostic chart: a transdiagnostic measure of personality organization, personality syndromes, mental functioning, and symptomatology. Psychoanal Psychol 2017. https://doi.org/10.1037/pap0000142.

Social Cognition and Borderline Personality Disorder

Splitting and Trust Impairment Findings

Eric A. Fertuck, PhD[a],*, Stephanie Fischer[a], Joseph Beeney, PhD[b]

KEYWORDS

- Social cognition • Borderline personality disorder • Splitting • Trust impairment
- Object relations • Emotion recognition • Trust • Borderline personality organization

KEY POINTS

- Borderline personality disorder (BPD) has its origins as a psychiatric diagnosis in the concept of borderline personality organization (BPO). BPO is rooted in psychoanalytic object relations theory (ORT).
- From the ORT theoretic perspective, BPD is characterized by 2 central features: (1) a propensity to view significant others as either idealized (eg, a savior) or persecutory (eg, a betrayer) and (2) a traitlike paranoid view of interpersonal relations, wherein those with BPD think that they will ultimately be betrayed, abandoned, or neglected by significant others, despite periodic idealizations.
- Although ORT is one of the oldest theoretic models of BPD, until recently there has been little empirical and experimental evaluation of this model, with most support coming from clinical observation, qualitative interviews, and self-report instruments. However, since 1967, there has been an accumulation of self-report, interview, laboratory, and translational neuroscience studies that have evaluated these two features.
- This empirical, scoping review evaluates the support for these two central facets of ORT of BPD from the perspective of experimental, social cognitive, and translational neuroscience research.
- This article synthesizes the extant literature, identifies avenues for further investigation, and discusses the relative promise of different methods to evaluate ORT compared with other models of BPD and related mental disorders.

[a] Department of Psychology, The City College of New York, The City University of New York, NAC Room 7/239, 160 Convent Avenue, New York, NY 10031, USA; [b] Department of Psychiatry, University of Pittsburgh, Western Psychiatric Institute & Clinic, Thomas Detre Hall, 3811 O'Hara Street, Pittsburgh, PA 15213, USA
* Corresponding author.
E-mail address: efertuck@ccny.cuny.edu

Psychiatr Clin N Am 41 (2018) 613–632
https://doi.org/10.1016/j.psc.2018.07.003
0193-953X/18/© 2018 Elsevier Inc. All rights reserved.

Interpersonal relationships in borderline personality disorder (BPD) are often chaotic, because people with BPD frequently cycle between love and hate feelings for significant others.[1] Accordingly, those with BPD maintain unstable social networks, because they fluctuate between establishing new relationships and ending them.[2] This social instability not only disrupts family and professional life but also disturbs the sense of self, or identity, of individuals with BPD. Furthermore, many of the Diagnostic and Statistical Manual of Mental Disorders, Fifth Edition (DSM-5), symptoms of BPD, such as self-injury, suicidality, intense and inappropriate anger, impulsivity, and heightened emotional sensitivity, are mediated by the quality of interpersonal bonds between persons with BPD and their significant others.[3] Overt and subtle cues within social situations are powerful precursors for affective instability and emotional arousal in BPD, and can generate the pervasive thought patterns that anticipate abandonment and rejection, and the tendency to alternate between extreme negative and positive evaluations of the self and others.[4–6] Consequently, the mechanisms that underlie these interpersonal impairments in BPD can aggravate interpersonal conflicts, lead to uncooperative exchanges in social interactions, threaten the formation of new relationships, and undermine long-term relationships.

OBJECT RELATIONS THEORY AND BORDERLINE PERSONALITY DISORDER

Historically, object relations theory (ORT) was the first to propose that impairments in the mental representations of others and the self are at the core of BPD.[1,7] In a generative body of theorizing and research that began more than 50 years ago, Kernberg and colleagues[9] proposed the concept of borderline personality organization (BPO). BPO is organized around mental representations of self and others that are split, or polarized, between idealized (highly positive personality attributes) and persecutory (highly negative personality attributes), and the capacity to integrate such negative and positive attributes causes the impairment of identity diffusion. Kernberg and colleagues[9] contrasted BPO with neurotic personality organization (a healthier organization in which there is some capacity to integrate positive and negative attributes in self and other), and psychotic personality organization (an organization of personality characterized by severe and pervasive deficits in social reality testing). Although BPO is a construct that encompasses most of the 10 DSM-5 personality disorders, BPD represents the DSM-5 disorder that is most emblematic of splitting of mental representations and BPO.

From the ORT theoretic perspective, BPD is characterized by 2 cardinal features:

1. A propensity to view the self and significant others as either idealized (eg, a savior) or persecutory (eg, a betrayer)
2. A traitlike paranoid view of interpersonal relations, wherein those with BPD think that they will ultimately be betrayed, abandoned, or neglected by significant others, despite periodic idealizations that are destined to result in disappointment.

In ORT, polarized evaluations of self and others, and a propensity to be suspicious of and mistrust others, are the core mechanisms of BPD and, more broadly, BPO. ORT now has a rich clinical tradition; however, the empirical study of these characteristics has been slow to develop and is scattered in different mental health literatures, ranging from the psychodynamic, social cognitive, personality assessment, and social neuroscientific. Because of the continued influence of ORT theory as a prominent model of BPD and an evidence-based treatment of BPD (ie, transference-focused psychotherapy[8,9] [TFP] is based on ORT), the authors conducted a scoping review[10] of the empirical research that has evaluated spitting and trustworthiness impairments in BPD. This scoping review endeavors to:

1. Evaluate the extent, characteristics, and variability of research in these features
2. Determine the eventual need to undertake a systematic review
3. Synthesize and communicate the extant research findings
4. Determine gaps and future directions identified in this research literature

This article summarizes and synthesizes the empirical literature that used reliable and valid psychometric instruments, assessing BPD using either semistructured clinical interviews or an established dimensional assessment of BPD features. Studies that did not meet these broad criteria were not included. The focus of this review is on the varied methods used to assess splitting (and conceptually related constructs such as dichotomous thinking [DT]) and trust impairments with the aim of identifying the consistency of findings, the relative merits and limitations of different methods, the sensitivity and specificity of the findings to BPD, and their potential clinical significance for elucidating the mechanisms of BPD and its treatment.

Empirical Studies of Splitting and Borderline Personality Disorder

Interpersonal relationships in BPD show rapid fluctuations between idealization and devaluation of others, with few "shades of gray" in between. This propensity to have a combination of black-and-white, paradoxic beliefs about the self and others is termed splitting or DT. These extreme shifts in BPD are marked by a heightened sense of vigilance and emotional instability within interpersonal relationships as individuals with BPD desperately attempt to evade either real or imagined abandonment and rejection.

There are 2 main theories for the contradictory shifts in evaluation patterns of self and other in BPD. First, the cognitive theory of BPD proposes that interpersonal issues are caused by dysfunctional cognitive schemas, which activate the cognitive distortion called DT.[11] These maladaptive cognitive schemas revolve around perpetual fears related to rejection, abandonment, incompetency, helplessness, vulnerability, and not being loved. Cognitive theorists, such as Beck and colleagues,[12] point out that a pervasive cognitive bias, or schemas, used by those with BPD to evaluate the world negatively, contributes to the belief that others have malevolent intentions and are untrustworthy. Beliefs about being incompetent, helpless, and vulnerable stimulate individuals with BPD to seek assistance and security from others, but clashing beliefs about being rejected, abandoned, and unworthy of love lead them to simultaneously fear others, to defend themselves from suffering and potential abuse. Furthermore, individuals with BPD who turn toward others for social connection, but doubt the support and love of others, rapidly oscillate between positive and negative evaluations of others. This process prompts the oscillation between seeking others and pushing them away as a result of mistrust. The mix between the irreconcilable cognitive schemas and DT patterns produces a dynamic pattern in BPD that can drive the unstable patterns of interpersonal behavior and affect in BPD.

Comparatively, ORT posits that organizing others into extreme classifications is a consequence of splitting. Splitting is the strict separation of positive affects and negative affects within the mind. It is an early stage of psychological development. As children develop, they are faced with the developmental task of overcoming splitting by integrating feelings of love and hate. As such, splitting initially serves a protective psychological function: protecting the loving feelings from the anger associated with the hating ones. However, if maintained into adolescence and adulthood, splitting engenders pathologic personality (or identity) formation that interferes with psychological and interpersonal growth. In BPD, this splitting defense becomes crystalized into an adult personality organization. This so-called paranoid-schizoid position of individuals with BPD is a term developed by Melanie Klein[13] and refers to the tendency of these individuals to be unaware of their angry and aggressive feelings and to mistakenly see, or project, these feelings onto others, who are then perceived as bad or threatening. A variant of splitting is that the other may be perceived as an idealized savior who can protect the individual from the threat of the anger and aggression.[13] ORT theorizes that splitting persists in BPD because of an aggressive genetic temperament and/or because of disturbances in the person's early social interactions, such as experiencing abuse, neglect, or trauma. Splitting actively prevents a person from combining disparate feelings into a composite and united experience. Instead, conceptual knowledge of the good and bad characteristics of others is separate in memory; when negative representations are active, positive models are more difficult to activate. Splitting as a defensive process serves to protect good experiences from being overwhelmed and spoiled by the powerful and threatening bad experiences, such as when a person senses social stress or a threat in the environment (eg, rejection, abandonment, or abuse). For example, patients with BPD who originally thought of their therapist as an all-good person might experience perceived negative behavior from the therapist, such as feeling criticized or judged, or misinterpreting subtle neutral or ambiguous facial cues as negative, and suddenly shift toward seeing them as all bad.

Despite the theoretic differences that aim to explain the tendency to evaluate people extremely in black and white terms, both splitting and DT suggest that specific impairments in social cognitions amplify interpersonal and affective instability. The prevailing themes that overlap between both cognitive and psychodynamic theory center on BPD-oriented issues of abandonment and rejection, with the psychodynamic view emphasizing the role of affect as well as cognition. People with BPD are often hypervigilant for social threat and react intensely to real or perceived threats. The cognitive theory addresses DT by highlighting distorted schemas and biased malevolent interpretations, whereas psychodynamic theory proposes the use of primitive defense processes that cause the person to split others and the self into simplistic and exaggerated idealized and persecutory categories. The empirical investigations of splitting from varying methodologies are summarized here.

Projective test investigations

Projective personality assessment uses ambiguous visual stimuli, such as an inkblot or interpersonal scenes (eg, the thematic apperception test [TAT]), to elicit a spontaneous, verbal description from the participant. This verbal description is subsequently scored based on an established protocol by trained raters. A pioneering study compared a group of BPD, depressed, and heathy control participants on ratings of TAT protocols.[14] Reliable raters assessed the TAT protocols for the quality of self-other differentiation. They used the complexity of representations scoring method, which assesses participants' psychological capacity to represent self and others in the TAT cards along a dimension from undifferentiation of self and others, to polarized, or split, representations along positive (good) and negative (bad) traits, or to integration of positive and negative attributes of self and others combined in a realistic but complex fashion. Poorly differentiated (ie, split) mental representations were characteristic of BPD compared with healthy and depressive controls. Splitting processes in this study were not a monolithic trait, because nearly half of the BPD group showed healthier self-other differentiation on some of the TAT cards.

A related study investigated inpatient women with BPD and nonsuicidal self-injury (NSSI) and women with BPD but no NSSI. The NSSI group showed a greater propensity for splitting and other indicators of more primitive object relations than the non-NSSI BPD group on the TAT.[15] Problems with this study include the lack of a healthy or psychiatric control group. However, using narrative material, it does support that splitting is predominant in BPD and more severe for more high-risk patients with NSSI BPD.

In another study, researchers compared Holtzman inkblot technique responses among individuals with BPD, healthy controls, participants characterized as neurotic, participants with acute schizophrenia, and participants with chronic schizophrenia.[16] Different forms of splitting (4 different types were described) were characteristic of BPD and patients with schizophrenia. Furthermore, splitting scales were correlated with assessments of identity diffusion, primitive psychological defenses, and other aspects of mental disorder. Weaknesses of this study were that the groups were not matched on demographics, and there was no interrater reliability for non-BPD diagnoses.

SELF-REPORT STUDIES

The splitting index (SI)[17] is a self-report scale that was developed based on Kernberg's theory of the defense mechanism of splitting of self and objection representations. This measure was proposed to serve as a clinical instrument to identify severe personality disorders and measure splitting as a defense mechanism. The study correlated SI with borderline syndrome index, a questionnaire designed to measure BPD features. In a set of 6 preliminary studies within a population of college students, researchers concluded that SI is a reliable measure and has high positive correlations with BPD features.

One study used the SI to evaluate processes of splitting in a rigorously diagnosed BPD population.[18] Researchers examined the relationship between splitting processes comparing groups of individuals with schizophrenia and BPD recruited from outpatient treatment programs. Using the SI, the mean score was significantly higher in the BPD compared with the schizophrenia group. This study suggests that SI scores are sensitive and specific to BPD.

Structured Interview Investigations of Splitting

Structured (or semistructured) interview approaches attempt to model a sophisticated clinical interview to establish reliability while retaining the capacity to make sophisticated clinical inferences used by expert clinicians to assess splitting phenomena in clinical practice. In one study, a BPD and a matched healthy control group were compared using a psychodynamic interview, which was then rated using the Defense Mechanism Rating Scale.[19] Defenses specifically associated with BPD compared with controls were action defenses (acting out, passive aggression, and hypochondriasis), borderline defenses (splitting of self and others' images, and projective identification), disavowal defenses (denial, rationalization, projection, and autistic fantasy), and narcissistic defenses. In discriminating BPD from controls, action and disavowal had the largest effect sizes, even more so than splitting, although splitting was more prominent in BPD than in comparison groups.

In another study, participants discussed a problem on the phone with 3 different confederates posing as mental health trainees. Each confederate mental health trainee was instructed to act rejecting, accepting, or neutral. After each discussion, participants completed ratings and a semistructured interview focused on soliciting the participants' perceptions of each trainee. Participant perceptions of the trainees were scored by judges on affect tone, differentiation, and complexity of attributions.

Individuals with BPD showed more DT (ie, others are viewed in extremes of good or bad, but there can be incongruence where the same other is seen as extreme in both good and bad traits simultaneously) than healthy controls or participants with a cluster-C personality disorder. However, the investigators found no evidence for group differences in splitting (seeing the same person as congruently all good or all bad across multiple trait attributions) in the ratings from the interview.[20] This study was innovative in its use of an ecologically valid approach to social assessment but limited by a large number of tests matched with a small sample size (n = 18 for each group).

Three studies have used the Semistructured Interview of Personality Organization (STIPO) to assess splitting processes, among other dimensions of personality organization, in BPD samples. Expert clinicians administer the STIPO, which is modeled after a sophisticated psychodynamic interview develop by Kernberg.[7] The first study used a clinical sample representing a broad spectrum of mental disorders. Most of the participants met criteria for at least 1 DSM personality disorder. The investigators found that cluster B and C personality disorders could be predicted by severity of identity diffusion, primitive defenses (such as splitting), and impaired reality testing.[21] A larger sample of 206 patients with BPD were administered the STIPO and the Structured Clinical Interviews for DSM-IV (SCID-I and SCID-II) in another study.[22] Severity of aggression; identity diffusion; use of more primitive, splitting-based defenses; and poorer reality testing were all associated with severity of DSM-IV BPD criteria. Although this study does not address the specificity of splitting phenomena to BPD, it supports the association between such processes and severity of DSM BPD symptoms. A smaller group of 50 outpatients with BPD were administered the STIPO in a later study. Identity diffusion (indicating polarization and lack of integration of the sense of self) was associated with poorer symptomatic and psychosocial functioning (as assessed by the Global Assessment of Functioning [GAF]).[23]

A related study investigated individuals diagnosed with BPD by DSM-IV Text Revision criteria.[24] Greater impairment in personality organization (including primitive, splitting-based defenses) correlated with an increased number of DSM-IV axis I and II diagnoses, indicating that increased splitting-based defenses may correspond with more polysymptomatic BPD disorder. Notably, in this BPD sample, the most severe impairment on the STIPO was in the domain of primitive (splitting-based) defenses, suggesting that this domain of personality organization is particularly emblematic of BPD severity.

Ecological Momentary Assessment Study

One innovative study used ecological momentary assessment (EMA) to investigate splitting phenomena in BPD.[25] EMA is an approach in which participants answer prompts at various points throughout a week or even within a day. The approach is a means to more validly sample sequences of experiences with self-reporting closer in time to the life events and reaction to them. This approach both allows for the examination of within-person processes (eg, increases in rejection are often followed by increases in rage) and provides increased validity by asking for reports on recent specific behaviors rather than remembered mental aggregates (eg, behaviors or emotions over the last week). These investigators used a well-characterized BPD and healthy control group using a 21-day EMA diary. All participants also made contemporaneous reports of their affective and relational experiences and high-risk (ie, impulsive) behaviors. Increased splitting (polarity) of emotional and interpersonal experiences was evident in the BPD compared with the healthy control group. Importantly, during moments of heighted relational stress, splitting increased and predicted a subsequent increase in risky and impulsive behaviors in the BPD group. Without a psychiatric control group, the specificity of these compelling findings to BPD was not investigated. The study is innovative for separately assessing affective and relational splitting within an EMA framework and for highlighting not just their diagnostic significance but their importance for predicting self-destructive behaviors in BPD.

Laboratory Tasks

In several laboratory studies, patients with BPD showed tendencies to appraise others in polarized ways using film characters as well as rating interactions with real people.

FILM CLIPS AND VISUAL ANALOG SCALES

One of the first studies to investigate DT in BPD in laboratory setting used characters from film clips which depicted emotional themes thought to prompt BPD schemas.[26] The investigators argued that though dichotomous thinking and splitting share many features, only DT can be multidimensional (ie, trait evaluations are extreme, but can feature a mix of both good and bad representations simultaneously of the same person). Splitting is conceived to be "all-good" or "all-bad" perceptions of others that is, unidimensional in nature (ie, extreme trait evaluations of 1 person having the same valence whether positive or negative). The investigators argue that only DT theory can capture incongruent trait evaluations on both positive and negative valances (eg, a person judged as both "totally reliable" and "totally lacking self-confidence" at the same time). Across 2 studies, the investigators have found support for higher scores on multidimensional versus unidimensional dichotomous thinking, which they have taken as support for DT being characteristic in BPD more so than splitting. However, the investigators may not appreciate that splitting can be multidimensional as well, because rapid changes (oscillations) in idealized and persecutory attributions in self and other are central to ORT of BPD. At the same time, though the idea that extreme scores on every valance may be an indicator of DT, it is not clear how such ratings translate into real life evaluations within close relationships with emotional intensity. Participants may make extreme evaluations on a trait like "unreliable," that may nonetheless be irrelevant in real social situations and social judgments. Thus, further research is needed to evaluate the real-world correlates of either style of DT. Within these 2 studies, the investigators also hypothesized that DT/splitting would be specifically activated by themes thought to be specific to BPD, such as rejection, abandonment, and abuse. They found support for this hypothesis in 1 study, but not the other.

INTERPERSONAL INTERACTIONS

Researchers had participants evaluate their interactions with supposed mental health worker trainees who assumed rejecting, accepting and neutral roles whereas/although discussing a problem on the phone.[20] A female sample of individuals with BPD, Cluster-C personality disorder, were recruited from a psychiatric center, and assessed with SCID-I and SCID-II, and compared with healthy controls. A structured response format (ie, visual analog scales with bipolar trait descriptions) and semistructured interviews (scored by trained raters on affect tone, differentiation, complexity of attributions, and extremity) was used. Participants spoke with 3 mental health trainees in each role about a recent personal problem for a fixed length of 10 minutes, exposing each participant equally to accepting-empathic, rejecting, and neutral partners. Across all conditions of interactions with trainees, the BPD group showed more DT than control groups. Researchers also found that splitting, negativity, and less complexity were more prominent in BPD but conclude that DT was most characteristic of BPD.

Empirical Studies of Trust Impairment and Borderline Personality Disorder

ORT posits that individuals with BPD develop mistrustful (paranoid) representations of others as a result of temperamental factors, early experiences with caregivers, and their interaction.[1] Clinical observations affirm this, because individuals with BPD interpret neutral and ambiguous cues in the social context with increased levels of vigilance and ultimately a negative bias.[27] The mechanism of mistrust among individuals with BPD is negative mental representations of self and others. That people with BPD tend to see others as threatening, hostile, rejecting, or untrustworthy has been supported by several lines of empirical research, including facial emotion recognition studies and social exchange/decision games. Although such aspects of BPD can be well described as mental representations and behaviors, looking to the neurobiological level can inform why such representations and behaviors are often entrenched and difficult to change, as well as highlighting the need to examine neurobiology and physiology as mechanisms of change in treatment.

Facial affect recognition

There has been a surge in studies examining the ability of individuals with BPD to recognize facial affect. At the same time, this body of studies is perplexing because of discrepant findings. In many studies, people with BPD have shown poorer emotion recognition accuracy, whereas, in others, researchers have found an enhanced ability for emotion recognition among people with BPD (see Ref.[28] for review). In a typical study of this kind, participants view facial expressions posed by actors, along with 6 emotional categories (happy, surprised, sad, angry, disgusted, fearful) and a neutral category. For each facial expression, the participant simply chooses the emotion category for the facial expression. In other variations of facial emotion recognition tasks,[29,30] or slowly morph photographs from neutral emotion to full emotional displays (eg, Ref.[31]). Emotion recognition studies assess whether people with BPD show diminished accuracy in reading facial emotion and whether they have biases in the ways they perceive the emotions of others. Such mistakes or biases are thought to be related to the problems that people with BPD have with social functioning,[32] although researchers have not given much attention to the real-world consequences of emotion recognition problems in BPD. However, it is plausible that a tendency to inaccurately read the emotions of others would lead to difficulties understanding the goals and intentions of others, which may lead a person to apply clichéd or rote interpretations. Such difficulty reading emotions could also lead to diffuse anxiety in navigating the social world, caused by a lack of clarity on social exchanges. Biases toward perceiving others' emotions as more negative than they are would likely lead to behavioral and emotional consequences, including perceiving others as malicious or rejecting.

Concerning ORT specifically, using Klein's[13] description of the paranoid-schizoid position, it might be hypothesized that individuals with BPD tend to misread neutral faces as bad or hostile. Within a research literature that includes contradictory findings, one of the most consistent findings is that people with BPD tend to misclassify neutral or ambiguous faces as negative.[30,32–36] People with BPD may often mistake neutral emotions for negative emotions. Such studies are consistent with the dynamics of the paranoid-schizoid stance and ORT's focus on aggression as a core emotion of BPD.[7] However, individuals with BPD experience a wide variety of increased negative emotions. A similar, but distinct, hypothesis of internal representations of others driving such mistakes is that, for individuals with BPD, their own increased emotions may color their perception of others' emotions, particularly when that emotion is neutral, ambiguous, or complicated. Thus, the literature suggests that people with BPD are likely to read negative emotional expressions on the faces of people who have no clear emotional expression. However, it is not yet clear what drives such biases; mental representations, extreme emotionality, the hyperactive function of the limbic system, or potentially the interplay of all three. Nonetheless, such dynamics are likely to affect the social lives of people with BPD, including within the therapeutic relationship.

In the few studies that have examined brain function during emotion recognition,[37–39] researchers tend to find evidence for increased activation in the amygdala and reduced activation in the orbital frontal cortex and other areas of the prefrontal cortex. Such a pattern of findings suggests greater limbic system activation in response to emotional faces and a lack of inhibition by prefrontal regions. The orbital frontal cortex (OFC) has many functions, including evaluation of the affective value of reward and punishment,[40] which may be involved in recognition of facial emotion.[41] It is also central to decision making and regulating negative emotions.[42] Greater amygdala activation and reduced OFC activation in these studies has often been paired with a tendency to show a negative bias in facial emotion activation, suggesting that more automatic affective processes bias more controlled decision making. In ORT's account of BPD, the focus is not on automatic and controlled processing but on the nature of conceptual memory (object relations dyads) in BPD.[1] At the same, considerable research has shown that activating attachment mental representations, even with subliminally presented stimuli, has effects on both behavior and neural activation (eg, Ref.[43]). Priming representations of others as unavailable or rejecting is associated with greater activation in the amygdala,[44] whereas priming attentive and responsive representations reduces this activation.[43] Thus, it is plausible that representations of malicious others among individuals with BPD could result in a tendency to see neutral faces as more negative and show corresponding neural activation associated with social threat.

Although results of studies of emotion recognition have been a confusing mix, studies directly related to the trait perception of trustworthiness from faces evince more coherent results. People make initial (but often enduring) judgments regarding other people from facial affect in as little as a tenth of a second.[45] Consistent with the notion that people with BPD perceive neutral people as bad, a series of studies have found reduced trust for others among individuals with BPD.[27,46,47] In one,[46] using facial stimuli morphed to show different degrees of trust and fear, people with BPD rated faces as less trustworthy across most degrees of trust but showed appraisal of fear that was not significantly different from healthy controls. The investigators described evidence that emotion appraisal (eg, reading fear) and trait appraisal (eg, reading trustworthiness) are distinct processes, and provided further support for this contention by finding that trustworthiness perception in BPD was biased, whereas fear perception was not. These results suggest that people with BPD have a response bias for evaluating others as less trustworthy, even when there is no clear evidence of bias in rating the intensity of fearful expressions. Moreover, response times for evaluating ambiguously trustworthy faces were longer for people with BPD compared with controls, suggesting increased mental effort in evaluating faces that were not readily identified at the extremes of trustworthiness (eg, the extremes of trustworthy or untrustworthy). These results may argue against emotion dysregulation as the source of bias in ratings regarding trustworthiness, given that ratings of emotional intensity were consistent with people without emotion regulation problems.

In addition to seeing lower trustworthiness in neutral faces, researchers have also found that rejection sensitivity mediates the relationship between mistrust and increased BPD symptoms.[27] This finding suggests the interesting possibility that fear of rejection of the self and mistrust of others are part of a similar process. One possibility is that rejection sensitivity and mistrust represent an object relations dyad of a deficient self and a rejecting, untrustworthy other, connected by fear/anxiety or anger/rage. Although individuals with BPD anxiously avoid rejection, substantial research has suggested that, once rejected, people with BPD tend to react with anger or rage (eg, Refs.[48,49]). Implicit in the concept of rejection sensitivity is the expectation that others will be unsupportive and overtly unkind. As a first strategy, people high in the trait avoid rejection. Although people experience rejection as painful, this experience has been found to be particularly painful and distressing to people with BPD.[50] The need to belong is critical for humans. Natural selection seems to have promoted social affiliation by using the neural architecture for physical pain.[51] Regions of the dorsal anterior cingulate, somatosensory cortex, anterior insula, and other regions involved in physical pain show higher activation when people are rejected. People high in rejection sensitivity, such as those with BPD, have an intense need for connection with others, partly because of a lack of confidence in their ability to cope with the stressors of life.[52,53] When they perceive others as rejecting, their experience of pain seems to be higher than in others.[54] It may be that, because of this increased sensitivity to rejection, people with BPD are more mistrustful of others. If a person is routinely hurt by others, because of real or perceived rejection, it makes sense to be cautious of others.[27]

One drawback of almost all studies of emotion recognition and trust appraisals in BPD published to date is that they use faces of strangers. Researchers make this choice in the service of standardization (each participant evaluates the same faces). However, theory and research suggest that people with BPD have particular difficulty in close attachment relationships, meaning that assessing such abilities in strangers may be less sensitive than examining performance for close others. Using a more ecologically valid approach, an innovative study recently asked heterosexual women diagnosed with BPD and controls to appraise the trustworthiness of their romantic partners following 3 different discussions. For the first, the participants were asked to talk about their favorite films. In the second, they were asked to discuss their personal fears. In the third, they were asked to focus on possible reasons for breaking up the relationship. These discussion topics were selected to represent a baseline condition, a discussion meant to activate a sense of personal threat, and a discussion meant to bring to mind the potential dissolution of the attachment bond. Although women with BPD did not differ from controls in trustworthiness ratings after the neutral condition, they had lower ratings following both the personal threat and relationship threat conditions. Also, ratings by women with BPD were lower for the relationship threat condition compared with the personal threat condition. These results seem to suggest that negative representations of romantic partners are more easily activated among women with BPD, particularly in response to a relationship threat. In addition, these findings may indicate that people with BPD struggle to put specific, immediate interpersonal experiences in a broader context of experiences. If mistrust is more easily generated by discussing relationship threats, it suggests that individuals with BPD may have difficulty contextualizing the current discord in the broader context of relationship experiences.

Hypermentalization

There has been steady and increasing interest in deficits in mentalization,[55,56] an imaginative form of social cognition characterized by seeing the behavior of others as driven by intentional mental states (eg, goals, intentions). Emotion recognition and trait appraisals are near neighbors to mentalization, because judgments on the emotional state and behavioral dispositions of others inform people's hypotheses about others' goals and intentions. Although there is some evidence of problems with mentalization in BPD, a series of studies[57,58] have characterized the social cognitive style of people with BPD as hypermentalization. The term hypermentalization refers to errors in mentalization that are the result of making interpretations or attributions that go well beyond the observable data. Explanations for others' behavior is described in terms of mental states, but the explanations are not plausible, given the data.[57] For instance, a man may receive a gift from his wife: a photograph of a lone tree on the plains. A hypermentalizing response would be for the man to interpret the wife as trying to covertly show him that he is a bad, neglectful partner. He sees her as trying to communicate to him that she is like the tree, which he sees as painfully alone. Given the data, a more reasonable interpretation may be that the wife selected the gift because she thought it was pretty and wanted to give her partner something nice. There is frequently a flavor of mistrust or paranoia evident in hypermentalization, as depicted earlier (in addition to a difficulty differentiating the boundaries between self and other). Sharp and Vanwoerden[59] argue that hypermentalization is the result of a lack of integration of more controlled-explicit social cognition and automatic-implicit cognition among people with BPD, which is particularly evident at higher levels of arousal. Their model of hypermentalization is consonant with ORT. In response to stressful interpersonal events, people with BPD may engage in more automatic-implicit cognition, in which internal representations of more malevolent others are evident, and, because of lowered explicit monitoring, the plausibility of these accounts, given the explicit data, is left unchecked. Hypermentalization may be evidence of a tendency to apply representations of malicious others onto new situations in which information is not fully available.

Trust in neuroeconomic games

In the past 15 years, researchers have been drawn to neuroeconomics games to study aspects of social decision making.[60] Trust is a major ingredient of social decision making, and making adaptive social exchanges often depends on the ability to know when to trust and when to withdraw trust flexibly.[61] However, individual differences in decisions to trust or mistrust may be caused by environmental contexts in which trust has been habitually rewarded or punished.[62] In the trust game, a multiround game used in several studies of individuals with BPD, participants play with another participant (typically a healthy control or computer algorithm presented as another person). One player acts as the investor and begins each round with an amount of money to invest. The investor keeps whatever they do not invest. Whatever the investor does invest triples and goes to the other player, called the trustee. The trustee then decides how much of this investment to keep and how much to return to the investor. The goal for both participants is to make as much money as they can. However, this is a game that tends to reward collaboration rather than greed. From the investors' viewpoint, they need to trust the trustee and invest, ideally, all of the amount allotted on each round. From the trustees' viewpoint, they need to maintain trust with the investor and respond with social cues if trust breaks down (the major way to repair trust and collaboration in the game is for the trustee to return a more generous amount of the investment).

There is evidence from studies using this game that people diagnosed with BPD mistrust others and send behavioral signals that lead to others mistrusting them. In one study, people with BPD reported less trust for others and repaid less money to investors in the trust game. In the game, after investors decide how much money to invest, that amount is revealed on the screen. The amount invested is an indication to the trustees of how much the investor currently trusts them. When healthy trustees learned that an investor invested a small amount of money, activation in their anterior insula increased. The amount of money invested seemed to be tightly indexed by insula activation in healthy trustees; larger investments were associated with lower insula activation and smaller investments with more. The anterior insula is a region involved in the integration of multiple modes of sensation and cognition and may also respond to norm violations. It seems that healthy trustees discern that they may have violated the other player's trust. It was not clear that individuals with BPD detected the same violations. There was no relationship between the investment and insula activation among people with BPD. In addition, consistent with this account, people with BPD typically failed to repair broken trust by returning more generous repayments on subsequent rounds. Thus, individuals with BPD struggle to maintain trust and collaboration with others. A likely long-term outcome of such struggles is to view others as withholding, a common perception among people with BPD. In addition, such difficulties collaborating with others are likely to severely limit the social, romantic, and work options of people with the disorder.

In a separate study, playing this time as the investor rather than the trustee, people with BPD showed less trust in their partners by investing less than either healthy controls or people with depression.[63] However, in a conceptually similar game in which the participants' investments went into a random lottery (nonsocial condition), people with BPD showed similar investments to other groups. Also, they were less optimistic about the amount of money that would be returned to them if they thought they were playing with a person versus a computer (in reality, both were computer controlled). This study seems to strongly support the idea that people with BPD mistrust people specifically. They were willing to invest more money in a lottery but less when another person would ostensibly decide how much to return. It seems, consistent with ORT, that they hold representations of people that lead to mistrust and pessimism, which does not generalize when considering nonsocial exchanges.

Oxytocin and borderline personality disorder

The serious interpersonal difficulties and mistrust of others have led some researchers to investigate the role of oxytocin in BPD.[64] Oxytocin is a neuropeptide that has been found to be involved in social approach, attachment distress, and pair bonding in animal studies,[65] and to modulate salience of social cues, increase prosocial behavior and trust, in addition to playing a role in emotion regulation among humans.[66] Oxytocin is thought to have effects on social behavior through modulation of the neural network supporting affiliative behavior, which includes the reward system and brain regions involved in social cognition, although a larger proportion of studies have focused on the effects of oxytocin on the amygdala.[67] Also, adverse developmental experiences are associated with endogenous oxytocin levels, with low cerebrospinal fluid levels found in women who experienced abuse or neglect as children.[68]

Some studies suggest oxytocin may be a factor in the interpersonal problems commonly experienced by people with BPD, such as hypervigilance to social threat and tendency toward mistrust of others.[69,70] Testing this hypothesis, a handful of studies have administered intranasal oxytocin and examined changes in social factors like trust, social threat, and cooperation.[71-74] In one study,[73] researchers used functional brain imaging and eye tracking while participants with and without BPD classified facial emotions. The gaze of participants with BPD was captured by angry faces faster and for a longer period relative to participants without BPD. Increased amygdala activation accompanied this greater attention to threatening stimuli. Both suggest hypervigilance for social threat. Both eye fixation changes and amygdala activation were no different from those of participants without BPD following oxytocin administration. The results suggest that exogenous oxytocin may decrease vigilance for social threat among people with BPD.

However, oxytocin administration has also shown some paradoxic effects for people with BPD. In another study,[72] using a neuroeconomic game similar to the trust game, the researchers found that, among participants with BPD, administration of oxytocin decreased trust and cooperation. However, results differed by attachment style. Participants with BPD who reported high attachment anxiety and rejection sensitivity were those who showed lower trust following oxytocin administration. Although other causes are plausible, this may mean that the effects of oxytocin are dependent on differences in internal working models of self and others that are thought to underlie differences in attachment styles.

When focusing at the biological level, or when describing automatic processes that occur within milliseconds, it can be easy to think only in terms causes or solutions only at the same level. However, research has shown that interpersonal variables and stress affect levels of oxytocin,[68,75] and it is plausible that changes in representations of self and others can affect both trust and oxytocin. However, neither theorists nor researchers have attempted to make such links. At the same time, theorists and researchers have been developing new neurobiological models of social interactions that could apply to ORT.[76] Coan and colleagues[77,78] propose within their social baseline theory that individual differences in representations of others are likely to affect peoples' ability for self-regulation and thus stress level and susceptibility to mental disorder. Representations of others as hostile, punitive, exploitative, untrustworthy, or simply unhelpful are likely to have interpersonal consequences (more conflict, less reliance on others for support), which are also likely to affect neurobiological systems, including the oxytocinergic system. Changes to more integrated and less negative views of self and others are, thus, likely to affect people's interpersonal behavior, brain function, and physiologic responses. Oxytocin activity in the hypothalamus, nucleus accumbens, ventral tegmental area, and amygdala have been associated with attachment security.[79]

One of the most provocative treatment studies of an ORT-informed treatment has found that a substantial number of people with BPD treated with TFP move from insecure to secure attachment over the course of a year of therapy.[80] Subsequent research could examine whether such changes are accompanied by changes to the oxytocinergic system. Research seems to show interactions between representations of self and others and the effects of oxytocin on social behavior, which makes the simple administration of oxytocin unlikely to be helpful for many people. Because of this, psychotherapy, or potentially psychotherapy combined with oxytocin administration, may be more promising for social rehabilitation among individuals with BPD than oxytocin alone because psychotherapy focuses on changing internal representations. Without such changes, oxytocin may have paradoxic effects.

Discussion and Future Directions

There has been a slow but steady evolution in the breadth and sophistication of splitting and trust impairment studies in BPD over the last 50 years. Consequently, even though it is the oldest model of BPD, ORT has sustained and robust scientific relevance. The accumulation and consistency of findings for trust impairment suggest that a systematic review of this literature is justified. However, the varied methods and largely unreplicated approaches used to study splitting suggest that it is premature to conduct a systematic review of this literature. Taken together, although support for splitting and trust impairment is scattered across the literature, there is a potential for convergence among methodologies and cross-fertilization across disciplines. Critically, and consistent with ORT, when both splitting and trust impairments have been concurrently investigated, evidence has suggested the two are linked. People who have impairments in trust judgments may resort to splitting as an automatic, but maladaptive, strategy to navigate interpersonal relations. Once instantiated, splitting may then perpetuate impairments in trust. The key themes and directions are synthesized here for future investigation.

Self-esteem and Borderline Personality Disorder

The extreme mental representations that are formed through DT and splitting may be partly driven by low self-esteem evident in BPD, a potentially fruitful avenue of research in BPD. Social psychologists define self-esteem as the quality of the subjective knowledge about the self, and the study of self-esteem can provide insight and understanding about the psychopathology in BPD. Previous studies that used assessments of splitting or DT found them to be related to low self-esteem levels.[17,81] One self-esteem study[82] found that people low in self-esteem segregate positive and negative information about others in memory (ie, DT or splitting), whereas those high in self-esteem are able to integrate both positive and negative information in memory. The investigators suggest that having a single composite memory store that contains both positive and negative trait-related information allows people to have a more balanced evaluation of others in which they have a cognitive representation of others as a combination of both good and bad, without the propensity to lean toward extreme appraisals. The opposite is having 2 distinct memory stores, which causes shifting back and forth between the two, resulting in fluctuating between simplistic evaluations at extreme poles of positive and negative. Because people low in self-esteem (similar to BPD) are specifically anxious to avoid rejection but also share an intense desire to form and maintain relationships, both individuals with low self-esteem and those with BPD are extra cautious about signs of interpersonal threat, and, once a threat is identified, these individuals split their mental representations to focus on the entirely bad aspects in the other person. This method has yet to be directly used in BPD but would provide a rigorous laboratory method to study splitting phenomena in this disorder.

With regard to the BPD diagnosis, the sensitivity of splitting and trust impairment is consistent, but the specificity of these constructs to BPD requires further study because of the lack of studies that have included psychiatric controls. The degree to which splitting and trust impairments are also present in non-BPD personality disorders (eg, paranoid and narcissistic personality disorders) and other mental disorders in which trust is impaired (eg, psychotic disorders) is an open question. A related psychometric challenge is that there is no gold standard for the measurement of splitting. The most promising candidate measures that use sophisticated raters who are experts in the mental disorder of splitting are the STIPO (cited previously) and the differentiation-relatedness (DR) scale (Diamond D, Blatt SJ, Stayner DA, et al. Manual for the differentiation–relatedness scale. Unpublished manual. 2014). Regrettably, with the exception of 1 dissertation report that found evidence of greater splitting phenomena in a sample diagnosed with BPD compared with healthy controls (Erbe J. Mental representations, social exclusion, and neurobiological processes in Borderline Personality Disorder: a multi-level study. Unpublished dissertation. City University of New York. 2016), the DR scale has not been specifically used in a DSM-diagnosed

BPD sample. Consensus regarding the most valid measure of splitting phenomena and trust impairments as a dependent variable is lacking in laboratory and neuroscience studies.

No studies have integrated the clinically sophisticated interview of splitting with laboratory or EMA methods. Convergent validity and multitrait method studies such as these are needed. Further, studies comparing ORT and other prominent models of BPD have not been conducted. For instance, do ORT studies of splitting and trust impairment add variance in predicting BPD status above and beyond the variance predicted by emotion dysregulation and mentalization-based/attachment-based models? Such studies would contribute to integration of various models toward empirically different integration and identification of potential subtypes of BPD.

Are state and trait dimensions in integrating splitting (which is state based; ie, perceptions of self and others can change rapidly from moment to moment) and trust impairments (which are frequently trait based; ie, stable over time) related dynamically? If splitting is improved, does the quality of trust in interpersonal relationships improve as well (as a trait), with concomitant functional improvement in BPD? There is a need for longitudinal studies to capture state fluctuations of self and others. Moreover, risk factors such as early adversity, abuse, neglect, trauma, attachment disturbance, and temperament need more study as predictors of splitting and trust impairment in adolescence and adulthood. Using the same methodology as Fertuck and colleagues,[46] a study of posttraumatic stress disorder (PTSD) compared a group with comparable traumatic histories but without PTSD and a healthy (not trauma) control group. PTSD was associated with a bias to be more trusting of neutral faces than the group exposed to trauma (but with no PTSD).[83] Early adversity and trauma may interact with dispositional factors to lead to differential trajectories of mental disorder,[84] such as PTSD versus BPD. Splitting and trust impairment may serve as mediators of the influence of these different trajectories.

Studies of splitting and trust as treatment targets are lacking. TFP, for one, can now be better evaluated in terms of mechanism of change. Federal funding agencies and psychotherapy research have moved away from studies that compare the efficacy of different treatments. The current gold-standard approach to psychotherapy research is to identify the mechanisms of the disorder, measure those mechanisms validly and reliably, and show change in these mechanisms as a result of treatment. For ORT, those mechanisms include splitting and interpersonal trust as well as mentalization/hypermentalization, reactivity to social threat, emotion recognition, and other interpersonal difficulties. Another sophisticated approach to such treatment studies would be to measure change in physiology or neural networks supporting the proposed mechanism. Improvements in functional neural connectivity analyses (eg, Ref.[85]) make examination of the strength and patterns of connectivity within neural networks an attractive choice for treatment studies.

Although trust impairment has received a focus in social neuroscience research, neuroscientific research in splitting is nonexistent. The major obstacle to more neuroscience research on this topic is identifying a task that isolates the phenomenon that can be conducted within the confines of a functional MRI (fMRI) scanner and other brain imaging methods. A task suitable for the context of neuroimaging has to be highly replicable (researchers average many instances of the same cognitive task) and cannot include movements, such as speaking. Recent advances in machine learning may open new opportunities for evaluating differences in conceptual knowledge among people with and without BPD. As an example, Just and colleagues[86] were able to correctly classify 91% of participants who had made a suicide attempt based on the neural signatures of death-related and life-related concepts. This study suggests that differences in concept representations can be made using machine learning algorithms. Such an approach could be a useful adjunct to studies of social appraisal among individuals with BPD. Establishing the differences in representations of self and others as a means to classify individuals with BPD versus those without the disorder could be a substantial first step toward revealing the nature of those representations.

In summary, empirical research is increasingly highlighting the interpersonal nature of BPD. To fully validate ORT, studies are needed that more directly examine the influence of representations of self and others on brain functioning and behavior in BPD. Although advances like machine learning (a type of artificial intelligence) have begun to allow detection of individual differences in concepts from patterns of functional brain activation, researchers also commonly affect internal representations by using stimuli that activate the representation. The attachment literature abounds with examples of this type of manipulation.[87] Often, researchers find effects even when participants are not conscious of the stimuli. It may be possible to detect the elements of the nature of representations of self and others using such an approach. Learning more about the characters of social representations among people with BPD, and the contexts and themes that are more likely to activate these representations, would go a long way to further validate ORT and advance the understanding of the disorder.

ACKNOWLEDGMENTS

This review was supported in part by grants from NIMH (MH077044) the American Psychoanalytic Association, the Neuropsychoanalysis Foundation and the City College of New York City Seeds grant to E.A. Fertuck.

REFERENCES

1. Kernberg O. Borderline personality organization. J Am Psychoanal Assoc 1967; 15:641–85.
2. Clifton A, Pilkonis PA, McCarty C. Social networks in borderline personality disorder. J Personal Disord 2007;21:434–41.
3. Brodsky BS, Groves SA, Oquendo MA, et al. Interpersonal precipitants and suicide attempts in borderline personality disorder. Suicide Life Threat Behav 2006; 36:313–22.
4. Downey G, Mougios V, Ayduk O, et al. Rejection sensitivity and the defensive motivational system: insights from the startle response to rejection cues. Psychol Sci 2004;15:668–73.
5. Ayduk O, Zayas V, Downey G, et al. Rejection sensitivity and executive control: joint predictors of borderline personality features. J Res Pers 2008;42:151–68.
6. Roepke S, Vater A, Preissler S, et al. Social cognition in borderline personality disorder. Front Neurosci 2012;6:195.
7. Kernberg OF. Borderline conditions and pathological narcissism. New York: Rowman & Littlefield; 1985.
8. Stoffers Jutta M, Völlm Birgit A, Rücker G, et al. Psychological therapies for people with borderline personality disorder. Cochrane Database Syst Rev 2012;(8):CD005652. John Wiley & Sons, Ltd.
9. Kernberg OF, Yeomans FE, Clarkin JF, et al. Transference focused psychotherapy: overview and update. Int J Psychoanal 2008;89:601–20.
10. Arksey H, O'Malley L. Scoping studies: towards a methodological framework. Int J Soc Res Methodol 2005;8:19 32.

11. Napolitano LA, McKay D. Dichotomous thinking in borderline personality disorder. Cognit Ther Res 2007;31:717–26.
12. Beck AT, Butler AC, Brown GK, et al. Dysfunctional beliefs discriminate personality disorders. Behav Res Ther 2001;39:1213–25.
13. Klein M. Envy and gratitude, and other works, 1946-1963. London: Hogarth Press and the Institute of Psycho-Analysis; 1975.
14. Westen D, Lohr N, Silk KR, et al. Object relations and social cognition in borderlines, major depressives, and normals: a thematic apperception test analysis. Psychol Assess 1990;2:355–64.
15. Whipple R, Fowler JC. Affect, relationship schemas, and social cognition: self-injuring borderline personality disorder inpatients. Psychoanal Psychol 2011;28: 183–95.
16. Leichsenring F. Splitting: an empirical study. Bull Menninger Clin 1999;63:520–37.
17. Gould JR, Prentice NM, Ainslie RC. The splitting index construction. J Pers Assess 1996;66:414–30.
18. Pec O, Bob P, Raboch J. Splitting in schizophrenia and borderline personality disorder. PLoS One 2014;9:e91228.
19. Kramer U, de Roten Y, Perry JC, et al. Beyond splitting: observer-rated defense mechanisms in borderline personality disorder. Psychoanal Psychol 2013;30:3–15.
20. Arntz A, ten Haaf J. Social cognition in borderline personality disorder: evidence for dichotomous thinking but no evidence for less complex attributions. Behav Res Ther 2012;50:707–18.
21. Stern BL, Caligor E, Clarkin JF, et al. Structured Interview of Personality Organization (STIPO): preliminary psychometrics in a clinical sample. J Pers Assess 2010;92:35–44.
22. Ferrer M, Andion O, Calvo N, et al. Clinical components of borderline personality disorder and personality functioning. Psychopathology 2018;51(1):57–64.
23. Esguevillas Á, Díaz-Caneja CM, Arango C, et al. Personality organization and its association with clinical and functional features in borderline personality disorder. Psychiatry Res 2018;262:393–9.
24. Fischer-Kern M, Buchheim A, Hörz S, et al. The relationship between personality organization, reflective functioning, and psychiatric classification in borderline personality disorder. Psychoanal Psychol 2010;27:395–409.
25. Coifman KG, Berenson KR, Rafaeli E, et al. From negative to positive and back again: polarized affective and relational experience in borderline personality disorder. J Abnorm Psychol 2012;121:668–79.
26. Veen G, Arntz A. Multidimensional dichotomous thinking characterizes borderline personality disorder. Cogn Ther Res 2000;24:23–45.
27. Miano A, Fertuck EA, Arntz A, et al. Rejection sensitivity is a mediator between borderline personality disorder features and facial trust appraisal. J Personal Disord 2013;27:442–56.
28. Mitchell AE, Dickens GL, Picchioni MM. Facial emotion processing in borderline personality disorder: a systematic review and meta-analysis. Neuropsychol Rev 2014;24:166–84.
29. Fertuck EA, Jekal A, Song I, et al. Enhanced 'Reading the Mind in the Eyes' in borderline personality disorder compared to healthy controls. Psychol Med 2009;39:1979–88.
30. Dyck M, Habel U, Slodczyk J, et al. Negative bias in fast emotion discrimination in borderline personality disorder. Psychol Med 2009;39:855–64.
31. Domes G, Czieschnek D, Weidler F, et al. Recognition of facial affect in borderline personality disorder. J Pers Disord 2008;22:135–47.

32. Domes G, Schulze L, Herpertz SC. Emotion recognition in borderline personality disorder-a review of the literature. J Pers Disord 2009;23:6–19.
33. Arntz A, Veen G. Evaluations of others by borderline patients. J Nerv Ment Dis 2001;189:513–21.
34. Meyer B, Pilkonis PA, Beevers CG. What's in a (neutral) face? Personality disorders, attachment styles, and the appraisal of ambiguous social cues. J Pers Disord 2004;18:320–36.
35. Daros AR, Zakzanis KK, Ruocco AC. Facial emotion recognition in borderline personality disorder. Psychol Med 2013;43:1953–63.
36. Wagner AW, Linehan MM. Facial expression recognition ability among women with borderline personality disorder: implications for emotion regulation? J Pers Disord 1999;13:329–44.
37. Donegan NH, Sanislow CA, Blumberg HP, et al. Amygdala hyperreactivity in borderline personality disorder: implications for emotional dysregulation. Biol Psychiatry 2003;54:1284–93.
38. Minzenberg MJ, Fan J, New AS, et al. Fronto-limbic dysfunction in response to facial emotion in borderline personality disorder: an event-related fMRI study. Psychiatry Res 2007;155:231–43.
39. Mier D, Lis S, Esslinger C, et al. Neuronal correlates of social cognition in borderline personality disorder. Soc Cogn Affect Neurosci 2013;8(5):531–7.
40. O'Doherty J, Rolls ET, Francis S, et al. Representation of pleasant and aversive taste in the human brain. J Neurophysiol 2001;85:1315–21.
41. Adolphs R. Neural systems for recognizing emotion. Curr Opin Neurobiol 2002; 12:169–77.
42. Bechara A, Tranel D, Damasio H. Characterization of the decision-making deficit of patients with ventromedial prefrontal cortex lesions. Brain 2000;123(Pt 1): 2189–202.
43. Norman L, Lawrence N, Iles A, et al. Attachment-security priming attenuates amygdala activation to social and linguistic threat. Soc Cogn Affect Neurosci 2015;10:832–9.
44. Lemche E, Giampietro VP, Surguladze Sa, et al. Human attachment security is mediated by the amygdala: evidence from combined fMRI and psychophysiological measures. Hum Brain Mapp 2006;27:623–35.
45. Willis J, Todorov A. First impressions: making up your mind after a 100-ms exposure to a face. Psychol Sci 2006;17:592–8.
46. Fertuck EA, Grinband J, Stanley B. Facial trust appraisal negatively biased in borderline personality disorder. Psychiatry Res 2013;207:195–202.
47. Miano A, Fertuck EA, Roepke S, et al. Romantic relationship dysfunction in borderline personality disorder—a naturalistic approach to trustworthiness perception. Personal Disord 2017;8(3):281–6.
48. Berenson KR, Downey G, Rafaeli E, et al. The rejection-rage contingency in borderline personality disorder. J Abnorm Psychol 2011;120:681–90.
49. Scott LN, Wright AGC, Beeney JE, et al. Borderline personality disorder symptoms and aggression: a within-person process model. J Abnorm Psychol 2017; 126(4):429–40.
50. Domsalla M, Koppe G, Niedtfeld I, et al. Cerebral processing of social rejection in patients with borderline personality disorder. Soc Cogn Affect Neurosci 2014; 9(11):1789–97.
51 Eisenberger NI, Lieberman MD, Williams KD. Does rejection hurt? An fMRI study of social exclusion. Science 2003;302:290–2.

52. Downey G, Feldman SI. Implications of rejection sensitivity for intimate relationships. J Pers Soc Psychol 1996;70:1327–43.
53. Downey G, Freitas AL, Michaelis B, et al. The self-fulfilling prophecy in close relationships: rejection sensitivity and rejection by romantic partners. J Pers Soc Psychol 1998;75:545–60.
54. Burklund LJ, Eisenberger NI, Lieberman MD. The face of rejection: rejection sensitivity moderates dorsal anterior cingulate activity to disapproving facial expressions. Soc Neurosci 2007;2:238–53.
55. Bateman A, Fonagy P. Psychotherapy for borderline personality disorder: mentalization-based treatment. Oxford (UK): Oxford University Press; 2004.
56. Choi-Kain LW, Gunderson JG. Mentalization: ontogeny, assessment, and application in the treatment of borderline personality disorder. Am J Psychiatry 2008;165: 1127–35.
57. Sharp C, Pane H, Ha C, et al. Theory of mind and emotion regulation difficulties in adolescents with borderline traits. J Am Acad Child Adolesc Psychiatry 2011;50: 563–73.e1.
58. Sharp C, Ha C, Carbone C, et al. Hypermentalizing in adolescent inpatients: treatment effects and association with borderline traits. J Pers Disord 2013;27: 3–18.
59. Sharp C, Vanwoerden S. Hypermentalizing in borderline personality disorder: a model and data. J Infant Child Adolesc Psychother 2015;14:33–45.
60. Kishida KT, King-Casas B, Montague PR. Neuroeconomic approaches to mental disorders. Neuron 2010;67:543–54.
61. King-Casas B, Tomlin D, Anen C, et al. Getting to know you: reputation and trust in a two-person economic exchange. Science 2005;308:78–83.
62. Pitula CE, Wenner JA, Gunnar MR, et al. To trust or not to trust: social decision-making in post-institutionalized, internationally adopted youth. Dev Sci 2017;20. https://doi.org/10.1111/desc.12375.
63. Unoka Z, Seres I, Áspán N, et al. Trust game reveals restricted interpersonal transactions in patients with borderline personality disorder. J Personal Disord 2009;23:399–409.
64. Herpertz SC, Bertsch K. A new perspective on the pathophysiology of borderline personality disorder: a model of the role of oxytocin. Am J Psychiatry 2015;172: 840–51.
65. Lim MM, Young LJ. Neuropeptidergic regulation of affiliative behavior and social bonding in animals. Horm Behav 2006;50:506–17.
66. Weisman O, Feldman R. Oxytocin effects on the human brain: findings, questions, and future directions. Biol Psychiatry 2013;74:158–9.
67. Insel TR. A neurobiological basis of social attachment. Am J Psychiatry 1997;154: 726–35.
68. Heim C, Young LJ, Newport DJ, et al. Lower CSF oxytocin concentrations in women with a history of childhood abuse. Mol Psychiatry 2009;14:954–8.
69. Kosfeld M, Heinrichs M, Zak PJ, et al. Oxytocin increases trust in humans. Nature 2005;435:673–6.
70. Baumgartner T, Heinrichs M, Vonlanthen A, et al. Oxytocin shapes the neural circuitry of trust and trust adaptation in humans. Neuron 2008;58:639–50.
71. Simeon D, Bartz J, Hamilton H, et al. Oxytocin administration attenuates stress reactivity in borderline personality disorder: a pilot study. Psychoneuroendocrinology 2011;36:1418–21.
72. Bartz J, Simeon D, Hamilton H, et al. Oxytocin can hinder trust and cooperation in borderline personality disorder. Soc Cogn Affect Neurosci 2011;6:556–63.

73. Bertsch K, Gamer M, Schmidt B, et al. Oxytocin and reduction of social threat hypersensitivity in women with borderline personality disorder. Am J Psychiatry 2013;170:1169–77.
74. Jobst A, Padberg F, Mauer M-C, et al. Lower oxytocin plasma levels in borderline patients with unresolved attachment representations. Front Hum Neurosci 2016; 10:1–11.
75. Heinrichs M, Baumgartner T, Kirschbaum C, et al. Social support and oxytocin interact to suppress cortisol and subjective responses to psychosocial stress. Biol Psychiatry 2003;54:1389–98.
76. Hughes AE, Crowell SE, Uyeji L, et al. A developmental neuroscience of borderline pathology: emotion dysregulation and social baseline theory. J Abnorm Child Psychol 2012;40:21–33.
77. Coan Ja, Schaefer HS, Davidson RJ. Lending a hand: social regulation of the neural response to threat. Psychol Sci 2006;17:1032–9.
78. Beckes L, Coan JA. Social baseline theory and the social regulation of emotion. In: Campbell L, La Guardia JG, Olson JM, et al, editors. The Ontario symposium on personality and social psychology: Vol. 12. The science of the couple. New York: Psychology Press; 2012. p. 81–93.
79. Coan JA. Chapter: toward a neuroscience of attachment. In: Handbook of attachment: theory, research, and clinical applications. 2nd edition. New York: Guilford Press; 2008. p. 241–65.
80. Levy KN, Meehan KB, Kelly KM, et al. Change in attachment patterns and reflective function in a randomized control trial of transference-focused psychotherapy for borderline personality disorder. J Consult Clin Psychol 2006;74:1027–40.
81. Watson DC. The relationship of self-esteem, locus of control, and dimensional models to personality disorders. J Soc Behav Pers 1998;13:399–420.
82. Graham SM, Clark MS. Self-esteem and organization of valenced information about others: The "Jekyll and Hyde"-ing. J Pers Soc Psychol 2006;90:652–65.
83. Fertuck EA, Jekal J, Song I, et al. Enhanced "Reading the Mind in the Eyes" in borderline personality disorder compared to healthy controls. Psychol Med 2009;39:1979–88.
84. Chesin M, Fertuck EA, Goodman J, et al. The interaction between rejection sensitivity and emotional maltreatment in borderline personality disorder. Psychopathology 2015;48(1):31–5.
85. Gates KM, Molenaar PCM. Group search algorithm recovers effective connectivity maps for individuals in homogeneous and heterogeneous samples. Neuroimage 2012;63:310–9.
86. Just MA, Pan L, Cherkassky VL, et al. Machine learning of neural representations of suicide and emotion concepts identifies suicidal youth. Nat Hum Behav 2017; 1:911–9.
87. Niedenthal PM, Brauer M, Robin L, et al. Adult attachment and the perception of facial expression of emotion. J Pers Soc Psychol 2002;82:419–33.

The Neurobiology of Borderline Personality Disorder

Maria Mercedes Perez-Rodriguez, MD, PhD[a],*,
Andrea Bulbena-Cabré, MD, PhD[a,b,c], Anahita Bassir Nia, MD[a],
Gillian Zipursky[a], Marianne Goodman, MD[a,b],
Antonia S. New, MD[a]

KEYWORDS

- Borderline personality disorder • Alexithymia • Genetics • Emotion dysregulation
- Impulsive aggression • Neuroimaging • Oxytocin • Opioids

KEY POINTS

- Evidence clearly suggests that borderline personality disorder (BPD) is substantially heritable and at least as heritable as other major psychiatric disorders.
- Brain imaging studies have suggested a dysregulation in top-down control of emotions and behavior in BPD; however, this model is also seen in other disorders, such as panic disorder.
- Abnormalities in the oxytocin and opioid systems may underlie the interpersonal dysfunction characteristic of BPD.
- An impairment in emotional interoception (a disconnect between heightened objectively measured emotional responses and blunted subjective appreciation of those responses) may be a core feature of BPD.

INTRODUCTION

The name borderline personality disorder (BPD) was coined at Mount Sinai in New York by Adolph Stern[1] and has its origins in a Freudian conceptualization of the mind, with BPD on the border between psychosis and neurosis. However, because

Disclosure Statement: None.
M.M. Perez-Rodriguez has received salary support from NIMH grant KL2TR001435, CDC/NIOSH grant U01 OH011473-01, NIH grant 1R01MH097799-01A1 (PI New), and NARSAD (PI Perez); M. M. Perez-Rodriguez is site-PI (Principal Investigator) of a study funded by Neurocrine Biosciences.
[a] Department of Psychiatry, Icahn School of Medicine at Mount Sinai, One Gustave L Levy Place, New York, NY 10029, USA; [b] Department of Psychiatry, Mental Illness Research Education and Clinical Centers, VA Bronx Health Care System, 130 W Kingsbridge Road, Bronx, NY 10468, USA; [c] Department of Psychiatry and Forensic Medicine, Autonomous University of Barcelona (UAB), Campus de la UAB, Plaça Cívica, 08193 Bellaterra, Barcelona, Spain
* Corresponding author. Department of Psychiatry, One Gustave L Levy Place, Box # 1230, New York, NY 10029.
E-mail address: mercedes.perez@mssm.edu

neurosis is no longer used in the language of clinical psychiatry, this name can lead to confusion. Rapid advances in understanding neurobiological features of BPD have also led to the view that this psychoanalytically grounded name seems obsolete. The surge in neurobiological studies of BPD emerged from evidence that BPD is a heritable illness.

There have been several reviews of the neurobiology of BPD, including very well written reviews of pharmacology, brain imaging findings, and candidate genes association studies. A comprehensive review of all recent empirical findings in brain imaging, genetics, heritability, and novel therapeutics would be very long and difficult to read. Instead, this article reviews the most salient neurobiological information available about BPD and presents a theoretic model grounded in those findings for what lies at the heart of BPD.

The empirical literature supports a coherent construct underlying the BPD diagnosis. Early studies showed 3 factors underlying BPD as defined in *Diagnostic and Statistical Manual of Mental Disorders*, 5th edition (DSM-5): disturbed relatedness (unstable relationships, identity disturbance, and chronic emptiness), behavioral dysregulation (impulsivity, suicidality, or self-mutilatory behavior), and affective dysregulation (affective instability, inappropriate anger, and efforts to avoid abandonment). However, subsequent analyses showed that these factors were highly correlated with each other ($r = .90, .94$, and $.99$) and these correlations suggest and underlying unifying construct.[2] The DSM-5 emphasizes a general characteristic of personality disorders and evidence suggests that this so-called g-factor maps particularly on to BPD.[3] What precisely that g-factor is has not been agreed on. Affective instability and, particularly, emotional reactivity in the context of interpersonal relationships, has been viewed as the essential core of BPD.[4] Although it is clearly a very central characteristic, this review focuses on a very specific and underappreciated characteristic of BPD that has only recently come under investigative scrutiny. This review explores several different models but posits that the core characteristic of BPD may be an impairment in emotional interoception or alexithymia.

The article begins with a review of the heritability and genetics of BPD, followed by biological models of BPD, including the neurobiology of affective instability, impaired interoception, opiate models of poor attachment, and structural brain imaging over the course of the development in BPD.

GENETICS, HERITABILITY, AND IMPLICATED GENES

Although family, twin, and adoption studies strongly and consistently suggest that BPD traits are heritable, the specific genetic underpinnings of BPD remain unknown.[5–7] Similar to most psychiatric disorders, BPD is believed to have a complex, multifactorial cause, resulting from the interaction of a genetic vulnerability with environmental factors.[8] The very limited understanding of the genetic architecture of BPD is a critical obstacle to advancing treatment and preventive efforts in BPD. Specifically, genetic research can help identify new treatment targets and develop preventive and disease-modifying treatments for BPD, which are not yet available.[9,10]

What follows is a brief overview of genetic studies of BPD and/or subclinical BPD traits, including most methodological approaches (eg, candidate gene association study, genome-wide association study [GWAS], gene-environment interactions, epigenetic modifications).

Most earlier genetic studies in BPD are candidate-gene association studies.[5,6] Most have very small sample sizes and positive results have not been confirmed by meta-analyses.[6] Most of the candidate association studies have focused on genes within the serotonergic, dopaminergic, and noradrenergic systems, which had been previously linked to BPD symptomatology. Only a few studies have examined other genes, such as those coding for the brain-derived neurotrophic factor; the vasopressin receptor 1A; and the sodium channel, voltage-gated, type IX, alpha subunit.[6]

As with other complex diseases, it is expected that the genetic vulnerability to BPD is the result of many individual risk variants, each with a very small effect on the risk of developing BPD. Because of the very small effect of each variant, very large samples are needed to identify risk variants using genome-wide approaches.[11] For example, in schizophrenia, successful GWASs have included tens of thousands of subjects.[12] In contrast, the only GWAS of the full BPD diagnosis to date included just fewer than 1000 BPD subjects.[13] Although no genetic variants reached genome-wide significance in this underpowered study, gene-based analysis yielded 2 significant genes: dihydropyrimidine dehydrogenase (DPYD) on chromosome 1 and Plakophilin-4 (PKP4) on chromosome 2. Moreover, the study also observed significant genetic overlap between BPD and bipolar disorder, major depressive disorder, and schizophrenia. There have also been 1 GWAS[14] and 1 genome-wide linkage study[15] of subclinical BPD traits, with significant results implicating the serine incorporator 5 (SERINC5) gene and chromosome 9, respectively.

Given the key role of trauma (objective or perceived) in traditional models of the genesis of BPD, it is surprising that there are very few studies examining gene-environment interactions in BPD subjects.[8] Most have small samples and have identified gene-environment interactions that have not been replicated. Research evidence has suggested that there is a gene–environment interaction in BPD, suggesting that those genetic factors that increase risk for BPD also increase risk for exposure to environmental stressors that may trigger BPD.[8] Although animal models of the interaction between genetic factors and early life experience can be very valuable, larger, longitudinal studies in humans are needed to elucidate the gene–environment interplay leading to BPD. Ideally, these studies will include large, prospective children cohorts.

Epigenetics is a relatively new field that opened a new avenue for exploring changes in gene expression caused by environmental conditions. Epigenetic modifications affect gene expression and include DNA methylation, histone remodeling, and noncoding RNA silencing.[16,17] Several studies have investigated patterns of epigenetic modifications in BPD.[18–28] Some of them have found DNA methylation abnormalities associated with BPD[18,24,27] and severity of childhood maltreatment.[19,21–25,28] One study suggests that methylation status can be modified through psychotherapy in BPD patients.[24]

In summary, despite the known heritability of BPD, no specific risk genes or molecular pathways have been identified to date.[5,6] It behooves the field to perform larger, better powered, genetic studies in BPD subjects. Advancing genetic research in BPD is a critical step toward the identification of new drug targets and the development of disease-modifying therapies against the core pathophysiological features of BPD, which are currently lacking. Moreover, other genetic research approaches, such as deep sequencing, induced pluripotent stem cells, and postmortem brain studies, which have not yet been used in BPD, may help uncover the neurobiological underpinnings of this disorder.

BIOLOGICAL MODELS
Alexithymia

The discovery of high levels of alexithymia in BPD emerged out of evidence that there is a disconnect between objectively measured emotional responses in BPD (which are heightened) and the subjective appreciation of those responses (which is blunted). This is called an impairment in emotional interoception. This view, grounded in neurobiology, may come closer to the description of this disorder as a disorder of the self.

The authors' interest in this idea came from an early study we did measuring emotional responsiveness in BPD subjects using affective startle. The simple hypothesis was that BPD subjects would be hyperresponsive to unpleasant emotional probes. Affective startle is a very well-studied approach for measuring affective arousal and valence.[29] Individuals often have a characteristic eye blink response to a loud sound burst. Providing a prepulse or a warning that such a sound is about to occur at a particular time can influence the intensity of the blink. Providing that prepulse with an affective valence can influence the intensity of the blink. For example, if the prepulse is the showing of a word such as *murder*, the blink is amplified compared with a prepulse of a neutral valence, such as the word *table*. Similarly, a word with a positive valence, such as *cuddle*, will decrease the amplitude of the blink in response to the sound blast. The prepulse need not be a word and is, in fact, often an emotional picture. This objective way of measuring emotional response has been shown to be reliable and is thought to reflect amygdala activity.[30]

Hazlett and colleagues[31] (including the current authors, Goodman and New) studied individuals with BPD compared with age-matched and sex-matched healthy controls using affective startle in response to negative and neutral words. As predicted, both the BPD and healthy control groups showed an increased startle response to negative compared with neutral words; however, the BPD group showed a heightened enhancement of startle response on average to negative words specifically compared with healthy controls. What was entirely unexpected was that when subjects were asked to report on how the words made them feel, the BPD subjects reported a more neutral response to the negative words than did the controls.

Since that initial study, Hazlett and colleagues[32] (including the current authors, Goodman and New) have gone on to find the same pattern of results in affective response comparing BPD subjects to healthy controls and to a clinical control group of schizotypal subjects using functional MRI blood oxygenation level-dependent (BOLD) response instead of affective startle. Subjects were shown pictures with positive, negative, and neutral valence. Again, BPD subjects showed a heightened objectively measured emotional response in the mean amygdala BOLD response to negative images and to positive images. Yet, BPD subjects showed a blunted (or more neutral) rating of their own responses to those emotional images and this was particularly pronounced in the negative valence. Other studies of responses to emotional probes in BPD have shown the same heightened emotional responses with blunted (or at least not heightened) subjective ratings.[32] These observations led New and colleagues[33] to measure a clinically observed psychological attribute called alexithymia or, examining the Greek etymology, difficulty reading emotions. Using the Toronto Alexithymia Scale, subjects with BPD had extremely high levels of alexithymia compared with healthy controls and, indeed, the effect size was very large. The difficulties for identifying and describing their own feelings were pronounced.

In Mannheim, Germany, Dr Christian Schmahl conducted a body of work on pain responses in BPD, which is related to the work on emotional responses. As in emotional responses, a similar disconnect between objectively measured and subjectively assessed is seen in relation to pain in BPD.[34] Schmahl and colleagues[35] did an elegant study that showed that BPD subjects have a heightened pain threshold, tolerating higher levels of pain than controls, while retaining an intact capacity for subtle sensory discrimination tasks using laser-evoked potentials (LEPs). This methodology permits assessment of very rapid response near the somatosensory cortex that precedes cortical response to stimuli. That study showed that, although pain thresholds were higher in subjects with BPD than in controls, the rapid LEP response, reflecting the immediate and preconscious neural signature of the sensory experience of pain, was normal or heightened in BPD. These data support a higher pain threshold (the experience of pain is diminished) although the evidence suggests that the neural signature of pain is intact. This is another instance of the discrepancy between objectively measured experience and subjective appraisal of that experience in BPD.

Further evidence of the impaired ability of patients to perceive or process their own emotional and even physical experiences emerged from a study of heartbeat-evoked potentials (HEPs), which are used as an indicator of the cortical processing of bodily signals from the cardiovascular system. Generally, there is a neural imprimatur of heart beats in the anterior insula. Subjects with BPD have been shown to have significantly reduced mean HEP amplitudes compared with healthy controls; subjects with BPD in remission have intermediate HEP.[36] Furthermore, HEP amplitudes were negatively correlated with emotional dysregulation.

This neurobiologically grounded model of impaired emotional interoception is particularly compelling for BPD because, as work progressed in laboratories studying this disorder, very effective evidence-based psychotherapies were being developed for BPD. These include, most famously, dialectical behavioral therapy, as well as mentalization-based therapy; transference-focused therapy; Systems Training for Emotional Predictability and Problem Solving; schema therapy; and, most recently, good psychiatric management for BPD.[37] What lies at the heart of these therapies is that they are focused, often time-limited, and emphasize practical approaches to present day problems.[38] What is central to teaching mentalization skills? Clinicians seem to have recognized that BPD patients are imperfect at knowing their own emotional experiences and so the treatments that have been most effective in this disorder are not those that focus on past experiences but rather those that teach patients to reflect on their own present emotions and how they come across to others. It is, therefore, a lovely synergy that is rare in psychiatric research that there is a convergence on the development of clinical treatments with understanding that has developed in the laboratory, each strengthening the importance of the other.

Emotion Dysregulation in Borderline Personality Disorder

Affective instability or disturbance is a feature found across multiple diagnoses,[39] including posttraumatic stress disorder, substance abuse, eating disorders, and BPD.[40] It is associated with considerable morbidity, including suicidality, aggression, and disrupted relationships.[41] Affective dysregulation is a primary feature of BPD, along with disturbed cognition, impulsivity, and intense unstable relationships.[42] The observed dysregulated affect includes hypersensitivity and hyperreactivity to emotional triggers[41]; rapid increases in depressed, anxious, and irritable affect; and impairments in emotion regulatory control.[43,44] The dysregulation of affect in BPD is quite different from the mood dysregulation seen in depression or bipolar disorder in which the mood disturbance is sustained for days, weeks, or months, and is relatively autonomous from environmental triggers. Here, the published evidence supporting abnormalities in emotion regulation in BPD is reviewed (behavioral, neuroimaging, and physiological studies).

From a behavioral standpoint, the emotional hyperreactivity in BPD may be more apparent for individually salient, or significant, emotional stimuli than a blanket hyperresponsiveness to all emotional stimuli.[45] BPD patients display greater mood variability in response to daily stress and may be particularly sensitive to affective triggers involving social rejection and abandonment, resulting in excessive emotional reactions.[46] Additionally, they experience greater negative affect and do not develop appropriate and adaptive emotion regulation strategies, engaging instead in maladaptive ways of coping. Some of these coping mechanisms include nonsuicidal self-injurious behaviors,[47] rumination,[48] thought suppression,[49] and impulsive suicidal behaviors.[50] They have low emotional awareness[51] and distress tolerance,[52] which likely contributes to the dysfunction exhibited in BPD (**Fig. 1**).

As previously noted, some physiologic measures, such as the affective startle modulation (ASM), have provided useful nonverbal metrics of affective valence, independently of arousal, which is useful in BPD. Hazlett and colleagues[31] (including the current authors, Goodman and New) showed that BPD subjects had exaggerated ASM during imagery of BPD-salient scripts describing rejection and abandonment but not during generally unpleasant scripts.[31] Recent data suggest that other factors, such as substance abuse or dissociative experiences, may modulate the ASM in BPD. A recent study that examined BPD subjects with and without a history of substance-use disorders (SUDs) showed lower startle modulation in the BPD-SUD group, suggesting that comorbid SUD may dampen the pattern of exaggerated ASM to unpleasant stimuli in BPD.[53] Other studies evaluating the effect of dissociative experiences in ASM in BPD found that greater dissociative symptoms reduced startle response magnitudes during imagery of idiographic aversive scripts in BPD subjects.[54] Dissociative experiences involve detachment from the overwhelming emotional aspects of trauma. According to the corticolimbic disconnection model,[55] dissociation is a mechanism that dampens affective reactivity to avoid emotional overstimulation. This model further suggests that during dissociation the medial prefrontal cortex inhibits processing of external emotional stimuli in the amygdala, thus attenuating emotional responses to these stimuli.[56] This concept is supported by a BPD study showing that subjects experiencing no dissociative symptoms showed larger startle response amplitude compared with subjects with high dissociative experiences.[57]

There is robust evidence from behavioral, neuroimaging, and physiologic studies that BPD patients are characterized by poor emotion regulation, hyperarousal state, and hyperreactivity to negative stimuli. Future lines of research should explore the biological basis of emotion dysregulation, as well as prevention; earlier treatment; and, especially, expansion of the therapeutic dimension.

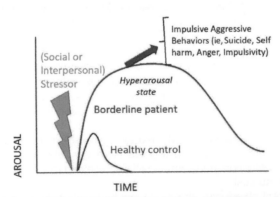

Fig. 1. Emotional dysregulation from a behavioral standpoint. When an individual with BPD encounters social or interpersonal stressors, they are unable to regulate their emotions and they enter a state of emotional hyperarousal, during which other state-potentiated vulnerabilities to impulsivity and aggression become overtly expressed, leading to impulsive, aggressive, and self-destructive behaviors.

BRAIN IMAGING

Functional neuroimaging has been the major tool used to study emotional processing in BPD. Affective instability in BPD has been associated with reduced top-down regulatory prefrontal cortex activity (orbitofrontal cortex, anterior cingulate cortex [ACC], and enhanced amygdala and insula activity while viewing emotional stimuli.[58–64] Additionally, some studies have suggested that patients with BPD have an impaired amygdala habituation, meaning that the amygdala is unable to decrease neural response when a negative stimulus is repeatedly presented.[32,44] Those studies found that amygdala activation increased in response to repeated negatively valenced pictures, whereas in healthy controls amygdala activation decreased. Failure to habituate correlates clinically with higher levels of trait anxiety,[65] aggression, and affective lability[32] (**Fig. 2**). BPD subjects, compared with controls, demonstrated enhanced coupling of the left amygdala with the dorsolateral prefrontal cortex and ventral striatum, suggesting a mechanism for abnormal top-down regulatory control.[66] Amygdala activity and habituation is a promising biomarker of treatment response, as shown by Goodman and colleagues[67] in a dialectical behavioral therapy trial.

Findings from structural MRI studies suggest that individuals with BPD, compared with healthy controls, have decreased volume in brain regions associated with emotion processing and regulation, which include the amygdala,[68–70] hippocampus,[68,69,71] orbitofrontal cortex,[72] and ACC.[61,72,73] A more recent meta-analysis showed that BPD subjects show "increased GM volume in bilateral supplementary motor area extending to right posterior cingulated cortex (PCC) and bilateral primary motor cortex, right middle frontal gyrus (MFG), and the bilateral precuneus extending to bilateral PCC. Decreased GM (Gray matter) was identified in bilateral middle temporal gyri, right inferior frontal gyrus extending to right insular, left hippocampus and left superior frontal gyrus extending to left medial orbitofrontal cortex," which encompasses frontolimbic circuits and the default mode network.[74]

Additional imaging methodologies used in BPD include diffusion tensor imaging (DTI), which permits visualization of white matter integrity. Although data on white

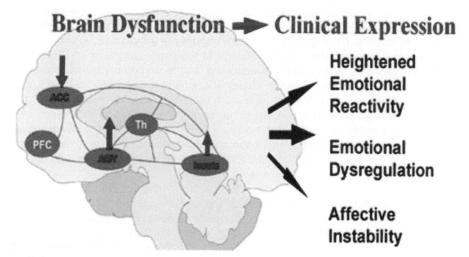

Fig. 2. This model posits that brain dysfunction is characterized by an underactive ACC and/or an over-reactive amygdala (AMY) and insula, and/or functional disconnectivity results in heightened emotional reactivity and difficulties regarding this affect, which is clinically expressed as affective instability. PFC, prefontal cortex; Th, thalamus.

matter integrity using DTI has been inconsistent, a study of adult BPD showed decreased axial diffusivity in the cingulum and inferior occipital and inferior longitudinal fasciculus.[75] Another study showed decreased fractional anisotropy (FA), a measure of white matter integrity, in the corpus callosum, corona radiata, and dorsal areas of the ACC in BPD.[76,77] Finally, another study showed decreased FA in the uncinated fasciculus in BPD subjects compared with controls,[78] as well as in the cingulum and fornix in BPD.[79] Studies in adolescent subjects with BPD show decreased FA in the Inferior Longitudinal Fasciculus using tractography,[80] as well as in the fornix and uncinate fasciculus.[81] Although no single region is definitively involved in BPD, abnormalities in central white matter structure and long tracts within the limbic system seem to be present in almost all DTI studies in BPD. This tends to support the fronto-limbic disconnectivity hypothesis by providing an anatomic substrate for abnormalities in the tracts connecting limbic areas to prefrontal cortex in BPD. These findings also underscore the possibility that abnormal maturation of white matter structures may play an important mechanistic role in BPD.

The newest imaging methodologies delineate topological organizations of brain networks. Such analyses use graph theory–based complex network analysis. Initial findings of this type of approach suggest abnormal topological properties and connectivity in BPD,[82] although this methodology is still considered exploratory.

NEUROPEPTIDE MODELS: OXYTOCIN AND OPIOIDS

Impulsivity and emotional dysregulation have been known as the core symptoms of BPD for decades. However, in 2010, Stanley and Siever[84] suggested that the main core factor of this disorder is interpersonal sensitivity,[4] which in turn triggers impulsivity and dysregulated affect.[41,83,84] It is proposed that this interpersonal dysfunction could be related to underlying neuropeptide dysregulation, including abnormalities in opioids, oxytocin, and vasopressin systems.[84] Here the evidence supporting the role of opioids and oxytocin in BPD is reviewed.

Opioids

Increasing evidence supports the dysregulation theory of BPD, which proposes low basal opioid levels and compensatory supersensitivity of μ-opioid receptors have an essential role in presentations of BPD. Some of the main symptoms of BPD, such as chronic dysphoria, lack of sense of wellbeing, and feeling empty inside, are manifestations of low basal opioid levels. Repetitive nonsuicidal self-injuries could be a result of an increase in opioid levels after such behaviors. Low levels of β-endorphin and met-enkephalin have been shown in the cerebrospinal fluid of individuals with cluster B personality disorder and history of self-injury.[85] On the other hand, naltrexone, an opioid antagonist, has been shown to reduce these nonsuicidal self-injury behaviors in BPD,[86] which may be a result of decreasing the rewarding effects of these behaviors by blocking opioid receptors.

Recent studies show that, similar to physical pain, intrapsychic pain, which is a main feature of BPD, is under the control of the opiate system and the same neural pathways are involved.[87] The endogenous opiate system, through μ-opioid receptors, has long been implicated in regulation of emotional and stress responses. Opioid dysfunction has been associated with attachment behavior deficits and anxiety-like responses in animal models.[88–90] In human beings, the opioid system is involved in normal and pathologic emotion regulation,[91,92] in addition to its more traditional role in modulating both the sensory and affective dimensions of pain.[93] While the notion that physical pain and emotional pain have common physiological mechanisms is well known,[94] more recently, evidence suggests that common neural substrates regulate pain of social rejection and physical pain.[87,95,96]

Empirical evidence supporting the endogenous opiate dysregulation theory of BPD is increasing. Beta-endorphin, which is the endogenous opioid peptide released during stress,[97] has a common precursor with adrenocorticotropin hormone (corticotropin),[98] the main hormone of stress response. Beta-endorphins are responsible for relieving pain in stressful situations to help the individual to survive.[98] Interestingly, individuals with BPD show increased pain threshold following acute painful stressors,[99,100] whereas they show lower tolerance for chronic pain[101] and more frequently report use of prescribed opioid analgesics.[102] One of the most compelling empirical reports supporting a definitive abnormality in opiate activity in patients with BPD comes from a recent PET imaging study that used the μ-opiate ligand, [^{11}C]carfentanil, to examine binding in the cerebral cortex of BPD subjects during induction of a neutral and sad sustained emotional state.[103] In the neutral state, BPD subjects showed more μ-opioid binding in regions of the prefrontal cortex, in the reward center (accumbens), and in the amygdala; and μ-opiate binding in prefrontal cortex correlated negatively with neuroticism in BPD. During sadness-induction, BPD subjects showed greater μ-opioid receptor-mediated neurotransmission compared with controls. The investigators interpreted the greater baseline μ-opiate receptor availability as perhaps reflecting deficits in endogenous circulating opiates. The mood induction seems to suggest that BPD subjects enhance endogenous opiate availability more than controls, which is convincing as a compensatory response.

Genetic studies suggest that the μ-opioid receptor gene is associated with attachment abnormalities and BPD. Polymorphism in the μ-opioid receptor gene (OPRM1 77G) in primates is associated with higher levels of attachment during early infancy and greater persistence of separation distress.[88] A more recent study demonstrated the role of μ-receptor genes in moderating the effects of social rejection on depression,[104] which may explain the severe reaction of BPD to interpersonal rejections. These data, although quite preliminary, raise the possibility that genetic variability in the opioid receptors may affect affective stability, attachment, and coherence of self-concepts.

Oxytocin

Interpersonal dysfunction is another feature of BPD[4,105] that has been proposed to serve as the main core component of this disorder.[84] One of the main regulators of social relationships is oxytocin, which plays an essential role in affiliation behaviors, such as parental caring and romantic partnering.[106,107]

Dysregulation of oxytocin has been shown in BPD and may explain the interpersonal hypersensitivity in this disorder.[108] Women with BPD had significantly lower plasma levels of oxytocin compared with a control group,[109] especially when they had a disorganized attachment style.[110] Oxytocin levels were negatively correlated with a childhood history of trauma.[109] Moreover, individuals with BPD show a reduction in oxytocin plasma levels after social exclusion.[111] Oxytocin abnormalities in BPD clinically manifest in misreading of social cues, difficulties in establishment of trust, and capacity for attachment in BPD.[84] Increasing evidence shows that individuals with BPD have a profound bias in facial emotion recognition toward identifying negative emotions in others, particularly anger.[112] Individuals with BPD also show an avoidant reaction to angry faces, which is correlated with their childhood history of trauma and diminishes after administration of intranasal oxytocin.[113] Brain imaging evaluations show increased and prolonged activation of the amygdala[114] and anterior insula[62] in response to negative emotional stimuli. Clinical studies show women with BPD exhibit more and faster initial fixation changes to the eyes of angry faces combined with increased amygdala activation in response to angry faces, which are normalized after intranasal oxytocin administration.[109]

Recently, it is shown that individuals with BPD also demonstrate a bias toward perceiving other people's faces as more untrustworthy compared with healthy volunteers.[115] Interestingly, intranasal administration of oxytocin has been shown to significantly enhance trustworthiness and attractiveness of male and female targets in healthy people.[116] However, oxytocin has a trust-lowering effect in individuals with BPD,[117,118] which is correlated with a history of childhood trauma.[118] In a study of nonverbal communications, oxytocin increased affiliative behaviors in healthy subjects but not individuals with BPD.[119] These findings suggest that oxytocin effects should be evaluated in the context of childhood experiences and attachment patterns and may have contradictory effects in BPD. It is suggested that oxytocin may promote prosociality when social cues are interpreted as safe; however, in unsafe interpretation of the environment, oxytocin may promote more defensive emotions and behaviors.[120]

Oxytocin also is known to diminish the stress response. In clinical studies, administration of intranasal oxytocin increases positive communication and decreases cortisol levels after couple conflicts[121] and other types of social stressors in individuals with impaired emotion regulation abilities.[122] In BPD, oxytocin significantly reduces the stress-related dysphoria, as well as cortisol levels.[123] Neuroimaging studies consistently found that amygdala responses to emotional stimuli are reduced by oxytocin administration, which could be a result of reduced uncertainty about the predictive values of emotional stimuli.[124]

In 2015, Herpertz and Bertsch[108] suggested that, in addition to abnormal bottom-up generation of emotions, individuals with BPD suffer from an abnormal top-down emotional regulation. Functional neuroimaging studies have revealed prefrontal hypometabolism during regulatory control processes,[125] and reduced activity in the subgenual ACC and dorsolateral prefrontal cortex in BPD.[62] Interestingly, oxytocin significantly attenuates the increased neuronal activity in the medial prefrontal cortex and the ACC in social anxiety disorder,[126] which has an important role in emotion regulation.

Genetic studies investigated the role of the oxytocin receptor gene in the formation of BPD symptoms, which seems to have interactions with gender and childhood trauma. A study of more than 1000 low-income children demonstrate that girls with at least 1 A-allele of the SNP rs53576 and history of childhood maltreatment had more BPD presentations, whereas maltreated boys were more vulnerable to developing BPD symptoms when homozygous for the G/G allele.[127] A study of more than 1000 low-income children demonstrate that girls with at least 1 A-allele of the oxytocin receptor gene (OXTR) single nucleotide polymorphism (SNP) rs53576 and history of childhood maltreatment had higher rates of BPD, whereas maltreated boys were more vulnerable to developing BPD symptoms when homozygous for the G/G allele.[128] It seems that SNP rs53576 in the oxytocin receptor gene (OXTR) moderates the relationship between childhood experiences and BPD presentations.

SUMMARY

Although this review presents data from disparate approaches to studying the neurobiology of BPD, it begins to suggest a theoretic framework that can form a coherent theory of BPD. Evidence clearly suggests that BPD is substantially heritable and is at least as heritable as other major psychiatric disorders. Brain imaging studies have suggested a dysregulation in top-down control of emotions in BPD; however, this model is also seen in other disorders, such as panic disorder. Thus the imaging may be of an upset brain. On the other hand, the structural and white matter abnormalities that are especially robust in adolescents suggest a developmental abnormality in neural circuitry underlying emotion regulation in BPD. The finding of impaired interoception is especially remarkable in BPD because it does seem to dovetail well with the focus on mentalization that underlies the evidence-based psychotherapies for this disorder and helps to explain the interpersonal difficulties in BPD. For example, if an individual with BPD is angry and manifests that in terms of their physiologic arousal but is unaware of that anger, then, when another person responds to the apparent anger, the individual is confused and hurt. This neurobiological model provides an explanation for the phenomenon that psychodynamic theory has described as projective identification. According to this model, in an interpersonal interaction, individuals with BPD may appear angry while being unaware of their feelings. The physiologic manifestations of anger then create anger in the person with whom they are interacting and the alexithymic BPD patients are not aware of their role in kindling anger in their interlocutor. This helps to explain why validation is so helpful; it is making explicit the perceived affect in the interaction about which the person with BPD may be unaware. The abnormalities in neuropeptides are somewhat contradictory in that some studies show improvement with oxytocin and others do not. Little is known about the opiate system in BPD but preliminary data suggest endogenous opiate deficits. This line of work is especially important and it holds the promise of a pharmacologic treatment of BPD, a tool that is unfortunately currently unavailable. Clearly further research into the neurobiology of BPD holds proximal promise of novel therapeutics and currently can help with psychoeducation of patients, family, and clinicians to enable more empathic contact with individuals with BPD.

REFERENCES

1. Stern A. Psychoanalytic investigation of and therapy in the borderline group of neuroses. Psychoanal Q 1938;7:467–89.
2. Sanislow CA, Grilo CM, McGlashan TH. Factor analysis of the DSM-III-R borderline personality disorder criteria in psychiatric inpatients. Am J Psychiatry 2000; 157(10):1629–33.
3. Sharp C, Wright AG, Fowler JC, et al. The structure of personality pathology: both general ('g') and specific ('s') factors? J Abnorm Psychol 2015;124(2): 387–98.
4. Gunderson JG. Disturbed relationships as a phenotype for borderline personality disorder. Am J Psychiatry 2007;164(11):1637–40.
5. Amad A, Ramoz N, Thomas P, et al. Genetics of borderline personality disorder: systematic review and proposal of an integrative model. Neurosci Biobehav Rev 2014;40:6–19.
6. Calati R, Gressier F, Balestri M, et al. Genetic modulation of borderline personality disorder: systematic review and meta-analysis. J Psychiatr Res 2013; 47(10):1275–87.
7. Siever LJ, Torgersen S, Gunderson JG, et al. The borderline diagnosis III: identifying endophenotypes for genetic studies. Biol Psychiatry 2002;51(12):964–8.
8. Carpenter RW, Tomko RL, Trull TJ, et al. Gene-environment studies and borderline personality disorder: a review. Curr Psychiatry Rep 2013;15(1):336.
9. Lieb K, Vollm B, Rucker G, et al. Pharmacotherapy for borderline personality disorder: Cochrane systematic review of randomised trials. Br J Psychiatry 2010; 196(1):4–12.

10. Stoffers J, Vollm BA, Rucker G, et al. Pharmacological interventions for border-line personality disorder. Cochrane Database Syst Rev 2010;(6):CD005653.
11. Bergen SE, Petryshen TL. Genome-wide association studies of schizophrenia: does bigger lead to better results? Curr Opin Psychiatry 2012;25(2):76–82.
12. Schizophrenia Working Group of the Psychiatric Genomics Consortium. Biological insights from 108 schizophrenia-associated genetic loci. Nature 2014; 511(7510):421–7.
13. Witt SH, Streit F, Jungkunz M, et al. Genome-wide association study of border-line personality disorder reveals genetic overlap with bipolar disorder, major depression and schizophrenia. Transl Psychiatry 2017;7(6):e1155.
14. Lubke GH, Laurin C, Amin N, et al. Genome-wide analyses of borderline person-ality features. Mol Psychiatry 2014;19(8):923–9.
15. Distel MA, Hottenga JJ, Trull TJ, et al. Chromosome 9: linkage for borderline per-sonality disorder features. Psychiatr Genet 2008;18(6):302–7.
16. Akbarian S. Epigenetic mechanisms in schizophrenia. Dialogues Clin Neurosci 2014;16(3):405–17.
17. Labonte B, Turecki G. The epigenetics of suicide: explaining the biological ef-fects of early life environmental adversity. Arch Suicide Res 2010;14(4):291–310.
18. Dammann G, Teschler S, Haag T, et al. Increased DNA methylation of neuropsy-chiatric genes occurs in borderline personality disorder. Epigenetics 2011; 6(12):1454–62.
19. Elbert T, Prados J, Stenz L, et al. Borderline personality disorder and childhood maltreatment: a genome-wide methylation analysis. Transl Psychiatry 2015; 14(2):177–88.
20. Prados J, Stenz L, Courtet P, et al. Borderline personality disorder and childhood maltreatment: a genome-wide methylation analysis. Genes Brain Behav 2015. https://doi.org/10.1111/gbb.12197.
21. Groleau P, Joober R, Israel M, et al. Methylation of the dopamine D2 receptor (DRD2) gene promoter in women with a bulimia-spectrum disorder: associations with borderline personality disorder and exposure to childhood abuse. J Psychiatr Res 2014;48(1):121–7.
22. Martin-Blanco A, Ferrer M, Soler J, et al. Association between methylation of the glucocorticoid receptor gene, childhood maltreatment, and clinical severity in borderline personality disorder. J Psychiatr Res 2014;57:34–40.
23. Perroud N, Paoloni-Giacobino A, Prada P, et al. Increased methylation of glucocorticoid receptor gene (NR3C1) in adults with a history of childhood maltreatment: a link with the severity and type of trauma. Transl Psychiatry 2011;1:e59.
24. Perroud N, Salzmann A, Prada P, et al. Response to psychotherapy in borderline personality disorder and methylation status of the BDNF gene. Transl Psychiatry 2013;3:e207.
25. Perroud N, Zewdie S, Stenz L, et al. Methylation of serotonin receptor 3a in ADHD, borderline personality, and bipolar disorders: link with severity of the dis-orders and childhood maltreatment. Depress Anxiety 2016;33(1):45–55.
26. Radtke KM, Schauer M, Gunter HM, et al. Epigenetic modifications of the gluco-corticoid receptor gene are associated with the vulnerability to psychopathology in childhood maltreatment. Transl Psychiatry 2015;5:e571.
27. Teschler S, Bartkuhn M, Kunzel N, et al. Aberrant methylation of gene associ-ated CpG sites occurs in borderline personality disorder. PLoS One 2013; 8(12):e84180.

28. Thaler L, Gauvin L, Joober R, et al. Methylation of BDNF in women with bulimic eating syndromes: associations with childhood abuse and borderline personality disorder. Prog Neuropsychopharmacol Biol Psychiatry 2014;54:43–9.

29. Cuthbert BN, Schupp HT, Bradley M, et al. Probing affective pictures: attended startle and tone probes. Psychophysiology 1998;35(3):344–7.

30. Pissiota A, Frans O, Michelgard A, et al. Amygdala and anterior cingulate cortex activation during affective startle modulation: a PET study of fear. Eur J Neurosci 2003;18(5):1325–31.

31. Hazlett EA, Speiser LJ, Goodman M, et al. Exaggerated affect-modulated startle during unpleasant stimuli in borderline personality disorder. Biol Psychiatry 2007;62(3):250–5.

32. Hazlett EA, Zhang J, New AS, et al. Potentiated amygdala response to repeated emotional pictures in borderline personality disorder. Biol Psychiatry 2012;72(6):448–56.

33. New AS, aan het Rot M, Ripoll LH, et al. Empathy and alexithymia in borderline personality disorder: clinical and laboratory measures. J Pers Disord 2012;26(5):660–75.

34. Niedtfeld I, Schulze L, Kirsch P, et al. Affect regulation and pain in borderline personality disorder: a possible link to the understanding of self-injury. Biol Psychiatry 2010;68(4):383–91.

35. Schmahl C, Greffrath W, Baumgartner U, et al. Differential nociceptive deficits in patients with borderline personality disorder and self-injurious behavior: laser-evoked potentials, spatial discrimination of noxious stimuli, and pain ratings. Pain 2004;110(1–2):470–9.

36. Muller LE, Schulz A, Andermann M, et al. Cortical representation of afferent bodily signals in borderline personality disorder: neural correlates and relationship to emotional dysregulation. JAMA Psychiatry 2015;72(11):1077–86.

37. Choi-Kain LW, Finch EF, Masland SR, et al. What works in the treatment of borderline personality disorder. Curr Behav Neurosci Rep 2017;4(1):21–30.

38. Choi-Kain LW, Albert EB, Gunderson JG. Evidence-based treatments for borderline personality disorder: implementation, integration, and stepped care. Harv Rev Psychiatry 2016;24(5):342–56.

39. Bradley B, DeFife JA, Guarnaccia C, et al. Emotion dysregulation and negative affect: association with psychiatric symptoms. J Clin Psychiatry 2011;72(5):685–91.

40. Aldao A, Nolen-Hoeksema S, Schweizer S. Emotion-regulation strategies across psychopathology: a meta-analytic review. Clin Psychol Rev 2010;30(2):217–37.

41. Koenigsberg HW, Harvey PD, Mitropoulou V, et al. Are the interpersonal and identity disturbances in the borderline personality disorder criteria linked to the traits of affective instability and impulsivity? J Pers Disord 2001;15(4):358–70.

42. Lieb K, Zanarini MC, Schmahl C, et al. Borderline personality disorder. Lancet 2004;364(9432):453–61.

43. Koenigsberg HW. Affective instability: toward an integration of neuroscience and psychological perspectives. J Pers Disord 2010;24(1):60–82.

44. Koenigsberg HW, Denny BT, Fan J, et al. The neural correlates of anomalous habituation to negative emotional pictures in borderline and avoidant personality disorder patients. Am J Psychiatry 2014;171(1):82–90.

45. Yen S, Zlotnick C, Costello E. Affect regulation in women with borderline personality disorder traits. J Nerv Ment Dis 2002;190(10):693–6.

46. Deckers JW, Lobbestael J, van Wingen GA, et al. The influence of stress on social cognition in patients with borderline personality disorder. Psychoneuroendocrinology 2015;52:119–29.

47. Zanarini MC, Frankenburg FR, Reich DB, et al. The 10-year course of physically self-destructive acts reported by borderline patients and axis II comparison subjects. Acta Psychiatr Scand 2008;117(3):177–84.

48. Baer RA, Sauer SE. Relationships between depressive rumination, anger rumination, and borderline personality features. Personal Disord 2011;2(2):142–50.

49. Rosenthal MZ, Cheavens JS, Lejuez CW, et al. Thought suppression mediates the relationship between negative affect and borderline personality disorder symptoms. Behav Res Ther 2005;43(9):1173–85.

50. Links PS, Eynan R, Heisel MJ, et al. Affective instability and suicidal ideation and behavior in patients with borderline personality disorder. J Pers Disord 2007; 21(1):72–86.

51. Leible TL, Snell WE. Borderline personality disorder and multiple aspects of emotional intelligence. Pers Indiv Differ 2004;37(2):393–404.

52. Gratz KL, Rosenthal MZ, Tull MT, et al. An experimental investigation of emotion dysregulation in borderline personality disorder. J Abnorm Psychol 2006;115(4): 850–5.

53. Baschnagel JS, Coffey SF, Hawk LW Jr, et al. Psychophysiological assessment of emotional processing in patients with borderline personality disorder with and without comorbid substance use. Personal Disord 2013;4(3):203–13.

54. Barnow S, Limberg A, Stopsack M, et al. Dissociation and emotion regulation in borderline personality disorder. Psychol Med 2012;42(4):783–94.

55. Sierra M, Berrios GE. Depersonalization: neurobiological perspectives. Biol Psychiatry 1998;44(9):898–908.

56. Sierra M, Senior C, Dalton J, et al. Autonomic response in depersonalization disorder. Arch Gen Psychiatry 2002;59(9):833–8.

57. Ebner-Priemer UW, Badeck S, Beckmann C, et al. Affective dysregulation and dissociative experience in female patients with borderline personality disorder: a startle response study. J Psychiatr Res 2005;39(1):85–92.

58. Brendel GR, Stern E, Silbersweig DA. Defining the neurocircuitry of borderline personality disorder: functional neuroimaging approaches. Dev Psychopathol 2005;17(4):1197–206.

59. Dell'Osso B, Berlin HA, Serati M, et al. Neuropsychobiological aspects, comorbidity patterns and dimensional models in borderline personality disorder. Neuropsychobiology 2010;61(4):169–79.

60. Minzenberg MJ, Fan J, New AS, et al. Fronto-limbic dysfunction in response to facial emotion in borderline personality disorder: an event-related fMRI study. Psychiatry Res 2007;155(3):231–43.

61. Minzenberg MJ, Fan J, New AS, et al. Frontolimbic structural changes in borderline personality disorder. J Psychiatr Res 2008;42(9):727–33.

62. Ruocco AC, Amirthavasagam S, Choi-Kain LW, et al. Neural correlates of negative emotionality in borderline personality disorder: an activation-likelihood-estimation meta-analysis. Biol Psychiatry 2013;73(2):153–60.

63. Schmahl C, Bremner JD. Neuroimaging in borderline personality disorder. J Psychiatr Res 2006;40(5):419–27.

64. Wingenfeld K, Rullkoetter N, Mensebach C, et al. Neural correlates of the individual emotional Stroop in borderline personality disorder. Psychoneuroendocrinology 2009;34(4):571–86.

65. Hare TA, Tottenham N, Galvan A, et al. Biological substrates of emotional reactivity and regulation in adolescence during an emotional go-nogo task. Biol Psychiatry 2008;63(10):927–34.

66. New AS, Hazlett EA, Buchsbaum MS, et al. Amygdala-prefrontal disconnection in borderline personality disorder. Neuropsychopharmacology 2007;32(7): 1629–40.

67. Goodman M, Carpenter D, Tang CY, et al. Dialectical behavior therapy alters emotion regulation and amygdala activity in patients with borderline personality disorder. J Psychiatr Res 2014;57:108–16.

68. Nunes PM, Wenzel A, Borges KT, et al. Volumes of the hippocampus and amygdala in patients with borderline personality disorder: a meta-analysis. J Pers Disord 2009;23(4):333–45.

69. Ruocco AC, Amirthavasagam S, Zakzanis KK. Amygdala and hippocampal volume reductions as candidate endophenotypes for borderline personality disorder: a meta-analysis of magnetic resonance imaging studies. Psychiatry Res 2012;201(3):245–52.

70. Tebartz van Elst L, Ludaescher P, Thiel T, et al. Evidence of disturbed amygdalar energy metabolism in patients with borderline personality disorder. Neurosci Lett 2007;417(1):36–41.

71. Brambilla P, Soloff PH, Sala M, et al. Anatomical MRI study of borderline personality disorder patients. Psychiatry Res 2004;131(2):125–33.

72. Tebartz van Elst L, Hesslinger B, Thiel T, et al. Frontolimbic brain abnormalities in patients with borderline personality disorder: a volumetric magnetic resonance imaging study. Biol Psychiatry 2003;54(2):163–71.

73. Hazlett EA, New AS, Newmark R, et al. Reduced anterior and posterior cingulate gray matter in borderline personality disorder. Biol Psychiatry 2005;58(8): 614–23.

74. Yang X, Hu L, Zeng J, et al. Default mode network and frontolimbic gray matter abnormalities in patients with borderline personality disorder: a voxel-based meta-analysis. Sci Rep 2016;6:34247.

75. Ninomiya T, Oshita H, Kawano Y, et al. Reduced white matter integrity in borderline personality disorder: a diffusion tensor imaging study. J Affect Disord 2018; 225:723–32.

76. Gan J, Yi J, Zhong M, et al. Abnormal white matter structural connectivity in treatment-naive young adults with borderline personality disorder. Acta Psychiatr Scand 2016;134(6):494–503.

77. Rusch N, Bracht T, Kreher BW, et al. Reduced interhemispheric structural connectivity between anterior cingulate cortices in borderline personality disorder. Psychiatry Res 2010;181(2):151–4.

78. Lischke A, Domin M, Freyberger HJ, et al. Structural alterations in white-matter tracts connecting (para-)limbic and prefrontal brain regions in borderline personality disorder. Psychol Med 2015;45(15):3171–80.

79. Whalley HC, Nickson T, Pope M, et al. White matter integrity and its association with affective and interpersonal symptoms in borderline personality disorder. Neuroimage Clin 2015;7:476–81.

80. New AS, Carpenter DM, Perez-Rodriguez MM, et al. Developmental differences in diffusion tensor imaging parameters in borderline personality disorder. J Psychiatr Res 2013;47(8):1101–9.

81. Kimmel CL, Alhassoon OM, Wollman SC, et al. Age-related parieto-occipital and other gray matter changes in borderline personality disorder: a meta-analysis of cortical and subcortical structures. Psychiatry Res 2016;251:15–25.

82. Xu T, Cullen KR, Mueller B, et al. Network analysis of functional brain connectivity in borderline personality disorder using resting-state fMRI. Neuroimage Clin 2016;18(11):302–15.

83. Brodsky BS, Groves SA, Oquendo MA, et al. Interpersonal precipitants and suicide attempts in borderline personality disorder. Suicide Life Threat Behav 2006; 36(3):313–22.

84. Stanley B, Siever LJ. The interpersonal dimension of borderline personality disorder: toward a neuropeptide model. Am J Psychiatry 2010;167(1):24–39.

85. Stanley B, Sher L, Wilson S, et al. Non-suicidal self-injurious behavior, endogenous opioids and monoamine neurotransmitters. J Affect Disord 2010;124(1–2): 134–40.

86. Sonne S, Rubey R, Brady K, et al. Naltrexone treatment of self-injurious thoughts and behaviors. J Nerv Ment Dis 1996;184(3):192–5.

87. Eisenberger NI, Lieberman MD, Williams KD. Does rejection hurt? An FMRI study of social exclusion. Science 2003;302(5643):290–2.

88. Barr CS, Schwandt ML, Lindell SG, et al. Variation at the mu-opioid receptor gene (OPRM1) influences attachment behavior in infant primates. Proc Natl Acad Sci U S A 2008;105(13):5277–81.

89. Moles A, Kieffer BL, D'Amato FR. Deficit in attachment behavior in mice lacking the mu-opioid receptor gene. Science 2004;304(5679):1983–6.

90. Panksepp J, Herman BH, Vilberg T, et al. Endogenous opioids and social behavior. Neurosci Biobehav Rev 1980;4(4):473–87.

91. Kennedy SE, Koeppe RA, Young EA, et al. Dysregulation of endogenous opioid emotion regulation circuitry in major depression in women. Arch Gen Psychiatry 2006;63(11):1199–208.

92. Zubieta JK, Ketter TA, Bueller JA, et al. Regulation of human affective responses by anterior cingulate and limbic mu-opioid neurotransmission. Arch Gen Psychiatry 2003;60(11):1145–53.

93. Zubieta JK, Smith YR, Bueller JA, et al. Regional mu opioid receptor regulation of sensory and affective dimensions of pain. Science 2001;293(5528):311–5.

94. Macdonald G, Leary MR. Why does social exclusion hurt? The relationship between social and physical pain. Psychol Bull 2005;131(2):202–23.

95. Eisenberger NI, Jarcho JM, Lieberman MD, et al. An experimental study of shared sensitivity to physical pain and social rejection. Pain 2006;126(1–3):132–8.

96. Panksepp J. Neuroscience. Feeling the pain of social loss. Science 2003; 302(5643):237–9.

97. Roth-Deri I, Green-Sadan T, Yadid G. Beta-endorphin and drug-induced reward and reinforcement. Prog Neurobiol 2008;86(1):1–21.

98. Bandelow B, Schmahl C, Falkai P, et al. Borderline personality disorder: a dysregulation of the endogenous opioid system? Psychol Rev 2010;117(2):623–36.

99. Bekrater-Bodmann R, Chung BY, Richter I, et al. Deficits in pain perception in borderline personality disorder: results from the thermal grill illusion. Pain 2015;156(10):2084–92.

100. Schmahl C, Meinzer M, Zeuch A, et al. Pain sensitivity is reduced in borderline personality disorder, but not in posttraumatic stress disorder and bulimia nervosa. World J Biol Psychiatry 2010;11(2 Pt 2):364–71.

101. Biskin RS, Frankenburg FR, Fitzmaurice GM, et al. Pain in patients with borderline personality disorder. Personal Ment Health 2014;8(3):218–27.

102. Frankenburg FR, Fitzmaurice GM, Zanarini MC. The use of prescription opioid medication by patients with borderline personality disorder and axis II comparison subjects: a 10-year follow-up study. J Clin Psychiatry 2014;75(4):357–61.

103. Prossin AR, Love TM, Koeppe RA, et al. Dysregulation of regional endogenous opioid function in borderline personality disorder. Am J Psychiatry 2010;167(8): 925–33.
104. Slavich GM, Tartter MA, Brennan PA, et al. Endogenous opioid system influences depressive reactions to socially painful targeted rejection life events. Psychoneuroendocrinology 2014;49:141–9.
105. New AS, Triebwasser J, Charney DS. The case for shifting borderline personality disorder to axis I. Biol Psychiatry 2008;64(8):653–9.
106. Francis DD, Champagne FC, Meaney MJ. Variations in maternal behaviour are associated with differences in oxytocin receptor levels in the rat. J Neuroendocrinol 2000;12(12):1145–8.
107. Grewen KM, Girdler SS, Amico J, et al. Effects of partner support on resting oxytocin, cortisol, norepinephrine, and blood pressure before and after warm partner contact. Psychosom Med 2005;67(4):531–8.
108. Herpertz SC, Bertsch K. A new perspective on the pathophysiology of borderline personality disorder: a model of the role of oxytocin. Am J Psychiatry 2015;172(9):840–51.
109. Bertsch K, Schmidinger I, Neumann ID, et al. Reduced plasma oxytocin levels in female patients with borderline personality disorder. Horm Behav 2013;63(3): 424–9.
110. Jobst A, Padberg F, Mauer MC, et al. Lower oxytocin plasma levels in borderline patients with unresolved attachment representations. Front Hum Neurosci 2016; 10:125.
111. Jobst A, Sabass L, Palagyi A, et al. Effects of social exclusion on emotions and oxytocin and cortisol levels in patients with chronic depression. J Psychiatr Res 2015;60:170–7.
112. Domes G, Czieschnek D, Weidler F, et al. Recognition of facial affect in borderline personality disorder. J Personal Disord 2008;22(2):135–47.
113. Brune M, Ebert A, Kolb M, et al. Oxytocin influences avoidant reactions to social threat in adults with borderline personality disorder. Hum Psychopharmacol 2013;28(6):552–61.
114. Herpertz S, Dietrich T, Wenning B, et al. Evidence of abnormal amygdala functioning in borderline personality disorder: a functional MRI study. Biol Psychiatry 2001;50(4):292–8.
115. Fertuck EA, Grinband J, Stanley B. Facial trust appraisal negatively biased in borderline personality disorder. Psychiatry Res 2013;207(3):195–202.
116. Theodoridou A, Rowe AC, Penton-Voak IS, et al. Oxytocin and social perception: oxytocin increases perceived facial trustworthiness and attractiveness. Horm Behav 2009;56(1):128–32.
117. Bartz J, Simeon D, Hamilton H, et al. Oxytocin can hinder trust and cooperation in borderline personality disorder. Soc Cogn Affect Neurosci 2011;6(5):556–63.
118. Ebert A, Kolb M, Heller J, et al. Modulation of interpersonal trust in borderline personality disorder by intranasal oxytocin and childhood trauma. Soc Neurosci 2013;8(4):305–13.
119. Brune M, Kolb M, Ebert A, et al. Nonverbal communication of patients with borderline personality disorder during clinical interviews: a double-blind placebo-controlled study using intranasal oxytocin. J Nerv Ment Dis 2015;203(2):107–11.
120. Olff M, Frijling JL, Kubzansky LD, et al. The role of oxytocin in social bonding, stress regulation and mental health: an update on the moderating effects of context and interindividual differences. Psychoneuroendocrinology 2013; 38(9):1883–94.

121. Ditzen B, Schaer M, Gabriel B, et al. Intranasal oxytocin increases positive communication and reduces cortisol levels during couple conflict. Biol Psychiatry 2009;65(9):728–31.
122. Quirin M, Kuhl J, Dusing R. Oxytocin buffers cortisol responses to stress in individuals with impaired emotion regulation abilities. Psychoneuroendocrinology 2011;36(6):898–904.
123. Simeon D, Bartz J, Hamilton H, et al. Oxytocin administration attenuates stress reactivity in borderline personality disorder: a pilot study. Psychoneuroendocrinology 2011;36(9):1418–21.
124. Domes G, Heinrichs M, Glascher J, et al. Oxytocin attenuates amygdala responses to emotional faces regardless of valence. Biol Psychiatry 2007; 62(10):1187–90.
125. O'Neill A, Frodl T. Brain structure and function in borderline personality disorder. Brain Struct Funct 2012;217(4):767–82.
126. Labuschagne I, Phan KL, Wood A, et al. Medial frontal hyperactivity to sad faces in generalized social anxiety disorder and modulation by oxytocin. Int J Neuropsychopharmacol 2012;15(7):883–96.
127. Cicchetti D, Rogosch FA, Hecht KF, et al. Moderation of maltreatment effects on childhood borderline personality symptoms by gender and oxytocin receptor and FK506 binding protein 5 genes. Dev Psychopathol 2014;26(3):831–49.
128. Hammen C, Bower JE, Cole SW. Oxytocin receptor gene variation and differential susceptibility to family environment in predicting youth borderline symptoms. J Pers Disord 2015;29(2):177–92.

Attachment and Borderline Personality Disorder

Anna Buchheim, PhD[a],*, Diana Diamond, PhD[b]

KEYWORDS

- Attachment representation • Unresolved trauma • Reflective functioning • Oxytocin
- Transference focused psychotherapy

KEY POINTS

- Borderline personality disorder has been associated with increased occurrence of insecure and especially unresolved attachment representations.
- Unresolved attachment has been linked to impaired cognitive functioning, trauma-related psychopathology, an impaired oxytocin system, and higher neural activations in the limbic system.
- Two randomized clinical trials on transference-focused psychotherapy have assessed attachment representations of patients with borderline personality disorder and how they change over the course of transference-focused psychotherapy.
- Results demonstrated that transference-focused psychotherapy was superior in showing significant improvements in attachment representations and reflective functioning compared with other treatments.
- A significant shift from unresolved to organized attachment suggests that transference-focused psychotherapy can be considered an effective treatment for traumatized patients.

INTRODUCTION TO THE ETIOLOGIC MODELS OF BORDERLINE PERSONALITY DISORDER FROM AN ATTACHMENT PERSPECTIVE

Borderline personality disorder (BPD) is characterized by affect dysregulation, behavioral dyscontrol, and interpersonal hypersensitivity with etiologic roots in insecure infant–parent attachment and adverse childhood experiences.[1] From a psychodynamic perspective based on the object relations model,[2,3] individuals with borderline personality organization are characterized by contradictory, maladaptive,

The authors do not have any relationship with a commercial company that has a direct financial interest in the subject matter or materials discussed in article or with a company making a competing product.
[a] Institute of Psychology, University of Innsbruck, Innrain 52, Innsbruck 6020, Austria; [b] City University of New York, Personality Disorders Institute, Weill Medical Center of Cornell University, New York University, New York, NY, USA
* Corresponding author.
E-mail address: anna.buchheim@uibk.ac.at

Abbreviations	
AAI	Adult Attachment Interview
AAP	Adult Attachment Projective Picture System
BPD	Borderline personality disorder
DBT	Dialectical behavior therapy
ECP	Experienced community psychotherapists
OT	Oxytocin
RCT	Randomized clinical trial
RF	Reflective functioning
TFP	Transference-focused psychotherapy

internalized representations of self and significant others that are highly polarized and affectively charged. These distorted perceptions of self and others are thought to contribute to disturbed interpersonal relationships and identity diffusion experienced by patients with BPD. The emerging consensus that the essential features of personality disorder involve difficulties with self-identity and interpersonal functioning[4,5] has long been a central tenet of object relations theory[2] and is now reflected in *Diagnostic and Statistical Manual of Mental Disorders*-5, section III.[6] Personality researchers and clinicians across diverse treatment orientations link self and interpersonal functioning to mental representations, for example, to schemata or internal working models of attachment.[7]

Attachment theory provides a powerful framework for understanding the links between close relationships, mental representations of attachment, and psychopathology and its neural correlates, and has widened and sharpened the lens through which we view personality development in general and personality disorders specifically.[8–13] The concept of adult attachment status covers a specific aspect of personality and measures an individual's current representational state with respect to early attachment relationships and their associated modes of defenses and affect regulation. In this article, we review the major contributions of attachment theory and research to understanding personality disorders, first introducing the research instruments that have been developed to assess mental representations of attachment in adults. Second, we present a model of BPD that integrates both attachment and neural correlates, with a focus on the significance of the lack of resolution of loss and trauma in individuals with BPD. Finally, we discuss the findings from several randomized clinical trials (RCTs) that have been used to assess attachment representations in patients with BPD, providing data on individual patients that demonstrates the nature and quality of the maladaptive attachment representations in this group.

The Assessment of Adult Attachment

In adults, there are 2 major approaches to assess attachment styles and attachment representations: self-reports measure an individual's subjective and conscious evaluations of attachment and assign individuals to attachment style categories or scores on 2 dimensions of insecurity, namely, anxiety and avoidance.[14] Narrative methods, including the Adult Attachment Interview (AAI; George C, Kaplan N, Main M. The adult attachment interview. University of California at Berkeley: Unpublished manuscript; 1985; and Main M, Goldwyn R. Adult attachment scoring and classification system, Version 6.0. University of California at Berkeley: Unpublished manuscript; 1998) and the Adult Attachment Projective Picture System (AAP)[15–17] enable an analysis of the mental organization of inner working models of attachment, including defensive processes. Both measures are designed to "surprise the unconscious" by introducing attachment-related stress using a semistructured interview format focusing on attachment relevant questions with concrete probes designed to elicit episodic memories (the AAI) or stories to attachment-related pictures (the AAP).

The AAI is a semistructured interview designed to elicit thoughts, feelings, and memories about early attachment experiences and to assess the individual's state of mind with respect to early attachment. Main and Goldwyn (Main M, Goldwyn R. Adult attachment scoring and classification system, Version 6.0. University of California at Berkeley: Unpublished manuscript; 1998) identified 3 major organized patterns of adult attachment:

- *Secure/autonomous*, characterized by open, seemingly honest, coherent discourse that gives the impression that individuals value the significance of attachment relationships;
- *Dismissing*, characterized by a constricted and distant discourse style in which all relationships are either idealized or devalued; and
- *Preoccupied*, characterized by a confused, angry, or passive discourse style that suggests that individuals are entangled in these relationships.

The 2 disorganized patterns include the *unresolved attachment status and cannot classify category*.

- The *unresolved category* is characterized by a global breakdown in discourse strategy around themes of loss or trauma
- The *cannot classify category* is characterized by a lack of any consistent discourse style, or by 2 distinct but diverse patterns.[18]

The AAP[16,17] provides attachment classifications based on the analysis of "story" responses to a set of theoretically derived attachment-related drawings of scenes depicting solitude, illness, separation, death, and potential maltreatment. Story coding reflects the evaluation of story content, defensive processes, and the inclusion of personal experience. Story content is evaluated to which there are integrated representations of self and attachment figure, and the degree to which narrative show an integration of the responsivity and sensitivity of self and other. The AAP narratives are evaluated using 2 dimensions: Agency of self, defined as the capacity for constructive thinking or action, and Connectedness, defined as the desire to be connected in close relationships.

Attachment classifications in the AAP are derived from the analysis of attachment narratives with 3 organized categories (secure, dismissing, preoccupied) and 1 unresolved status with respect to trauma, loss, or attachment-related threats. Individuals, who are unresolved regarding experiences of loss or trauma, report in their narratives content or process markers of unintegrated, traumatic, or threatening story characteristics. These individuals, overwhelmed by trauma or loss, may therefore become dysregulated during the attachment task. Dysregulation can be momentary or prolonged, but in either case the individual is unable to use defensive processes to remain organized and to exclude distressing thoughts and feelings from consciousness.[17]

With respect to borderline pathology, all studies using interview measures (Main M, Goldwyn R. Adult attachment scoring and classification system, Version 6.0. University of California at Berkeley: Unpublished manuscript; 1998)[18,19] reported a strong association between BPD and indices of unresolved attachment.[9,10,12,19–23] Similarly, approximately one-half of the attachment-style studies, which use self-report measures, reported a strong association between BPD and indices of fearful or preoccupied and angry/hostile attachment.[24,25]

Insecure/disorganized attachment patterns impart greater risk for the maladaptive personality traits underlying BPD,[26] although a range of insecure states of mind have been linked to BPD.[22] However, there is increasing evidence that patients with

BPD, particularly those who have been hospitalized and/or are suicidal and/or chronically self-injurious (parasuicidal), have failed to integrate or resolved attachment traumata, particularly sexual and physical abuse by caretakers.[23,27,28] In several studies, BPD has been associated with an increased occurrence of insecure and especially disorganized/unresolved attachment representations.[9,10,12,20,21,29]

Hence, particularly important for understanding attachment in clinical groups is the distinction between secure versus insecure and organized versus disorganized attachment states of mind. Those with disorganized attachment (either unresolved or cannot classify) tend show multiple, unintegrated, and contradictory states of mind with respect to attachment, and thus not surprisingly are more highly represented in clinical groups and particularly in those with personality disorders. It should be noted that in the 2 RCTs on transference-focused psychotherapy (TFP), more than one-half the patients had a primary attachment classification of disorganized. In the US Weill Cornell RCT that included patients with borderline and some narcissistic disorders, 31.7% of patients with BPD were classified as unresolved with respect to attachment and 18.3% were classified in the cannot classify category, with 30% of patients classified as dismissing with respect to attachment and 15% of patients were classified as preoccupied.[10,22]

NEUROBIOLOGICAL CORRELATES OF DISORGANIZED/UNRESOLVED ATTACHMENT

Unresolved attachment has been linked to psychological disorders, impaired cognitive functioning, and trauma-related psychopathology.[10,30,31] In a study by Buchheim and colleagues,[10] patients with unresolved BPD (n = 52) compared with organized patients (n = 40) showed lower scores in psychosocial functioning (Global Assessment of Functioning; $P = .003$), more impairment of borderline personality organization (Structured Interview of Personality Organization; $P < .001$), and revealed more borderline symptoms (Structured Clinical Interview for DSM-IV-II; $P = .012$) at the beginning of treatment. There was an association between the post traumatic stress disorder diagnosis lifetime and unresolved trauma, which was observed by 21 of 25 patients (84%) with this experience and only by 31 of 67 patients (46%) without this experience (exact Fisher test, $P < .002$). Because this subgroup of patients with BPD were significantly more impaired with respect to psychopathology, and psychosocial functioning experiences of more trauma in their history, Buchheim and colleagues[10] suggested that unresolved attachment might constitute an aggravating factor in BPD and be an important target of change in psychotherapy.

Moreover, unresolved/disorganized attachment status in individuals with BDP, as measured with the AAP,[17] has been associated with significantly lower plasma levels of the neuropeptide oxytocin (OT) than was the case with patients with BPD with organized attachment representations.[32] The neuropeptide OT has been hypothesized to play a crucial role in attachment because it is involved in the regulation of human social behaviors such as mother–infant interaction, pair bonding, affiliative behavior, trust, and trustworthiness.[33–35] The findings that lower levels of OT are found in patients with BPD with disorganized attachment than in those with organized (secure and insecure) attachment extended previous findings of impaired OT regulation in BPD. These findings provided the first evidence of that the association between OT and the breakdown of emotional regulation may be linked to attachment threat, stemming from disorganized/unresolved attachment representations in patients with BPD.[32] Indeed recent theoretic models of BPD suggest from a neurobiological perspective that impaired interpersonal functioning in BPD seem to be related to alterations in the (social) reward and empathy networks,[35,36] which has been strongly associated with a life history of early maltreatment.[37] Decades of research have shown that early experiences of maltreatment, such as sexual and physical abuse and emotional neglect, are implicated in the etiology of BPD.[25,38–40] There is also increasing evidence that the oxytocinergic system may be involved in these domains of dysfunction and may, thus, contribute to borderline psychopathology.[35] The association of interpersonal hypersensitivity and history of early maltreatment were supported by data showing lower OT concentrations in individuals with BPD with insecure/unresolved attachment or a history of early traumatization.[32,41,42]

A recent study using the AAP explored the neural correlates of emotional dysregulation during the activation of the attachment system in patients with BPD compared with healthy controls using functional MRI.[20] Unresolved attachment was associated with increasing amygdala activation over the course of the attachment task in patients as well as controls. Unresolved controls, but not patients, showed activation in the right dorsolateral prefrontal cortex and the rostral cingulate zone. The authors interpreted this as a neural signature of the inability patients with BPD to exert top-down control under conditions of attachment distress. These findings pointed to neural mechanisms for underlying affective dysregulation in BPD in the context of attachment trauma and fear.[20,35]

THE ROLE OF MENTALIZATION IN THE DEVELOPMENT OF BORDERLINE PERSONALITY DISORDER

Deficits in mentalization are also linked to the development of insecure/disorganized attachment in individuals with BPD. Mentalization involves the psychological capacity to envision the affects and behaviors of self and others in terms of their underlying mental states (thoughts, wishes, beliefs, and motivations)[43,44] and, as such, is fundamental to both self-regulation and affect regulation as well as to interpersonal functioning. OT is also implicated in the development of mentalization because its receptors are found in areas of the brain involved with social, affiliative behaviors such as reading facial expressions, establishing trust, or managing stress during social interactions.[45]

Although the concept of mentalization has dual roots in attachment theory and research, as well as in neurocognitive concepts of cognitive empathy and theory of mind,[46] it should be noted that, in more recent formulations, Fonagy and colleagues have decoupled the origins of mentalization from its exclusive evolution through interfamilial attachment relationships. Fonagy and colleagues emphasize that attachment and mentalization are separate systems and that theory of mind as a mechanism aimed at understanding and predicting the actions and behaviors of others is not necessarily related to the attachment system in which full mentalization develops. Rather, deficits in mentalization are thought to be indicative of epistemic hypervigilance, distrust, and a lack of resilience that involve failures to learn from social communication at the group or cultural level with roots in both genetic and environmental factors.

Deficient coregulation and social communication in infancy are purported to underpin emotional dysregulation and social cognition deficits across development.[47,48] Socially oriented models of BPD place epistemic trust and social communication as central to the early development of BPD. In families with abusive or hostile caregivers, epistemic mistrust becomes entrenched in an adaptive process. Across development, epistemic hypervigilance may manifest as an overinterpretation (ie, hypermentalization) of the motives of others and personality dysfunction will be maintained in a self-perpetuating cycle of social dysfunction and mentalization difficulties, that is, deficits in the ability to perceived and interpret human behavior in terms of intentional mental states.[48] Deficits in mentalization in turn lead to emotional dysregulation, further disrupting the ability to mentalize.[49] Difficulties with mentalization are related to a history of unresolved attachment, which also leads to problems with affect regulation, attention, and self-control.[50]

Fonagy and colleagues (Fonagy P, Target M, Steele H, et al. Reflective[51] functioning manual: version 5, for application to adult attachment interviews. Unpublished manuscript; 1998) established the concept of mentalization or reflective functioning (RF) on the basis of the AAI transcripts, having developed the idea that the interviewees showed different forms and levels of thinking about mental states such as thoughts, feelings, desires, and beliefs as underlying one's own and others' behaviors. Mentalization has been shown to be severely impaired in patients with BPD.[22,52] Recent studies examined the interplay of attachment and RF in patients with BPD and confirm the theoretic assumption that RF mediates the relationship between attachment disturbances and BPD symptom severity.[13,53] Both attachment representation and mentalization (RF) have been used as moderator, mediator, and outcome variables in psychotherapy studies.[13,24,54,55]

The RF Scale (Fonagy P, Target M, Steele H, et al. Reflective functioning manual: version 5, for application to adult attachment interviews. Unpublished manuscript; 1998). Deficits in mentalization are assessed through the RF scale and Fonagy developed the RF scale to capture "the psychological processes underlying the capacity to mentalize" in the context of attachment relationships. Designed for use with the AAI, the RF scale is an 11-point scale that assesses individual differences in the capacity to mentalize. Mentalization in the RF system includes a number of dimensions, including that mental states have a developmental trajectory and may shift and change with maturation, are subject to change with change in life circumstances or relationships, and are relatively opaque and subject to limitations, including on the part of the interviewer who may not intuit or understanding the formulations of the speaker or have discrepant views of things. The RF scale ranges from −1 (negative RF, in which interviews are antireflective, totally barren of mentalization, or grossly distorting of the mental states of self and others) to 9 (exceptional RF in which interviews show unusually complex, elaborate, or original reasoning about mental states). Those with personality disorders typically score at level 3 or below that is characterized by a simplistic, naïve, and formulated view of mental states or by hyperactive or over analytical RF, in which the individual claims infallible knowledge of mental states with little evidence to corroborate this conviction and lack of awareness of the separateness of mind of self and others (Fonagy P, Target M, Steele H, et al. Reflective functioning manual: version 5, for application to adult attachment interviews. Unpublished manuscript; 1998).

Using the RF scale, an accretion of studies has now linked the deficits in mentalization to the development of personality disorders. Individuals with a history of abuse are less likely to develop BPD if they had high RF on the AAI, (Fonagy P, Target M, Steele H, et al. Reflective functioning manual: version 5, for application to AAIs. Unpublished manuscript; 1998), although the capacity for RF may moderate the negative impact of a traumatic early attachment history and potentially guard against the transgenerational transmission of insecure disorganized attachment patterns. Slade[56] has suggested that RF may be "the core capacity" that differentiates secure from insecure states of mind and that attachment categories may "be proxies" for an underlying organizing psychological capacity of mentalization. Just as deficits in mentalization are fundamental to severe personality disorders, several studies have shown that improvements in mentalization are a key mechanism of change in psychodynamic psychotherapy with such patients.[22,13,52]

In sum, patients with BPD with unresolved attachment are significantly more impaired with respect to psychopathology, psychosocial functioning, and neuropeptide modulation and have reported not necessarily more attachment trauma in their history, but rather a lack of resolution of traumatic loss and abuse. Moreover, unresolved attachment is associated with a variety of neural and social cognitive correlates that mediate the affective dysregulation. Taken together this suggests that low RF and insecure, unresolved attachment are important targets of change in psychotherapy.

RANDOMIZED, CONTROLLED STUDIES DEMONSTRATING CHANGE OF ATTACHMENT STATUS AND REFLECTIVE FUNCTIONING IN THE COURSE OF TRANSFERENCE-FOCUSED PSYCHOTHERAPY
Targets of Transference-Focused Psychotherapy

Psychotherapy is recommended as the primary treatment for BPD with evidence-based psychotherapy programs having common and differential treatment targets.[57] TFP is 1 of the 4 evidence-based treatments for BPD and constitutes a manualized psychoanalytic psychotherapy designed for patients with severe personality disorders organized at the borderline level.[58] TFP focuses not only on improving symptoms and containing self-destructive behavior, but also aims to improve personality organization and functioning. Major parts of the concept of personality functioning have recently been adopted by the alternative *Diagnostic and Statistical Manual of Mental Disorders*-5 model for personality disorders.[6] TFP has the goal of integrating mental representations of self and significant others, modification of lower level (primitive) defensive mechanisms, and resolution of identity diffusion by analysis of the transference within the therapeutic relationship. The aim of TFP is thus to promote the development of increasingly integrated, differentiated, and mature representations of self and others, and in so doing to improve tolerance of negative affects (eg, aggression, anxiety, envy, guilt) that are interlinked with the split polarized internal world and concomitant primitive defenses characteristic of BPD.[59] Another way to think about this process in terms of attachment theory and research is that the treatment situation in TFP, with its dyadic intimacy and intensity, activates primary internal working models of attachment that, in the case of more severely disturbed patients, are likely to be insecure, multiple, contradictory, and conflictual in nature with the goal of moving the patient toward increased attachment security.[13] It should be noted that, in contrast with attachment models, however, TFP is based on the idea that mental representations that organize the transference are linked to a broad array of motivational systems, including sexuality, aggression, play, affiliation, and fear/attachment.[60–62] However, the emphasis in attachment theory and research and in the AAI in particular on the individual's current state of mind with respect to attachment representations is consistent with the emphasis in TFP on the way self–object–affect dyads are activated in the here and now of the transference relationship. In addition, by asking about specific experiences of trauma, loss, and abuse, the AAI interview reveals to what extent individuals have integrated and mastered past attachment losses and traumas. Although it was originally developed on a normative sample, the latter set of questions make it particularly useful for investigating the representational world of clinical groups such as those with BPD who are likely to have endured experiences of neglect, loss, and/or trauma, about which they remain unresolved.

Studies on Attachment in Transference-Focused Psychotherapy

Several studies, including 2 RCTs, one conducted at the Personality Disorders Institute at the Weill-Cornell Medical College (the Cornell-NY RCT), and another conducted independently by the Vienna-Munich TFP group (the V-M RCT), have demonstrated the effectiveness and efficacy of TFP for borderline pathologies. A full description of the method and findings from the 2 RCTs can be found elsewhere.[10,22,52,63,64] In this summary, we focus on the changes in from insecure to secure attachment and mentalization observed in both studies, with a particular focus on the shift from disorganized to organized attachment status after 1 year of TFP that was observed only in the Vienna-Munich study. The latter study is described in greater detail with case material presented to illustrate these changes.

The Cornell New York Randomized Controlled Study

In the Cornell-NY RCT, conducted by Clarkin and colleagues,[63] a total of 90 patients diagnosed with BPD were randomly assigned for 1 year to 1 of the 3 manualized outpatient treatments: twice weekly TFP, dialectical behavior therapy (DBT[65]), or supportive psychodynamic therapy.[66] Results showed that all 3 groups had significant improvement in both global and social functioning and significant decreases in depression and anxiety. Both patients treated in TFP and DBT, but not supportive psychodynamic therapy, showed significant improvement in suicidality, depression, anger, and global functioning. Only the TFP-treated group demonstrated significant improvements in verbal assault, direct assault, and irritability.[63] Further, changes in attachment organization and reflective function were evaluated as putative mechanisms of change in treatment[22] with the hypotheses that increased integration and coherence in the representational world, as measured by AAI classification (Main M, Goldwyn R. Adult attachment scoring and classification system, Version 6.0. University of California at Berkeley: Unpublished manuscript; 1998) and RF (Fonagy P, Target M, Steele H, et al. Reflective functioning manual: version 5, for application to adult attachment interviews. Unpublished manuscript; 1998) would be found in TFP but not the other treatments. In fact, after 12 months there was a significant (3-fold) increase in the number of patients classified as secure with respect to attachment for individuals in TFP but not the other 2 treatments. In addition, significant changes were found in the AAI subscale of narrative coherence, that is, in the organization, clarity, and credibility of discourse, the best predictor of attachment security among the AAI subscales (Waters E, Treboux D, Fyffe C, et al. Secure versus insecure and dismissing versus preoccupied attachment representation scored as continuous variables from AAI state of mind scales. Stony Brook, State University of New York: Unpublished manuscript; 2001). Significant changes in RF were also found as a function of treatment, with those in TFP showing increases in both constructs during the course of therapy.

Vienna-Munich Randomized Controlled Study

The V-M RCT conducted independently by Doering and colleagues[64] in Germany and Austria provided further data establishing TFP as an efficacious treatment. Doering and colleagues conducted an RCT with 104 female patients with BPD comparing 1 year of TFP with treatment by experienced community psychotherapists (ECP) that was largely supportive therapy as usual. Although patients improved in both treatment groups, patients randomly assigned to TFP evidenced lower drop-out and showed significantly greater decreases in the number of patients attempting suicide, number of inpatient admissions, and BPD symptoms, and significantly greater improvements in personality organization and psychosocial functioning after 1 year of treatment. Both groups improved significantly in depression and anxiety and the TFP group improved in general psychopathology, all without significant group differences. Self-harming behavior did not change in either group.

In this study by Buchheim and colleagues,[10] 92 patients were administered the AAI at the beginning and 63 after 1 year of treatment, The AAI interviews were transcribed verbatim and scored by 2 certified raters, blind to time and treatment condition, scored the transcripts to assign the individual to 1 of 4 attachment classifications: secure/autonomous, dismissing, preoccupied, and unresolved. A subset of transcripts (n = 36) was double rated by both judges showing agreement on 89% of the 4 categorical classifications (kappa = 0.84), and on 94% of the 2 classifications (organized vs unresolved; kappa = 0.89). Moreover, Buchheim and colleagues[10] focused on the coherence continuous subscale (range, 1–9). The AAI was additionally scored with the RF Scale (Fonagy P, Target M, Steele H, et al. Reflective functioning manual: version 5, for application to adult attachment interviews. Unpublished manuscript; 1998). Coders for the RF scale were trained at the Anna Freud Center in London. Coders were blind to treatment condition. The 2 coders coded a subset of each other's transcripts (n = 25) and showed a good interrater reliability (κ = 0.79).

Data on Reflective Functioning

Analyzing RF, there were no differences between the groups with regard to sociodemographic and clinical variables at baseline.[52] Baseline RF was 2.77 (standard deviation, 1.27) in the TFP and 2.66 (standard deviation, 0.93) in the ECP group. TFP group improved significantly with regard to RF (effect size d = 0.34), whereas the ECP group remained unchanged (d = 0.07).[52] RF at baseline was about 2.7 with no difference between the 2 groups. This result confirmed former studies reporting questionable or low mentalizing capacity in patients with BPD.[67] A score of 3 is characterized by either naïve/simplistic or overanalytic/hyperactive reflections on the mental states of self and others (Fonagy P, Target M, Steele H, et al. Reflecting functioning manual: version 5, for application to adult attachment interviews. Unpublished manuscript; 1998). The findings[52] revealed significant within-group differences of RF in the TFP group, although no changes occurred in the ECP group.

Changes in Reflective Functioning and Attachment After 1 Year of Transference-Focused Psychotherapy Case Example of Reflective Functioning at the Beginning of Transference-Focused Psychotherapy Treatment

RF depicts a specific structural aspect of the personality, namely, the ability of the individual to understand and interpret one's own and others' behaviors and actions as expressions of various intentional mental states in the context of attachment relationships. Thus, improvements in RF are expected to go hand in hand with changes in attachment representations, which is illustrated in this section.

Why do you think your parents behaved as they did during your childhood?

Because my mother loved me more than anything, that's why.

This statement is characterized by self-serving, coded as an RF of 1, a very low RF.

And my father? Well, I don't really know why my father was so brutal. Well, he grew up without a father. His father was an alcoholic too, so could this have influenced him? But why he was more friendly toward me than to the others, the other children, I don't really know.

This statement is characterized by disavowal, coded as an RF of 1, a very low RF.

Case Example of Reflective Functioning with the Same Patient After 1 Year of Transference-Focused Psychotherapy Treatment

> Why do you think your parents behaved as they did during your childhood?
>
> *Well, I think my father was so aggressive because, I think that maybe this is also in the family, his father was an alcoholic, too, and was so aggressive and apparently his mother was also aggressive toward him and hit him, and, but I also think that my father was desperate some way, because he had imagined his life to be different, I think, than to be sitting in a small apartment with 3 children.*
>
> *And why my mother, ok, she had 3 children to take care of and she was dependent on, at that time, the husband bringing home the money. I think that my mother was so, well, busy with herself, with her illnesses and all that, that she could not bear it at all that I was feeling unwell.*
>
> This statement is characterized by an accurate if ordinary attribution of mental states, coded as an RF of 5, or ordinary RF.

This shift from low to moderate RF in the study by Fischer-Kern and colleagues[52] was in line with the New York-Cornell RCT, which yielded a significant increase of RF only in TFP, but not in dialectic behavior therapy and psychodynamic supportive therapy.[22]

Based on Kernberg's[2] developmentally based theory of BPD, the central mechanisms of change in TFP stem from the integration of polarized affect states and split-off mental representations of self and others, which gradually enables the patient to think more coherently and reflectively. Several studies on process and outcome in psychodynamic therapies have shown enhancement in RF as a long-term goal. A study on psychodynamic, hospitalization-based treatment for patients with personality disorder revealed no increases in RF during 1 year of treatment[68] and 2 single case studies revealed improvements of RF only after 5 years of outpatient psychodynamic treatment.[69,70] Therefore, the findings that show improvement in RF in patients with BPD after 1 year of TFP are particularly impressive. The study by Fischer-Kern and colleagues,[52] coupled with the work of Levy and colleagues[22] (2006) has shown that TFP is not only efficacious as a treatment for BPD with respect to symptom change but also with regard to improvements in mentalization, and as illustrated in the following section in improvements in the security of attachment representations.

Data on the Adult Attachment Interview

Buchheim and colleagues (2017)[10] found that at baseline both treatment groups (n = 45 ECP patients and n = 47 TFP patients) were characterized by the prevalence of unresolved trauma and near total absence of secure attachment (ECP group: 4 F, 6 Ds, 9 E, 26 U; TFP group: 2 F, 12 Ds, 7 E, 26 U) [F- Secure; Ds- Dismissing; E- Preoccupied; U- Unresolved]. The generalized exact Fisher test did not show significant differences in distributions of attachment classifications between the TFP and ECP groups ($P = .436$). Interestingly, the second administration of the AAI after 1 year of treatment was completed by 56% of the ECP and 81% of the TFP participants, indicating a higher compliance of patients from the TFP group to participating in the follow-up. The difference of proportions was statistically significant (Fisher exact test: $P = .013$).

Case Example of Unresolved Attachment at the Beginning of Transference-Focused Psychotherapy Treatment

---

I'd like you to try to describe your relationship with your parents as a young child if you could start from as far back as you can remember?

I was abused by my father when I was 6 years old, I think until I was 10 years old. I told once my mother and she terribly rejected me. (Pause) I think it was not too dramatic anyway that time, I think I was provoking it somehow. I always tried to keep it away from me for a long time, maybe it would be better to be a boy, I really don't know.

This statement represents an unresolved state of mind based on evaluations of the interviewee's transient mental disorientation when describing experiences of sexual abuse. This discourse pattern suggests that these experiences are accessible to memory, but not yet integrated to create a whole sense of self–other representation. In this example, we can identify descriptions containing irrational convictions of the interviewee's own guilt and confusion between self and other (Main M, Goldwyn R. Adult attachment scoring and classification system, Version 6.0. University of California at Berkeley: Unpublished manuscript; 1998). In sum, the existence of unprocessed traumas is evident in the discourse characteristics communicated in the structure of the language, even when they are not verbalized directly, but just alluded to in the content, alerting the therapist to their existence.

The numbers of patients in the study[10] who improved versus worsened in their secure (F) or insecure (Ds + E + U) attachment status were compared by the exact McNemar test. No significant improvements in attachment representations were found within the ECP group. On the contrary, highly significant improvements were found within the TFP group (exact McNemar test; $P < .001$). Comparing both groups, the proportion of TFP patients (12 of 38) who improved in their attachment security was significantly higher than the proportion (0 of 25) in the ECP group (Fisher exact test; $P = .002$). Fully analogous results were obtained for the changes between the organized (F + Ds + E) and disorganized/unresolved (U) status. No significant shifts from disorganized to organized were found within the ECP group, although significant shifts from disorganized to organized were found within the TFP group (exact McNemar test; $P < .001$). Comparing both groups, the proportion of patients with improved organization (17 of 38) was significantly higher in the TFP group than that of the patients in the ECP group (3 of 25; Fisher exact test; $P = .012$).[10]

Case Example of Unresolved Attachment with the Same Patient After 1 Year of Transference-Focused Psychotherapy Treatment

---

I'd like you to try to describe your relationship with your parents as a young child if you could start from as far back as you can remember?

I was abused by my father when I was 6 years old, I think until 10 years. Now I realize how much that affected me, especially that I was not able to talk to my mother about it. She denied it and I did also. It is still very hard to talk about it. And I still have sometimes troubles not to accuse myself, but I know better now, that it was possibly not my fault.

This statement demonstrates that the patient does not deny the abusive experiences anymore and is able to reflect in a coherent manner how hurtful it was to grow up with a mother, who was not able to protect her.

Consistent with the findings described previously for the Cornell-NY RCT, the improvement of coherence was considerably higher in the TFP group (Cohen's d = 1.27) than in the ECP group (d = 0.32).[10]

In sum, as expected, attachment status did not differ between the 2 patients groups at baseline, showing a predominance of unresolved attachment representations. This result confirmed previous studies on attachment in BDP[9,21,29,71] and various psychological models agree on childhood traumatization as one risk factor for the development of BPD.[40] Moreover, the study by Buchheim and colleagues[10] found that unresolved patients with BPD were significantly more impaired with respect to psychopathology and psychosocial functioning, and have reported greater levels of traumatic abuse and loss in their history, suggesting that unresolved attachment might constitute an aggravating factor in BPD and thus an important target of change in psychotherapy.

These findings revealed significant within-group changes of attachment status (insecure to secure and unresolved to organized) in the TFP group, although no significant changes occurred in the ECP group. This finding was in line with a former study yielding a significant increase of attachment security only in TFP, but not in DBT and psychodynamic supportive therapy.[22] This study confirmed that improvements in borderline symptomatology accompany improvement in attachment representations and a significant increase of coherence and RF in the patients' narratives treated with TFP. The significant shift from insecure to a secure attachment status in many of patients with BPD in the TFP treatment group implied that TFP treatment was able to enhance the patients' capacity to internalize a secure base, attachment related autonomy and capacity for flexible integration. Adding to the findings of Levy and colleagues,[22] Buchheim and colleagues[10] found a significant shift from unresolved to organized attachment representations in the TFP group, suggesting that TFP can be considered an effective treatment for traumatized patients. In TFP, the actual genetic origins of traumatic experience are less significant and usually not taken up and explored until later in the treatment. Rather, the focus is on how trauma is embedded in the interplay of self–other dyads (eg, victim, victimizer or sufferer/savior), and modes of defense and affect regulation as they are activated in the therapeutic arena.[72] During the first year of treatment, TFP is designed to diminish self-destructive behaviors by clarifying the dual experience of self as victim and victimizer through the here-and-now transference relationship. These findings are consistent with the putative mechanisms of change in TFP, which are assumed to result from the integration of polarized affect states and representations of self and other into a more coherent whole.[13,63] Moreover, a greater number of patients who continued their participation in the AAI interview after 1 year of treatment were in the TFP group, suggesting greater compliance of these patients, which may itself indicate a greater capacity to reflect on and tolerate a reevaluation of attachment experiences, including those that involve traumatic abuse or loss.

Speaking to this point, a recent analysis by Tmej and colleagues (Tmej A, Fischer-Kern M, Doering S, et al. Changes in attachment representation in psychotherapy: is reflective functioning the crucial factor? Unpublished manuscript) from the same dataset showed that higher RF level before psychotherapy proved to be a moderator for change in attachment representation. Patients with unresolved attachment and low-level RF at the outset had the least chance for representational change during the first year of psychotherapy.

SUMMARY

Although an increasing number of studies have examined attachment in BPD, there have been relatively few psychotherapy studies that have explored change in attachment representations over the course of treatment.[54,55] This is somewhat surprising given the convergent evidence that disturbed relationships may be one endophenotypic expression of BPD and the value of targeting interpersonal relations and the patient's sense of self and significant others in treatment.[73] In contrast with the general agreement about the importance of mental representations in driving interpersonal behavior, the manner in which psychotherapeutic treatments address these cognitive/affective units vary in important ways.[59] For example, DBT[65] uses an instructional approach to help the patient learn and use skills. Mentalization-based treatment [43] emphasizes the need to temper the patient's affect dysregulation in therapy sessions, through fostering the patients' reflective capacities. In contrast, the TFP model provides a treatment framework that acknowledges the inevitability of affect arousal in a safe setting that provides the opportunity to modify extreme cognitions and related affects in the emotionally 'hot' and immediate experience of others.[59]

The findings of higher impairment levels and worse psychosocial functioning in patients with unresolved BPD suggest that unresolved attachment might constitute an aggravating factor in BPD and thus constitutes an important target of change in psychotherapy. Replicating the findings of Levy and colleagues,[22] TFP was superior in revealing changes from insecure to secure attachment. However, no previous study had shown that patients in TFP achieve a change from disorganized/unresolved to organized attachment, suggesting its effectiveness in treating patients with consequences of severe maltreatment, abuse and loss.[10] The significant shift from insecure to a secure attachment status in many of patients with BPD in TFP implies that this treatment was able to enhance the patients' coherence, attachment-related autonomy, and flexible integration, a capacity called earned security (Main M, Goldwyn R. Adult attachment scoring and classification system, Version 6.0. University of California at Berkeley: Unpublished manuscript; 1998). In comparison with the ECP group, the highly structured, interactive, but neutral stance of the TFP therapist, in which the therapist does not side with any aspect of the patient's internal experience or representational world, may provide a safer setting for reflecting on attachment relationships and experiences including split off or dissociated experiences of traumatic loss and abuse.[58] Thus, the change from disorganized to organized attachment in this study[10] is noteworthy because it indicates that TFP may be an effective treatment for patients with borderline structure and a severe trauma history, who have been noted not to respond to short-term CBT trauma treatment models that emphasize psychoeducation or exposure (eg, focal reconstruction of trauma narratives).[72]

It should be noted that TFP is designed to diminish and contain self-destructive and suicidal behaviors by mobilizing and clarifying the dominant and opposing object relational patterns that fuel them (eg, the representations of victimized self and abusing other along with linking affects of rage and fear) as they emerge in the here and now experience of the transference. Instead, the emphasis in TFP is not on the reconstruction of past experiences of trauma and abuse as much as on the identification and exploration of how past traumatic experiences have configured the maladaptive representations of self and others that underlie the difficulties with self and interpersonal functioning in the present in those with BPD. The information that unfolds within the patient's relation with the therapist provides the most direct access to understanding the makeup of the patient's internal world for 2 reasons:

1. It has immediacy and is observable by both therapist and patient simultaneously so that differing perceptions of the shared reality can be discussed in the moment, and
2. It includes the affect (feelings) that accompanies the perceptions, in contrast to discussion of historical material that can have an intellectualized quality.

As Draijer and Van Zon[72] point out, "in extremely traumatized patients there may be aggressive and oppressive inner parts that want control" (p. 170), and these may vie with vulnerable and fearful aspects of the self. Further these opposing representations are seen to be a mélange of objective and subjective experiences colored by the BPD patient's own extreme and polarized affect states. These opposing and contradictory aspects of self may contend with each other. The self as victim fearing attack from an abusive other oscillating with an enraged self-attacking a helpless other, with the latter often split off and dissociated. All of these highly polarized, contradictory aspects of self and others are mobilized, explored, and then interpreted as they emerge through the experience in the transference, leading to their modulation and integration. Our findings are thus consistent with the putative mechanisms of change in TFP, that might result from the integration of polarized affect states and self-other representations into a more coherent whole.[58] Such intrapsychic changes might be relevant for long-term treatment benefits.[57,73] In sum, so far TFP is the only evidence-based treatment demonstrating changes in attachment representations (from insecure to secure and disorganized to organized), and in RF after 1 year of treatment in individuals with BPD.

REFERENCES

1. Leichsenring F, Leibing E, Kruse J, et al. Borderline personality disorder. Lancet 2011;377:74–84.
2. Kernberg OF. Severe personality disorders: psychotherapeutic strategies. Yale University Press; 1984.
3. Kernberg OF, Caligor E. A psychoanalytic theory of personality disorders. In: Lenzenweger MF, Clarkin JF, editors. Major theories of personality disorder. 2nd edition. New York: Guilford Press; 2005. p. 114–56.
4. Bender DS, Skodol AE. Borderline personality as self-other representational disturbance. J Pers Disord 2007;21:500–17.
5. Gunderson JG, Lyons-Ruth K. BPD's interpersonal hypersensitivity phenotype. J Pers Disord 2008;22:22–41.
6. American Psychiatric Association (APA). Diagnostic and statistical manual of mental disorders. 5th edition. Arlington (VA): American Psychiatric Publishing; 2013. p. 761–81.
7. Clarkin JF, Cain NM, Lenzenweger MF. Advances in transference-focused psychotherapy derived from the study of borderline personality disorder: clinical insights with a focus on mechanism. Curr Opin Psychol 2018;21:80–5.
8. Westen D, Nakash O, Thomas C, et al. Clinical assessment of attachment patterns and personality disorder in adolescents and adults. J Consult Clin Psychol 2006;74:1065–85.
9. Bakermans-Kranenburg MJ, van IJzendoorn MH. The first 10,000 adult attachment interviews: distributions of adult attachment representations in clinical and non-clinical groups. Attach Hum Dev 2009;11:223–63.
10. Buchheim A, Hörz-Sagstetter S, Doering S, et al. Change of unresolved attachment in borderline personality disorder: RCT study of transference-focused psychotherapy. Psychother Psychosom 2017;86:314–6.
11. Buchheim A, George C, Gündel H, et al. Editorial: neuroscience of human attachment. Front Hum Neurosci 2017;11:136.
12. Diamond D, Levy KN, Clarkin JF, et al. Attachment and mentalization in female patients with comorbid narcissistic and borderline personality disorder. Personal Disord 2014;5:428–33.

13. Diamond D, Clarkin JF, Levy KN, et al. Change in attachment and reflective function in borderline patients with and without comorbid narcissistic personality disorder in transference focused psychotherapy. Contemp Psychoanal 2014; 50(1–2):175–210.
14. Ravitz P, Maunder R, Hunter J, et al. Adult attachment measures: a 25-year review. J Psychosom Res 2010;69:419–32.
15. George C, West M, Pettem O. The adult attachment projective: disorganization of adult attachment at the level of representation. In: Solomon J, George C, editors. Attachment disorganization. New York: Guilford; 1999. p. 462–507.
16. George C, West M. The development and preliminary validation of a new measure of adult attachment: the adult attachment projective. Attach Hum Dev 2001;3:30–61.
17. George C, West ML. The Adult Attachment Projective Picture System: attachment theory and assessment in adults. New York: Guilford Press; 2012.
18. Hesse E. The adult attachment interview: protocol, method of analysis and empirical studies. In: Cassidy J, Shaver P, editors. Handbook of attachment. 2nd edition. New York: Guilford Press; 2008. p. 718–44.
19. Buchheim A, Erk S, George C, et al. Neural correlates of attachment trauma in borderline personality disorder: a functional magnetic resonance imaging study. Psychiatry Res Neuroimaging 2008;16:223–35.
20. Buchheim A, Erk S, George C, et al. Neural response during the activation of the attachment system in patients with borderline personality disorder: an fMRI study. Front Hum Neurosci 2016;10:389.
21. Buchheim A, George C. Attachment disorganization in borderline personality disorder and anxiety disorder. In: Solomon J, George C, editors. Disorganized attachment and caregiving. New York: Guilford Press; 2011. p. 343–83.
22. Levy KN, Meehan KB, Kelly KM, et al. Change in attachment patterns and reflective function in a randomized control trial of transference-focused psychotherapy for borderline personality disorder. J Consult Clin Psychol 2006;74:1027–240.
23. Patrick M, Hobson RP, Castle D, et al. Personality disorder and the mental representation of early social experience. Dev Psychopathol 1994;6:375–88.
24. Levy K, Ellison WD, Scott LN. Attachment style. J Clin Psychol 2011;67:193–203.
25. Frías Á, Palma C, Farriols N, et al. Anxious adult attachment may mediate the relationship between childhood emotional abuse and borderline personality disorder. Personal Ment Health 2016;10:274–84.
26. Scott LN, Levy KN, Pincus AL. Adult attachment, personality traits, and borderline personality disorder features in young adults. J Pers Disord 2009;23:258–80.
27. Adam KS. Suicidal behavior and attachment: a developmental model. In: Sperling MB, Berman WH, editors. Attachment in adults. New York: Guilford Press; 1994. p. 275–98.
28. Fonagy P, Leigh T, Steele M, et al. The relation of attachment status, psychiatric classification and response to psychotherapy. J Consult Clin Psychol 1996;64: 22–31.
29. Agrawal HR, Gunderson J, Holmes BM, et al. Attachment studies with borderline patients: a review. Harv Rev Psychiatry 2004;12:94–104.
30. Nakash-Eisikovits O, Dutra L, Westen D. Relationship between attachment patterns and personality pathology in adolescents. J Am Acad Child Adolesc Psychiatry 2002;41:1111–23.
31. Joubert D, Webster L, Hackett RK. Unresolved attachment status and trauma-related symptomatology in maltreated adolescents: an examination of cognitive mediators. Child Psychiatry Hum Dev 2012;43:471–83.

32. Jobst A, Padberg F, Mauer MC, et al. Lower oxytocin plasma levels in borderline patients with unresolved attachment representations. Front Hum Neurosci 2016; 10:125.

33. Meyer-Lindenberg A, Kohn PD, Kolachana B, et al. Midbrain dopamine and prefrontal function in humans: interaction and modulation by COMT genotype. Nat Neurosci 2005;8:594–6.

34. Buchheim A, Heinrichs M, George C, et al. Oxytocin enhances the experience of attachment security. Psychoneuroendocrinology 2009;34:1417–22.

35. Weinstein L, Perez-Rodriguez MM, Siever L. Personality disorders, attachment and psychodynamic psychotherapy. Psychopathology 2014;47:425–36.

36. Herpertz SC, Bertsch K. A New perspective on the pathophysiology of borderline personality disorder: a model of the role of oxytocin. Am J Psychiatry 2015;172: 840–51.

37. Teicher MH, Samson JA. Childhood maltreatment and psychopathology: a case for ecophenotypic variants as clinically and neurobiologically distinct subtypes. Am J Psychiatry 2013;170:1114–33.

38. Bandelow B, Krause J, Wedekind D, et al. Early traumatic life events, parental attitudes, family history, and birth risk factors in patients with borderline personality disorder and healthy controls. Psychiatry Res 2005;134:169–79.

39. Zanarini MC, Frankenburg FR, Hennen J, et al. Prediction of the 10-year course of borderline personality disorder. Am J Psychiatry 2006;163:827–32.

40. Keinänen MT, Johnson JG, Richards ES, et al. A systematic review of the evidence based psychosocial risk factors for understanding of borderline personality disorder. Psychoanal Psychother 2012;26:65–9.

41. Heim C, Young LJ, Newport DJ, et al. Lower CSF oxytocin concentrations in women with a history of childhood abuse. Mol Psychiatry 2009;14:954–8.

42. Bertsch K, Schmidinger I, Neumann ID, et al. Reduced plasma oxytocin levels in female patients with borderline personality disorder. Horm Behav 2012;63:424–9.

43. Bateman A, Fonagy P. Psychotherapy for borderline personality disorder: mentalization-based treatment. Oxford (England): Oxford University Press; 2004.

44. Fonagy PG, Jurist G, Target EM. Affect regulation, mentalization, and the development of the self. New York: Other Press; 2002. p. 203–51.

45. Van IJzendoorn MH, Bakermans-Kranenburg MJ. A sniff of trust: meta-analysis of the effects of intranasal oxytocin administration on face recognition, trust to ingroup, and trust to out-group. Psychoneuroendocrinology 2012;37:438–43.

46. Choi-Kain LW, Gunderson JG. Mentalization: ontogeny, assessment, and application in the treatment of borderline personality disorder. Am J Psychiatry 2008;165: 1127–35.

47. Winsper C. The aetiology of borderline personality disorder (BPD): contemporary theories and putative mechanisms. Curr Opin Psychol 2018;21:105–10.

48. Fonagy P, Luyten P, Allison E, et al. What we have changed our minds about, part 2: borderline personality disorder, epistemic trust and the developmental significance of social communication. Borderline Personal Disord Emot Dysregul 2017; 4:9.

49. Sharp C, Pane H, Ha C, et al. Theory of mind and emotion regulation difficulties in adolescents with borderline traits. J Am Acad Child Adolesc Psychiatry 2011;50: 563–73.

50. Hallquist MN, Hipwell AE, Stepp SD. Poor self-control and harsh punishment in childhood prospectively predict borderline personality symptoms in adolescent girls. J Abnorm Psychol 2015;124:549.

51. Fonagy P, Target M, Steele H, et al. Reflective-functioning manual, version 5.0, for application to adult attachment interviews. London: University College London; 1998. p. 161–2.
52. Fischer-Kern M, Doering S, Taubner S, et al. Transference-focused psychotherapy for borderline personality disorder: change in reflective function. Br J Psychiatry 2015;207:173–4.
53. Badoud D, Prada P, Nicastro R, et al. Attachment and reflective functioning in women with borderline personality disorder. J Pers Disord 2018;32:17–30.
54. Steele H, Steele M, Murphy A. Use of the adult attachment interview to measure process and change in psychotherapy. Psychother Res 2009;19:633–43.
55. Taylor P, Rietzschel J, Danquah A, et al. Changes in attachment representations during psychological therapy. Psychother Res 2014;25:222–38.
56. Slade A. Parental reflective functioning: an introduction. Attach Hum Dev 2005;7: 269–81.
57. Stoffers JM, Völlm BA, Rücker G, et al. Psychological therapies for people with borderline personality disorder. Cochrane Database Syst Rev 2012;(8):CD005652.
58. Clarkin JF, Yeomans FE, Kernberg OF. Psychotherapy for borderline personality: focusing on object relations. Washington, DC: American Psychiatric Publishing; 2006.
59. Yeomans FE, Clarkin J, Kernberg OF. Transference-focused psychotherapy for borderline personality disorder: a clinical guide. Washington, DC: American Psychiatric Publishing; 2015.
60. Panksepp J. At the interface of the affective, behavioral, and cognitive neurosciences: decoding the emotional feelings of the brain. Brain Cogn 2003;52:4–14.
61. Panksepp J, Biven L. The archaeology of mind: neuroevolutionary origins of human emotions. WW Norton & Company; 2012. Available at: https://www.amazon.com/Archaeology-Mind-Neuroevolutionary-Interpersonal-Neurobiology/dp/B00MXDW3XO.
62. Auerbach JS, Diamond D. Mental representation in the thought of Sidney Blatt: developmental processes. J Am Psychoanal Assoc 2017;65:509–23.
63. Clarkin JF, Levy KN, Lenzenweger MF, et al. Evaluating three treatments for borderline personality disorder: a multiwave study. Am J Psychiatry 2007;164: 922–8.
64. Doering S, Hörz S, Rentrop M, et al. Transference-focused psychotherapy v. treatment by community psychotherapists for borderline personality disorder: randomized controlled trial. Br J Psychiatry 2010;196:389–95.
65. Linehan MM, Armstrong HE, Suarez A, et al. Cognitive-behavioral treatment of chronically parasuicidal borderline patients. Arch Gen Psychiatry 1991;48: 1060–4.
66. Appelbaum AH. Supportive psychotherapy. In: Oldham J, Skodol A, Bender D, editors. The American psychiatric publishing textbook of personality disorders. Washington, DC: American Psychiatric; 2005. p. 311–26.
67. Fischer-Kern M, Buchheim A, Hörz S, et al. The relationship between personality organization, reflective functioning, and psychiatric classification in borderline personality disorder. Psychoanal Psychol 2010;27:395–409.
68. Vermote R, Lowyck B, Luyten P, et al. Process and outcome in psychodynamic hospitalization-based treatment for patients with a personality disorder. J Nerv Ment Dis 2010;2:110–5.
69. Szecsödy I. A single-case study on the process and outcome of psychoanalysis. Scand Psychoanal Rev 2008;31:105–13.

70. Gullestad FS, Wilberg T. Change in reflective functioning during psychotherapy: a single-case study. Psychother Res 2011;21:97–111.
71. Mosquera D, Gonzalez A, Leeds AM. Early experience, structural dissociation, and emotional dysregulation in borderline personality disorder: the role of insecure and disorganized attachment. Borderline Personal Disord Emot Dysregul 2014;1:15.
72. Draijer N, Van Zon P. Transference-focused psychotherapy with former child soldiers: meeting the murderous self. J Trauma Dissociation 2013;14: 170–83.
73. Høglend P. Exploration of the patient-therapist relationship in psychotherapy. Am J Psychiatry 2014;171:1056–66.

Adolescence as a Sensitive Period for the Development of Personality Disorder

Carla Sharp, PhD*, Salome Vanwoerden, MA, Kiana Wall, BA

KEYWORDS

- Borderline disorder • Personality disorder • Adolescence • Sensitive period

KEY POINTS

- Adultlike personality disorder has its onset in adolescence.
- Rank order stability of personality disorder is moderate in adolescence and increases with age.
- Personality disorder is preceded by internalizing and externalizing disorder, but not the other way around.
- Personality disorder is comorbid with, but distinct from, internalizing and externalizing disorder throughout development.
- It is not until an agentic, self-determining author of the self emerges in adolescence that personality disorder can be detected.

The assessment, diagnosis, and treatment of personality disorder in adolescents were regarded as highly controversial until very recently. Arguments against the clinical management of personality disorder in adolescents have included the belief that:

1. Psychiatric nomenclature does not allow for the diagnosis of personality disorder in adolescence.
2. Certain features of personality disorder (eg, impulsivity, affective instability, or identity disturbances) are normative and not particularly symptomatic of personality disturbance.
3. The symptoms of personality disorder are better explained by internalizing and externalizing disorders.
4. Adolescent personalities are still developing and therefore too unstable to warrant a personality disorder diagnosis.

Conflicts of Interest: The authors declare that they have no conflicts of interest.
Department of Psychology, University of Houston, 126 Heyne Street, Houston, TX 77204, USA
* Corresponding author.
E-mail address: csharp2@uh.edu

Psychiatr Clin N Am 41 (2018) 669–683
https://doi.org/10.1016/j.psc.2018.07.004
0193-953X/18/© 2018 Elsevier Inc. All rights reserved.

5. Because personality disorder is long lasting, treatment resistant, and unpopular to treat, it would be stigmatizing to label an adolescent with personality disorder.[1]

Over the last 15 years, controversies over many of these concerns have been laid to rest because of accumulating empirical evidence challenging these beliefs. This evidence has been reviewed and evaluated in multiple recent reviews[2–4] and is not be repeated here. Instead, 4 key findings have been selected from the literature on borderline disorder in adolescents for discussion, with the ultimate goal of building an argument to support the idea that adolescence is a sensitive period for the development of personality disorder, here defined as maladaptive self-other relatedness. In reviewing this literature, this article focuses on borderline disorder for both pragmatic and substantive reasons. Pragmatic, simply because enough empirical research has been conducted on adolescent borderline personality disorder (BPD) to draw meaningful conclusions; and substantive, because recent evidence suggests that borderline disorder may be a proxy (or heuristic) for personality disorder in general.[5] BPD therefore serves as an appropriate paradigmatic disorder for evaluating adolescence as sensitive period for the development of personality disorder in general.

ADULTLIKE PERSONALITY DISORDER ONSETS IN ADOLESCENCE

The first finding relevant to the argument that adolescence is a sensitive period for developing personality disorder relates to the overwhelming evidence that personality disorder onsets in adolescence. This finding was first shown in the Children in the Community (CIC[6]) study, which evaluated the development and course of personality disorder in approximately 800 youth over 20 years. Child participants were initially assessed for personality disorders in late childhood (youngest age 9 years) and followed up thereafter during early adolescence (m_{age} = 14 [m- mean]), midadolescence (m_{age} = 16), and early adulthood (m_{age} = 22). Because of the longitudinal nature of the CIC study, tools chosen for the measurement of personality disorders varied over time as needed, but followed Diagnostic and Statistical Manual of Mental Disorders (DSM)-defined clusters and symptoms. Results of the CIC study suggest that personality disorder onsets in early adolescence, peaks in mid-adolescence, and subsequently declines into early adulthood. However, a large minority of participants (21% of the CIC sample) showed an increase in personality disorder into adulthood, suggesting that findings about the relative stability of personality disorder across the lifespan may extend to adolescent personality disorders.

Results of other community-based studies confirm and support findings of the CIC study. De Clerq and colleagues[7] assessed the maladaptive personality traits of 477 children (m_{age} = 10.67 years) using the Dimensional Personality Symptom Item Pool (DIPSI[8]), a dimensional measure of age-specific personality traits. Over a 1-year and 2-year follow-up, levels of the maladaptive personality traits disagreeableness, emotional instability, and compulsivity declined as the children entered early adolescence. However, this decline was less substantial in children who showed high scores. Over the course of 4 years, in a sample of 250 subjects ($m_{initialage}$ = 18.88 years), Wright and colleagues[9] assessed the stability of personality disorder features in late-adolescents and young adults. The International Personality Disorder Examination (IPDE[10]) assessed participants' personality disorder criteria at each of the study's 3 time points. The Revised Interpersonal Adjectives Scale–Big 5 (IASR-B5[11]) was included to measure the 3 personality factors (conscientiousness, neuroticism, and openness) of the 5-factor model in each participant. Results indicate that the development of adaptive personality traits such as affiliation, conscientiousness, and openness, as well as a decrease in neuroticism, is associated with a decrease in personality disorder symptoms over time. In contrast, as personality disorders developed, the development of adaptive personality traits ceased or even regressed.

The summation of these findings suggests onset of personality disorder in adolescents coupled with a general decline in personality disorder and an increase in adaptive personality traits as youth enter young adulthood. However, within these samples there seems to be a subset of adolescents who have diverged from the norm and whose personality problems persist or increase into adulthood. The question then arises whether the subset of adolescents for whom personality problems persists meet the threshold for a DSM-defined personality disorder.

To investigate this query, valid and reliable tools for assessing DSM criteria in BPD had to be developed and evaluated in adolescents. Studies have shown the validity and reliability of diagnostic tools such as the Structured Clinical Interview for DSM-III-R Personality Disorders (SCID-II[12]), Childhood Interview for DSM-IV Borderline Personality Disorder (CI-BPD[13]), the Personality Disorder Examination (PDE[14]), and the McLean Screening Instrument for Borderline Personality Disorder (MSI-BPD[15]) (see Ref.[4] for a review). Moreover, several self-report measures have also been found to be valid and reliable, including the Minnesota Multiphasic Personality Inventory – Adolescent version (MMPI-A[16]), Borderline Personality Questionnaire (BPQ[17]), Borderline Personality Disorder Features Scale for Children (BPFSC[18]), Personality Assessment Inventory Borderline subscale (PAI-BOR[19]), Dimensional Personality Symptom Item Pool (DIPSI[8]), and the Personality Inventory for DSM-5 (PID-5[20]). For the BPFSC,[18] BPFSP,[21] BPFSC-11,[22] and PAI-BOR,[19] studies of sensitivity and specificity have been conducted that showed good clinical utility for these measures. Together, these tools have been used to show that a subsample of teens meet full criteria for adultlike BPD in adolescents, with prevalence rates of 11% in outpatient[23] and 33%[24] and 43% to 49%[25] in inpatient samples; around 3% in UK,[26] 1% in US,[27,28] and 2% in Chinese[29] population-based studies; and a cumulative prevalence rate of 3%,[27] mirroring prevalence rates in adult samples.

RANK ORDER STABILITY IS MODERATE IN ADOLESCENCE AND INCREASES WITH AGE

The CIC study laid the groundwork for the understanding of the course and trajectory of personality disorder in adolescence and was also the first to report stability coefficients for adolescent personality disorders in the 0.4 to 0.7 range, similar to ranges reported for normal personality traits in both adults and children.[6] Stability coefficients for cluster B personality disorders (borderline, narcissistic, and histrionic personality disorders), as measured by the CIC study over the course of 9 years, were 0.63 for boys and 0.69 for girls. Analysis of the stability of BPD in adolescents, conducted on data from the Minnesota Twin Family Study (MTFS[30]), mirrored findings of the CIC study. Bornovalova and colleagues[31] showed a rank order stability of 0.53 to 0.73 in the MTFS sample of adolescent female twins, assessed over a period of 10 years from ages 17 to 24 years. Results from an outpatient sample in a study by Chanen and colleagues[23] show a BPD stability index of 0.54 over the course of 2 years in a sample of 101 adolescents, aged 15 to 18 years.

Overall, as found in adult samples, it seems that adolescents' ranking among peers in personality disorder is moderately stable over time. Moreover, prospective studies have shown that rank order stability of personality traits increases throughout the lifespan.[32] In addition, although only moderately stable, personality disorder seems to be more stable than internalizing or externalizing mental disorders. Internalizing mental disorder is characterized by negative emotionality, such as depressive and anxiety symptoms. Externalizing disorder encompasses disruptive or impulsive behavioral symptoms, such as delinquent or dangerous behaviors. For example, the CIC study[6] found that the stability of internalizing and externalizing symptoms was consistently lower than the consistency of cluster B personality disorder symptoms. This finding suggests that, during adolescence, borderline disorder and other cluster B symptoms can be expected to be more enduring and long lasting than periods of internalizing and externalizing symptoms. De Clerq and colleagues[7] found that, across 3 years and 3 time points, externalizing symptoms, as measured by the Dutch version of the Child Behavior Checklist (CBCL[33,34]), showed steeper and continued decline beyond those of maladaptive personality traits. These data point to normative developmental maturation processes wherein children grow out of externalizing behaviors, whereas maladaptive personality may be more persistent or may have functional impairment that persists beyond the normative decline of DSM-based symptoms.[35,36]

PERSONALITY DISORDER IS PRECEDED BY INTERNALIZING AND EXTERNALIZING DISORDER BUT NOT THE OTHER WAY AROUND

Stepp and colleagues[37] systematically reviewed the antecedents of BPD, identifying 39 studies that considered risk factors for BPD. Nineteen of these studies examined internalizing and externalizing mental disorders as a predictor of BPD, and 16 reported either internalizing or externalizing disorder as a significant predictor. For instance, Belsky and colleagues[38] found that borderline personality traits, measured in adolescents at age 12 years, were more common in those who had shown more behavioral and emotional problems at the age of 5 years. Stepp and colleagues[39] also showed that both internalizing (depression and suicidality) and externalizing (substance use disorder) mental disorder are associated with later BPD symptoms in adolescence. Based on findings of additive and interactive effects of internalizing and externalizing symptoms on borderline disorder over time, Bornovalova and colleagues[40] suggested that BPD traits measured in adulthood may be best understood as preceded by an inherited vulnerability for internalizing and externalizing disorders.

Internalizing symptoms have also been independently shown to predict later BPD. Krabbendam and colleagues[41] found that posttraumatic stress, depressive symptoms, and dissociation increased the risk for BPD in adulthood among detained, adolescent girls. In addition, internalizing constructs such as experiential avoidance have been shown to be predictive of borderline features in adolescents.[42] Similarly, externalizing symptoms, particularly attention-deficit/hyperactivity disorder (ADHD) and oppositional defiant disorder (ODD), have also been independently shown to predict BPD. An early study of the antecedents of personality disorder by Rey and colleagues[43] showed that young adults who had been diagnosed with a disruptive/ externalizing disorder in adolescence showed higher rates of personality disorders than those diagnosed with emotional/internalizing disorders, at rates of 40% and 12% respectively. In a clinical sample of male patients, initially aged 7 to 12 years, Burke and Stepp[44] found that ADHD and ODD significantly predicted BPD symptoms at age 24 years, even when accounting for substance abuse, other personality disorders, and physical punishment. Complementing this finding, in a large sample of girls aged 8 to 13 years from the Pittsburgh Girls Study, Stepp and colleagues[45] also identified ADHD and ODD as unique predictors of BPD symptoms at age 14 years.

Results of the aforementioned studies cumulatively suggest that both internalizing and externalizing disorders in childhood and adolescence are significant predictors of BPD, or an increase in BPD symptoms, in adolescence and adulthood. In contrast, borderline features seem not to precede internalizing and externalizing disorders. For instance, Lazarus and colleagues[46] and Bornovalova and colleagues[40] both showed, in samples of adolescents aged 14 to 17 and 14 to 18 years respectively, that, after accounting for cross-sectional relations and temporal stability between substance use problems and borderline features, the latter were not a causal antecedent to the former. More specifically, although BPD symptoms were associated with contemporaneous increases in alcohol use, the lagged and sustained effects of BPD on alcohol use were not significant, whereas the reverse was significant.[40,46] However, it is notable that most studies that examined longitudinal associations between BPD and internalizing and externalizing disorders either did not measure BPD symptoms before adolescence or did not explicitly test the hypothesis that BPD precedes internalizing and externalizing disorders, which is an important area for future research. As discussed later, based on developmental considerations, the authors think it unlikely that personality disorder (defined as maladaptive self-other relatedness) would precede internalizing and externalizing disorders even if it were measured.

PERSONALITY DISORDER IS COMORBID WITH, BUT DISTINCT FROM, INTERNALIZING AND EXTERNALIZING DISORDERS THROUGHOUT DEVELOPMENT

In addition to being antecedents of BPD in adolescents, internalizing and externalizing mental disorders are highly comorbid with BPD throughout adolescence and into adulthood. Similar to adult samples, comorbidities in adolescents with BPD range from 50% in a community sample[6] to 86% in a clinical sample.[47,48] For example, in a sample of 177 adolescent outpatients, Chanen and colleagues[49] found that subjects with BPD showed the highest levels of psychiatric severity and comorbidity, followed by adolescents with no BPD but another personality disorder, and finally adolescents with no personality disorder. Similarly, Ha and colleagues[24] found that inpatient adolescents with BPD had higher rates of comorbidity than their psychiatric control peers for mood disorders (70.6% vs 39.2%), anxiety disorders (67.3% vs 45.5%), and externalizing disorders (60.2% vs 34.4%). In addition, adolescents with BPD scored higher on the Youth Self-Report (YSR[50]), a dimensional measure of internalizing and externalizing mental disorder, than controls. In addition, Sharp and colleagues[51] report that adolescents with BPD showed significantly higher rates of complex comorbidity, as defined by Zanarini and colleagues,[52] wherein individuals must have any mood or anxiety disorder plus a disorder of impulsivity (ie, BPD).

Although evidence for comorbidity between internalizing, externalizing, and personality disorders is unequivocal, there is also strong evidence that BPD is not fully subsumed by internalizing and externalizing mental disorders. James and Taylor[53] as well as Eaton and colleagues[54] factor analyzed internalizing, externalizing, and borderline disorders (at the level of diagnosis) and showed that although BPD was a confluence of both internalizing and externalizing disorders (ie, loaded onto both internalizing and externalizing latent factors), there was enough variance not captured by these latent factors to suggest that BPD cannot be fully explained by these disorders. These findings were replicated in a study by Sharp[51] in adolescence.

That borderline disorder seems to denote unique disorder beyond internalizing and externalizing disorders despite high rates of comorbidity is further supported by longitudinal studies in adolescents. For example, Wright and colleagues[35] used data from the Pittsburgh Girls Study to further elucidate the understanding of within-person change, as well as outcomes, associated with adolescent BPD. Latent growth trajectories, based on 2450 adolescent girls aged 14 to 17 years, revealed that BPD symptoms were at least moderately associated with every aspect of psychosocial functioning measured, but, when internalizing and externalizing disorders were controlled for, BPD was related to poorer outcomes in social skills, self-perception, and sexual activity. Other functional domains that did not remain significant outcomes for borderline disorder once internalizing and externalizing disorders were controlled for include academic performance, extracurricular activities, and global functioning. That functional impairment in the interpersonal domain seems to be uniquely and more persistently associated with borderline disorder beyond that of general relations to internalizing and externalizing disorders is an important finding and begins to point to the possibility that personality disorder is particularly important for understanding and predicting functional outcomes in the interpersonal domain. Moreover, borderline disorder may be particularly important for predicting severity of mental disorder, as shown in a sample of 177 adolescent outpatients in whom BPD significantly predicted general mental disorder as measured by the YSR[50] and the Young Adult Self-Report (YASR[55]) peer relationships, self-care, and family and relationship functioning, beyond other personality disorders or axis I disorders.[49] Similarly, Sharp and colleagues[56] found that BPD provided incremental predictive value for both suicidal ideation and deliberate self-harm, relative to major depressive disorder, in a sample of 156 adolescent inpatients.

In summary, borderline disorder is comorbid with, but not fully explained by, internalizing and externalizing mental disorders across the lifespan.[54] Internalizing and externalizing disorders seem to be developmental antecedents of BPD[37] and the risk factors for borderline disorder are also nonspecific to the disorder and shared with internalizing and externalizing disorders.[37] The risk profile for borderline disorder is almost identical to that of various other internalizing[57–59] and externalizing disorders.[60,61] These conclusions may suggest that, in the developmental path to borderline disorder, internalizing and externalizing disorders are a stepping stone, as indicated by their antecedence to, comorbidity with, and shared risk factors for borderline disorder.

ADOLESCENCE AS A SENSITIVE PERIOD

The evidence presented thus far naturally raises the question of whether adolescence poses a sensitive period for the development of personality disorder. As discussed earlier, personality disorder onsets in adolescents and although some adolescents adhere to the normative decline in personality disorder through early adulthood, a subset of adolescents' symptoms increase or stagnate. This article has discussed how this subset likely meets clinical threshold for adultlike personality disorder categorically defined. It has also shown that personality disorder after onset in adolescence remains moderately stable, and more stable than internalizing and externalizing disorders, which are antecedents (but not consequences) of personality disorder. In addition, although internalizing and externalizing disorders are comorbid with personality disorder, personality disorder seems to uniquely associate with dysfunction (specifically in the domains on interpersonal function) and psychiatric severity. It therefore seems that something special happens in adolescence that allows internal and external mental disorders to ripen into personality disorder given the right circumstances. This article argues that adolescence represents a unique developmental period for the onset of personality disorder if internalizing and externalizing disorders are left untreated and in the context of biological vulnerability and stressful life events, because it is during adolescence that an agentic, self-determining author of the self emerges.[62]

It has long been noted that a key developmental task of adolescence is the emergence of a mature sense of self or identity, which can be identified by intrapersonal and interpersonal continuity along with the presence of an autonomous self.[63] However, to understand the process of self-maturation that consolidates during adolescence and how this leads to a sensitive period in the development of personality disorder, it is important to consider the typical trajectory of self and identity development. Harter[64] described the self as both a cognitive and social construction. As cognitive skills continuously emerge and mature through early adulthood, the organization and structure of the self are constrained by which developmental tasks an individual has achieved. Similarly, social interactions, which change form across development, have an influence on the content and valence of individuals' self-representations. Although the term identity is often used synonymously with self-related constructs such as self-representations or self-concept,[65] investigators have conceptualized identity to be the way an individual makes sense or meaning from their self-concepts.[66] Thus, identity is often studied with autobiographical narratives in which people are evaluated in their ability to integrate their autobiographical past and imagined future in a coherent way.[67] Although impairments in various aspects of the self may emerge, depending on the stage of development, it is proposed that it is a disruption in identity that characterizes the core of personality disorder.[68] The typical developmental trajectories of self-processes are described here, as well as how it is not until adolescence that an integrated and coherent identity is able to emerge.

Self-development emerges in infancy with basic functions; infants show body awareness by physical self-recognition,[69] and an early sense of agency is apparent with children as young as 6 months old carrying out and understanding others' goal-directed behavior.[70] In the second year of life, children start to show the use of personal pronouns (eg, saying "me"[71]). Very young children are able to label characteristics of themselves, suggesting a metarepresentation of the self, or the idea of "me."[72] Also beginning in early childhood, understanding of intent (both for the self and other) and theory of mind (mentalizing) is apparent, with children able to describe emotional experiences of the self and other as well as imitating and following behavioral intent of others.[73] Self-awareness is further apparent after age 3 years, with children developing the capacity for autobiographical memory and narratives, which, although largely facilitated by caregivers, represent a base by which children come to understand themselves within the greater social context.[74] These normative achievements may be disrupted by maladaptive caregiving experiences, such as abuse or neglect, which can further impair the ongoing development of the self at later ages.[75] However, because of cognitive limitations, self-representations remain largely positive, often unrealistically, and social comparison for the purpose of self-evaluation is not present, which also serves a protective function for the early self.[64] These developmental processes also play out similarly in the brain. Developmental neuroimaging studies have found that the dorsal medial prefrontal cortex (MPFC), which supports self-reflection, is one of the brain regions that develops last and comes on line in adolescence.[76] Until the MPFC matures in adolescence, social evaluation is not interpreted in any self-referential way and is unlikely to lead to self-conscious emotions and autonomic arousal.[77] Similarly, cognitive constraints on mentalizing ability in early childhood are associated with reduced awareness of others' appraisals of the self and social comparison is not used to build the concept of self.[78]

Through childhood these early emerging self-processes continue to develop with the support of increased perspective-taking skills and greater sense of self-agency.[64] As children increase in their self-understanding through middle childhood, they more spontaneously and thoughtfully begin to use this information for social comparison and self-evaluation.[79] Further, children internalize information regarding cultural values, which guide choices and interests with regard to roles, institutions, and values as well as informing self-evaluation.[80] By late childhood, self-evaluation has become more realistic, leading to a decrease in the egocentrism characteristic of early childhood and a parallel decrease in self-esteem, which can be expressed verbally.[81] This decrease in egocentrism occurs because the perspectives of others are starting to be internalized and self-evaluations are based on the standards of others.[82] Increased cognitive skills lead to children's autobiographical memories showing continuity and greater complexity as both positive and negative attributes begin to be integrated.[64] Also, as children move through the school system, social comparison becomes more salient and frequent.[83]

By early adolescence, these changes reach a peak with expanded cognitive skills, including self-consciousness and concern about the appraisal of others.[84] Social awareness has increased dramatically, particularly with regard to others' perspectives about the adolescent. This increase is caused by more mature perspective-taking abilities that are developing in the context of adolescents forming more intimate relationships with peers. The joint result of these 2 developments is shared reflection with peers such that the individual's personal goals become integrated the goals of close others.[64] Further, adolescents develop an imaginary audience, referring to the perception that others are as preoccupied with their behavior as the adolescents are, which is hypothesized to be a result of increased perspective taking and social awareness.[85] It has been suggested that the imaginary audience phenomenon is a function of the separation-individuation process of adolescence such that constructing an imaginary audience creates a sense of closeness and importance among peers as adolescents renegotiate relationships with parents, which is a reflection of the expansion of intimacy and close relationships beyond the family system into peers and potential romantic partners.[86]

Selman[87] described the ability acquired during early adolescence of stepping outside the social dyad to view the self as a social object that is observed by others. With this ability, young adolescents move to introspection to try to determine which perspectives to internalize as defining features of their identity. This process has the potential of leading to doubt and uncertainty as adolescents consider multiple perspectives and opinions.[88,89] In addition, because expanded cognitive skills mean that adolescents are able to form more abstract representations of themselves, there is a liability that self-representations become more removed from concrete behavioral evidence and therefore may be inaccurate.[90] In addition, although preadolescents' unreflective self-acceptance buffers them from potential negative self-image,[91] adolescence is a time when individuals become able and begin to examine multiple self-hypotheses that not only may be negative but also may be overwhelming based on the numerous context-dependent or relationship-dependent roles.[90] In addition, although the tendency to compartmentalize different selves from other contexts during preadolescence acted as a buffer against negative outcomes by reducing the possibility that negative attributes in one sphere may generalize to others, this is no longer the case. Another developmental advance is the ability to directly compare and contrast these different self-images that often seem contradictory to one another.[92] It is not until late adolescence that adolescents are able to integrate these various self-representations to resolve apparent contradictions; this means that adolescence is largely characterized by intrapersonal conflict, confusion, distress, and potential instability in self-representation.[93]

In addition to cognitive advancements that open the door for potential disruptions in self-development, environmental changes during this phase of life represent additional strain. Not only is high school generally a new social environment but teachers and parents hold more stringent expectations for adolescents. These environmental changes set the stage for new dimensions of social comparison (eg, academics, extra-curricular activities, appearance), with the environment placing greater emphasis on social comparison (eg, posting grades or accomplishments publicly at schools[80]). In addition, consequences of academic achievement gain greater weight with adolescents starting to consider possible future selves, such as college and potential occupations. Considering both cognitive and environmental changes that take place during adolescence, it is not surprising that individual differences in self-esteem are much more apparent during this age,[81] largely dependent on perceived adequacies in certain domains as well as perceptions of approval from others.

Despite the increased cognitive skills developed during adolescence, there remains an underdeveloped prefrontal control over these new capacities. Therefore, extreme or ineffectively applied use of these new cognitive capacities may be observed.[64] However, by late adolescence, the ability for causal coherence is developed, which allows adolescents to develop narratives that explain how chronologic events in their life are linked.[94] In addition, by midadolescence to late adolescence, individuals are able to identify overarching themes, values, or principles that integrate different events in their lives, called thematic coherence.[94] Both causal and thematic coherence are caused by the adolescent's newly acquired ability for higher-order abstractions, which is used to meaningfully integrate previous seeming contradictions in self-representations, allowing identity to consolidate. In addition, by late adolescence, individuals start to normalize potential contradictions in self-representations, which serves to reduce internal conflict.[93] As adolescents move into young adulthood, they gain a greater sense of agency as they take steps to become their future selves. Although the described developmental tasks are largely a result of cognitive development through adolescence, it is also suggested that higher level acquisitions require greater social scaffolding. Therefore, others assist adolescents in fostering new skills in order to integrate contradictory self-images and normalize potential contradictions.[95,96]

The monumental achievement of developing an agentic, self-determining author of the self during adolescence is offset by the significant vulnerability associated with failure of achieving such integration, consolidation, and coherence. It is only in the context of the normative emergence of the agentic self that disturbed self-other function can develop and be observed and diagnosed. The authors suggest that adolescence poses for the first time a developmental opportunity for DSM-5 section III criterion A (impaired function in self-other relatedness) to emerge as a qualitatively different level of mental disorder beyond internalizing and externalizing disorders, and on the severity pathway toward psychotic disorders.[97] As described elsewhere,[97] correlated but distinct internalizing and externalizing problems begin to emerge in preadolescence in the form of anxiety and depressive symptoms predominantly in girls, and ADHD and conduct problems predominantly in boys. If these disorders are left untreated, and in the context of predisposing biological vulnerabilities and interacting stressful life events, internalizing and externalizing problems form a platform for the development of personality disorder during adolescence, characterized by a qualitatively different levels of mental disorder in the form of maladaptive self-other relatedness; qualitatively different because this new level of mental disorder cannot be adequately captured by dispositional traits associated with internalizing and externalizing problems (ie, temperamental traits are insufficient to describe personality disorder because they constitute merely one component of the personality system).[98] Personality, and therefore personality disorder, is integrated and organized in nature[99] and the task of organizing traits into a coherent whole becomes a major focus of adolescence. Just as the Big Five can readily be observed in preadolescent children, so can maladaptive dispositional traits (DSM-5 section III, criterion B; eg, neuroticism, antagonism, disagreeableness, and psychoticism), which can be readily evaluated by assessing internalizing and externalizing mental disorders.[100] With the emergence of an agentic, self-determining actor, self-narrative becomes a vehicle by which traits are made sense of in the context of past, current, and future events. Although this process of identity formation proceeds smoothly for most adolescents, for some this process is characterized by incoherence, inconsistency, confusion, and distress, ultimately resulting in a personality structure resembling DSM-5 section III criterion A personality function. The progression from internalizing/externalizing to a next level of mental disorder characterized by maladaptive self-other function brings with it increases in psychiatric severity (p factor[101]), more persistence and stability, and lower population-based prevalence rates of disorder.[97] Kernberg's[102] model shares features with the proposed developmental model in that borderline disorder is identified as having heuristic value in representing what is common to all personality disorders (criterion A) and it lies on the severity pathway between internalizing/externalizing and psychotic mental disorders. This article reinterprets Kernberg's[102] original model in the light of developmental mental disorder data from the last decade and proposes that criterion A (personality disorder beyond maladaptive traits) cannot be diagnosed in any meaningful way until children reach adolescence to begin the task of integrating disparate representations into a coherent whole in the service of identity formation.

REFERENCES

1. Sharp C. Bridging the gap: the assessment and treatment of adolescent personality disorder in routine clinical care. Arch Dis Child 2017;102(1):103–8.
2. Chanen AM, Kaess M. Developmental pathways to borderline personality disorder. Curr Psychiatry Rep 2012;14(1):45–53.
3. Chanen AM, Sharp C, Hoffman P, et al, Global Alliance for Prevention and Early Intervention for Borderline Personality Disorder. Prevention and early intervention for borderline personality disorder: a novel public health priority. World Psychiatry 2017;16(2):215–6.
4. Sharp C, Fonagy P. Practitioner review: borderline personality disorder in adolescence - recent conceptualization, intervention, and implications for clinical practice. J Child Psychol Psychiatry 2015;56(12):1266–88.
5. Sharp C, Wright AGC, Fowler JC, et al. The structure of personality pathology: both general ('g') and specific ('s') factors? J Abnorm Psychol 2015;124(2): 387–98.
6. Cohen P, Crawford TN, Johnson JG, et al. The children in the community study of developmental course of personality disorder. J Pers Disord 2005;19(5): 466–86.
7. De Clercq B, Van Leeuwen K, van den Noortgate W, et al. Childhood personality pathology: dimensional stability and change. Dev Psychopathol 2009;21(3): 853–69.
8. De Clercq B, De Fruyt F, Mervielde I. Construction of the dimensional personality symptom item pool in children (DIPSI). Unpubl Manuscr Ghent Univ Belg. 2003.
9. Wright AGC, Pincus AL, Lenzenweger MF. Modeling stability and change in borderline personality disorder symptoms using the revised interpersonal adjective scales–big five (IASR–B5). J Pers Assess 2010;92(6):501–13.
10. Loranger AW, Sartorius N, Andreoli A, et al. The International Personality Disorder Examination: the World Health Organization/Alcohol, Drug Abuse, and

Mental Health Administration international pilot study of personality disorders. Arch Gen Psychiatry 1994;51(3):215–24.
11. Trapnell PD, Wiggins JS. Extension of the interpersonal adjective scales to include the big five dimensions of personality. J Pers Soc Psychol 1990;59(4): 781–90.
12. Spitzer RL, Williams JB, Gibbon M, et al. Structured clinical interview for DSM-III-R personality disorders (SCID-II). New York: New York State Psychiatric Department; 1989.
13. Zanarini MC. Childhood interview for DSM-IV borderline personality disorder (CI-BPD). Belmont (MA): McLean Hosp; 2003.
14. Loranger AW, Susman VL, Oldham JM, et al. The personality disorder examination: a preliminary report. J Pers Disord 1987;1(1):1–13.
15. Zanarini MC, Vujanovic AA, Parachini EA, et al. A screening measure for BPD: the McLean screening instrument for borderline personality disorder (MSI-BPD). J Pers Disord 2003;17(6):568–73.
16. Butcher JN, Williams CL, Graham JR, et al. Minnesota multiphasic personality inventory-adolescent (MMPI-A): manual for administration, scoring, and interpretation. Minneapolis (MN): University of Minnesota Press; 1992.
17. Poreh AM, Rawlings D, Claridge G, et al. The BPQ: a scale for the assessment of borderline personality based on DSM-IV criteria. J Pers Disord 2006;20(3): 247–60.
18. Crick NR, Murray-Close D, Woods K. Borderline personality features in childhood: a short-term longitudinal study. Dev Psychopathol 2005;17(4):1051–70.
19. Morey LC. The personality assessment inventory - adolescent professional manual. Odessa (FL): Psychological Assessment Resources; 2007.
20. Krueger RF, Derringer J, Markon KE, et al. Initial construction of a maladaptive personality trait model and inventory for DSM-5. Psychol Med 2012;42(9): 1879–90.
21. Sharp C, Mosko O, Chang B, et al. The cross-informant concordance and concurrent validity of the borderline personality features scale for children in a community sample of boys. Clin Child Psychol Psychiatry 2011;16(3):335–49.
22. Sharp C, Steinberg L, Temple J, et al. An 11-item measure to assess borderline traits in adolescents: refinement of the BPFSC using IRT. Personal Disord 2014; 5(1):70–8.
23. Chanen AM, Jackson HJ, McGorry PD, et al. Two-year stability of personality disorder in older adolescent outpatients. J Pers Disord 2004;18(6):526–41.
24. Ha C, Balderas JC, Zanarini MC, et al. Psychiatric comorbidity in hospitalized adolescents with borderline personality disorder. J Clin Psychiatry 2014;75(5): e457–64.
25. Levy KN, Becker DF, Grilo CM, et al. Concurrent and predictive validity of the personality disorder diagnosis in adolescent patients. Am J Psychiatry 1999; 156(10):1522–8.
26. Zanarini MC, Horwood J, Wolke D, et al. Prevalence of DSM-IV borderline personality disorder in two community samples: 6,330 English 11-year-olds and 34,653 American adults. J Pers Disord 2011;25(5):607–19.
27. Johnson JG, Cohen P, Kasen S, et al. Cumulative prevalence of personality disorders between adolescence and adulthood. Acta Psychiatr Scand 2008; 118(5):410–3.
28. Lewinsohn PM, Rohde P, Seeley JR, et al. Axis II psychopathology as a function of axis I disorders in childhood and adolescence. J Am Acad Child Adolesc Psychiatry 1997;36(12):1752–9.

29. Leung S-W, Leung F. Construct validity and prevalence rate of borderline personality disorder among Chinese adolescents. J Pers Disord 2009;23(5):494–513.

30. Iacono WG, Carlson SR, Taylor J, et al. Behavioral disinhibition and the development of substance-use disorders: findings from the Minnesota Twin Family Study. Dev Psychopathol 1999;11(4):869–900.

31. Bornovalova MA, Hicks BM, Iacono WG, et al. Stability, change, and heritability of borderline personality disorder traits from adolescence to adulthood: a longitudinal twin study. Dev Psychopathol 2009;21(4):1335–53.

32. Roberts BW, DelVecchio WF. The rank-order consistency of personality traits from childhood to old age: a quantitative review of longitudinal studies. Psychol Bull 2000;126(1):3–25.

33. Achenbach TM. Integrative guide for the 1991 CBCL/4-18, YSR, and TRF profiles. Vermont (MA): Department of Psychiatry, University of Vermont; 1991.

34. Verhulst FC. Manual for the CBCL/4-18 (in Dutch). Rotterdam (the Netherlands): Department of Child and Adolescent Psychiatry, Erasmus University; 1996.

35. Wright AGC, Zalewski M, Hallquist MN, et al. Developmental trajectories of borderline personality disorder symptoms and psychosocial functioning in adolescence. J Pers Disord 2016;30(3):351–72.

36. Zanarini MC, Frankenburg FR, Reich DB, et al. Attainment and stability of sustained symptomatic remission and recovery among patients with borderline personality disorder and axis II comparison subjects: a 16-year prospective follow-up study. Am J Psychiatry 2012;169(5):476–83.

37. Stepp SD, Lazarus SA, Byrd AL. A systematic review of risk factors prospectively associated with borderline personality disorder: taking stock and moving forward. Personal Disord 2016;7(4):316–23.

38. Belsky DW, Caspi A, Arseneault L, et al. Etiological features of borderline personality related characteristics in a birth cohort of 12-year-old children. Dev Psychopathol 2012;24(1):251–65.

39. Stepp SD, Olino TM, Klein DN, et al. Unique influences of adolescent antecedents on adult borderline personality disorder features. Personal Disord 2013; 4(3):223–9.

40. Bornovalova MA, Hicks BM, Iacono WG, et al. Longitudinal-twin study of borderline personality disorder traits and substance use in adolescence: developmental change, reciprocal effects, and genetic and environmental influences. Personal Disord 2013;4(1):23–32.

41. Krabbendam AA, Colins OF, Doreleijers TA, et al. Personality disorders in previously detained adolescent females: a prospective study. Am J Orthop 2015; 85(1):63–71.

42. Sharp C, Kalpakci A, Mellick W, et al. First evidence of a prospective relation between avoidance of internal states and borderline personality disorder features in adolescents. Eur Child Adolesc Psychiatry 2015;24(3):283–90.

43. Rey JM, Morris-Yates A, Singh M, et al. Continuities between psychiatric disorders in adolescents and personality disorders in young adults. Am J Psychiatry 1995;152(6):895–900.

44. Burke JD, Stepp SD, Hipwell AE, et al. Adolescent disruptive behavior and borderline personality disorder symptoms in young adult men. J Abnorm Child Psychol 2012;40(1):35–44.

45. Stepp SD, Burke JD, Hipwell AE, et al. Trajectories of attention deficit hyperactivity disorder and oppositional defiant disorder symptoms as precursors of borderline personality disorder symptoms in adolescent girls. J Abnorm Child Psychol 2012;40(1):7–20.

46. Lazarus SA, Beardslee J, Pedersen SL, et al. A within-person analysis of the association between borderline personality disorder and alcohol use in adolescents. J Abnorm Child Psychol 2017;45(6):1157–67.
47. Kaess M, von Ceumern-Lindenstjerna I-A, Parzer P, et al. Axis I and II comorbidity and psychosocial functioning in female adolescents with borderline personality disorder. Psychopathology 2013;46(1):55–62.
48. Speranza M, Revah-Levy A, Cortese S, et al. ADHD in adolescents with borderline personality disorder. BMC Psychiatry 2011;11(1):158–67.
49. Chanen AM, Jovev M, Jackson HJ. Adaptive functioning and psychiatric symptoms in adolescents with borderline personality disorder. J Clin Psychiatry 2007; 68(2):297–306.
50. Achenbach TM. Manual for the Youth Self-Report and 1991 profile. Burlington (NJ): Department of Psychiatry, University of Vermont; 1991.
51. Sharp C. Locating BPD within the internalizing-externalizing spectrum in adolescents. Presented at the Annual meeting for the North American Society for the Study of Personality Disorder (NASSPD). Boston (MD), April 2014
52. Zanarini MC, Frankenburg FR, Dubo ED, et al. Axis I comorbidity of borderline personality disorder. Am J Psychiatry 1998;155(12):1733–9.
53. James LM, Taylor J. Revisiting the structure of mental disorders: borderline personality disorder and the internalizing/externalizing spectra. Br J Clin Psychol 2008;47(4):361–80.
54. Eaton NR, Krueger RF, Keyes KM, et al. Borderline personality disorder comorbidity: relationship to the internalizing-externalizing structure of common mental disorders. Psychol Med 2011;41(5):1041–50.
55. Achenbach TM. Manual for the Young Adult Self-Report and Young Adult Behavior checklist. Burlington (NJ): Department of Psychiatry, University of Vermont; 1997.
56. Sharp C, Green KL, Yaroslavsky I, et al. The incremental validity of borderline personality disorder relative to major depressive disorder for suicidal ideation and deliberate self-harm in adolescents. J Pers Disord 2014;26(6):927–38.
57. Hankin BL. Adolescent depression: description, causes, and interventions. Epilepsy Behav 2006;8(1):102–14.
58. Murray L, Creswell C, Cooper PJ. The development of anxiety disorders in childhood: an integrative review. Psychol Med 2009;39(9):1413–23.
59. Sander JB, McCarty CA. Youth depression in the family context: familial risk factors and models of treatment. Clin Child Fam Psychol Rev 2005;8(3):203–19.
60. Deater-Deckard K, Dodge KA, Bates JE, et al. Multiple risk factors in the development of externalizing behavior problems: group and individual differences. Dev Psychopathol 1998;10(3):469–93.
61. Shaw DS, Owens EB, Vondra JI, et al. Early risk factors and pathways in the development of early disruptive behavior problems. Dev Psychopathol 1996; 8(4):679–99.
62. McAdams DP, Olson BD. Personality development: continuity and change over the life course. Annu Rev Psychol 2010;61:517–42.
63. Erikson EH. Identity, youth and crisis. New York: Norton Company; 1968.
64. Harter S. Emerging self-processes during childhood and adolescence. In: Leary MR, Tangney JP, editors. Handbook of self and identity. 2nd edition. New York: Guilford Press; 2012. p. 680–715.
65. Swann WB, Bosson JK. Self and identity. In: Fiske ST, Gilbert DT, Lindzey G, editors. Handbook of social psychology. 5th edition. Hoboken (NJ): John Wiley.; 2010. p. 589–628.

66. McLean KC, Pratt MW. Life's little (and big) lessons: identity statuses and meaning-making in the turning point narratives of emerging adults. Dev Psychol 2006;42(4):714–22.
67. McAdams DP, McLean KC. Narrative identity. Curr Dir Psychol Sci 2013;22(3): 233–8.
68. Schmeck K, Schluter-Muller S, Foelsch PA, et al. The role of identity in the DSM-5 classification of personality disorders. Child Adolesc Psychiatry Ment Health 2013;7(1):27–37.
69. Rochat P. Five levels of self-awareness as they unfold early in life. Conscious Cogn 2003;12(4):717–31.
70. Biro S, Leslie AM. Infants' perception of goal-directed actions: development through cue-based bootstrapping. Dev Sci 2007;10(3):379–98.
71. Lewis M, Ramsay D. Development of self-recognition, personal pronoun use, and pretend play during the 2nd year. Child Dev 2004;75(6):1821–31.
72. Lewis M. The emergence of consciousness and its role in human development. Ann N Y Acad Sci 2003;1001(1):104–33.
73. Bosacki SL. Children's theory of mind, self-perceptions, and peer relations: a longitudinal study. Infant Child Dev 2015;24(2):175–88.
74. Reese E, Yan C, Jack F, et al. Emerging identities: narrative and self from early childhood to early adolescence. In: McLean KC, Pasupathi M, editors. Narrative development in adolescence: creating the storied self. Boston: Springer US; 2010. p. 23–43.
75. Cicchetti D, Toth SL. Developmental Psychopathology and Preventive Intervention. In: Renninger KA, Sigel IE, Damon W, et al, editors. Handbook of child psychology: Child psychology in practice. Hoboken (NJ): John Wiley & Sons Inc; 2006. p. 497–547.
76. Shaw P, Kabani NJ, Lerch JP, et al. Neurodevelopmental trajectories of the human cerebral cortex. J Neurosci 2008;28(14):3586–94.
77. Somerville LH, Jones RM, Ruberry EJ, et al. The medial prefrontal cortex and the emergence of self-conscious emotion in adolescence. Psychol Sci 2013;24(8): 1554–62.
78. Sebastian C, Burnett S, Blakemore S-J. Development of the self-concept during adolescence. Trends Cogn Sci 2008;12(11):441–6.
79. Thompson RA. The development of the person: social understanding, relationships, conscience, self. In: Eisenberg N, Damon W, Lerner RM, editors. Handbook of child psychology: Social, emotional, and personality development. Hoboken (NJ): John Wiley & Sons Inc; 2007. p. 24–98.
80. Nelson K, Fivush R. The emergence of autobiographical memory: a social cultural developmental theory. Psychol Rev 2004;111(2):486–511.
81. Harter S. The development of self-esteem. In: Kernis MH, editor. Self-esteem issues and answers: a sourcebook of current perspectives. New York: Psychology Press; 2006. p. 144–50.
82. Connell JP, Wellborn JG. Competence, autonomy, and relatedness: a motivational analysis of self-system processes. In: Gunnar MR, Sroufe LA, editors. Self processes and development: the Minnesota symposia on child psychology, vol. 23. Hillsdale (NJ): Lawrence Erlbaum Associates; 1991. p. 43–77.
83. Eccles JS, Roeser RW. Schools, academic motivation, and stage-environment fit. In: Lerner RM, Steinberg L, editors. Handbook of adolescent psychology: individual bases of adolescent development. New York: John Wiley; 2009. p. 404–34.
84. Lerner RM, Brentano C, Dowling EM, et al. Positive youth development: thriving as the basis of personhood and civil society. New Dir Youth Dev 2002,(95):11–33.

85. Schwartz PD, Maynard AM, Uzelac SM. Adolescent egocentrism: a contemporary view. Adolescence 2008;43(171):441–8.
86. Lapsley DK. Toward an integrated theory of adolescent ego development: the "new look" at adolescent egocentrism. Am J Orthop 1993;63(4):562–71.
87. Selman RL. The promotion of social awareness: powerful lessons from the partnership of developmental theory and classroom practice. New York: Russell Sage Foundation; 2003.
88. Luyckx K, Goossens L, Soenens B. A developmental contextual perspective on identity construction in emerging adulthood: change dynamics in commitment formation and commitment evaluation. Dev Psychol 2006;42(2):366–80.
89. Meeus W, van de Schoot R, Keijsers L, et al. On the progression and stability of adolescent identity formation: a five-wave longitudinal study in early-to-middle and middle-to-late adolescence. Child Dev 2010;81(5):1565–81.
90. Harter S. Distinguished contributions in psychology. The construction of the self: a developmental perspective. New York: Guilford Press; 1999.
91. Thomaes S, Brummelman E, Sedikides C. Why most children think well of themselves. Child Dev 2017;88(6):1873–84.
92. Lichtwarck-Aschoff A, van Geert P, Bosma H, et al. Time and identity: a framework for research and theory formation. Dev Rev 2008;28(3):370–400.
93. Harter S, Monsour A. Development analysis of conflict caused by opposing attributes in the adolescent self-portrait. Dev Psychol 1992;28(2):251–60.
94. Bluck S, Habermas T. Extending the study of autobiographical memory: thinking back about life across the life span. Rev Gen Psychol 2001;5(2):135–47.
95. Fischer KW, Bidell TR. Dynamic development of action, thought, and emotion. In: Damon W, Lerner RM, editors. Theoretical models of human development. Handbook of child psychology. 2006. p. 313–99.
96. Kuhn D, Franklin S. The Second Decade: What Develops (and How). In: Kuhn D, Siegler RS, Damon W, editors. Handbook of child psychology: Cognition, perception, and language. Hoboken (NJ): John Wiley & Sons Inc; 2006. p. 953–93.
97. Sharp C, Wall K. Personality pathology grows up: adolescence as a sensitive period. Curr Opin Psychol 2018;21:111–6.
98. Livesley WJ, Jang KL. Toward an empirically based classification of personality disorder. J Pers Disord 2000;14(2):137–51.
99. McAdams DP. A conceptual history of personality psychology. In: Hogan R, Johnson JA, Briggs SR, editors. Handbook of personality psychology. San Diego (CA): Academic Press; 1997. p. 3–39.
100. De Clercq B, Decuyper M, De Caluwé E. Developmental manifestations of borderline personality pathology from an age-specific dimensional personality disorder trait framework. In: Sharp C, Tackett JL, editors. Handbook of borderline personality disorder in children and adolescents. New York: Springer New York; 2014. p. 81–94.
101. Caspi A, Houts RM, Belsky DW, et al. The p factor: one general psychopathology factor in the structure of psychiatric disorders? Clin Psychol Sci 2014;2(2):119–37.
102. Kernberg OF. The couch at sea: psychoanalytic studies of group and organizational leadership. Int J Group Psychother 1984;34(1):5–23.

The Longitudinal Course of Borderline Personality Disorder

Christina M. Temes, PhD*, Mary C. Zanarini, EdD

KEYWORDS

- Borderline personality disorder • Course • Longitudinal research • Remission
- Recovery

KEY POINTS

- Long-term follow-up studies indicate that most patients with borderline personality disorder (BPD) experience a remission of the disorder, and many have a recovery.
- Predictors of good outcomes include factors related to personal capacity and competence, psychosocial history, chronicity of illness, comorbidity, and levels of normal personality traits.
- Predictors of poor outcomes include factors related to greater severity and chronicity of illness, higher degrees of comorbidity, and history of childhood adversity.
- Acute symptoms (eg, self-mutilation) remit more rapidly and recur more rarely than temperamental symptoms (eg, chronic depressed affect).
- Never achieving recovery from BPD is associated with vocational impairment and physical health problems.

Prior to advances in research and treatment development in the last 30 years, borderline personality disorder (BPD) was historically viewed as a chronic, if not lifelong, disorder that was not amenable to change. Since this time, several small- and large-scale studies of the naturalistic course of BPD have been conducted. Generally, findings from these studies, reviewed herein, suggest that the course of BPD is much more variable and that many patients experience promising outcomes.

STUDIES OF THE COURSE OF BORDERLINE PERSONALITY DISORDER: REMISSION AND GLOBAL OUTCOMES
Small-Scale Studies of Borderline Personality Disorder Course

The earliest studies of the course of BPD were small, short-term prospective studies that were conducted before the Diagnostic and Statistical Manual of Mental Disorders,

Disclosure Statement: The authors have no conflicts of interest to disclose.
Department of Psychiatry, McLean Hospital, Harvard Medical School, 115 Mill Street, Belmont, MA 02478, USA
* Corresponding author.
E-mail address: ctemes@mclean.harvard.edu

Psychiatr Clin N Am 41 (2018) 685–694
https://doi.org/10.1016/j.psc.2018.07.002
psych.theclinics.com

Third Edition (DSM-III) criteria for the disorder were established.[1-5] Generally, these studies found that up to 2.5 years following index admission, most patients with BPD remained functionally impaired,[2,4] with 1 study finding that levels of functional impairment in patients with BPD were the same as in patients with schizophrenia.[4] Additionally, most patients with BPD were employed but working in low-level jobs and/or had impoverished social lives.[2,4] When the length of follow-up was extended to 5 to 7 years, similar functional outcomes were observed,[3,5] although patients with BPD were found to be functioning better socially than patients with schizophrenia, for whom social relationships had deteriorated.[5]

After DSM criteria for BPD were defined, many smaller-scale studies were conducted in the 1980s and 1990s to examine the course of the disorder.[6] These studies included both prospective follow-up studies[7-18] and follow-back studies.[19-21] The range of follow-up duration was 6 months to 7 years and generally included only 1 follow-up assessment, although 1 study added additional waves of follow-up.[22,23]

Findings from these studies were mixed, although many of these studies found that patients with BPD continued to meet criteria for BPD and to be impaired across a variety of domains, particularly in vocational and social realms.[8,12,17,20,21] Additionally, many of the studied patients continued to struggle with symptoms of comorbid conditions, particularly mood, anxiety, and substance use disorders, over the course of follow-up.[7-10,12,13,21] That being said, many of these studies also found that patients with BPD experienced reductions in several symptomatic outcomes (eg, impulsivity or self-harm) and/or exhibited significant improvements in psychosocial functioning over follow-up.[10,11,14,16,18] It should be noted that there was considerable methodological variability in these studies, including several design limitations that limit the generalizability of some findings. These limitations include the use of small samples, unstandardized diagnostic procedures (eg, chart review or clinical diagnosis), varying lengths of follow-up within the same study, high attrition rates, and having only 1 follow-up wave.

Large-Scale Follow-Back Studies

In the 1980s, 4 larger-scale, longer-term follow-back studies[24-27] were conducted. Findings from these studies were more optimistic regarding the long-term course for BPD than the previous longitudinal studies. Three of the 4 studies used samples treated at long-term residential facilities.[24,26,27] McGlashan[24] studied patients who were initially treated at the Chestnut Lodge, a small, private psychiatric hospital. These patients were identified and diagnosed by retrospective chart review and then were located and assessed on average 15 years after discharge. In general, 80% of borderline patients (more than comparison groups) had a reasonable outcome (ie, with moderate symptoms) at follow-up; many had a good outcome, and a few had a full recovery. Most borderline patients were eventually able to work full time and had regular social contact. In a similar study, Plakun[26] examined symptom course in patients with BPD who were initially inpatients at Austen Riggs, a small, private, long-term stay psychiatric hospital. Patients were assessed via questionnaire on average 14 years following index admission. Results from this study indicated that borderline patients' functioning improved significantly over time, with patients functioning similarly to those with major affective disorder (MAD) on follow-up. That being said, borderline patients with comorbid MAD functioned worse at follow-up than those without this comorbidity. Stone[27] traced and assessed 502 patients (206 of whom were diagnosed with BPD via retrospective chart review) who had been treated on a long-term, intensive therapy unit at the

New York State Psychiatric Institute. He found that two-thirds of the patients with BPD had a good outcome at the time of follow-up, further noting that 40% had a quick trajectory to a good global outcome.

In an effort to examine the long-term course of BPD in patients recruited from a more representative treatment setting, via chart review, Paris and colleagues[25] identified and diagnosed patients (mostly inpatients) treated at the Jewish General Hospital in Montreal and located/assessed these patients on average 15 years after discharge. A subset of these patients was again located and reassessed 12 years later, on average 27 years after discharge.[28] Findings from these studies were largely consistent with those found in the other long-term follow-back studies. At the 15-year follow-back interview, most patients evidenced significant improvements in functioning and reductions in symptoms, with 75% no longer diagnosable as borderline. By the 27-year assessment,[28] patients had continued to improve; they functioned generally in the normal range across a broad number of functioning measures, and 92% were remitted for BPD.

In general, results from the longer-term follow-back studies suggest that when followed for longer periods, borderline patients exhibit significant reductions in symptoms and improvements in functioning, with most patients functioning at least moderately well. Specifically, across these studies, patients exhibited mean scores of 63 to 67 on the Global Assessment Score (GAS[29]) or the Health Sickness Rating Scale (HSRS[30]), precursors of the Global Assessment of Functioning (GAF[1]).

Prediction of Outcome in Follow-Back Studies

In addition to course, predictors of good and poor global outcome were examined in each of the large-scale follow-back studies.[24–27] Good global outcome in these studies was predicted by a variety of factors related to personal capacity, psychosocial history, comorbidity, and levels of normal personality traits. Predictors of good outcome included being unusually talented or (if female) physically attractive,[27] having a higher IQ,[24,27] not having a history of parental divorce,[31] absence of narcissistic entitlement,[31] presence of physically self-destructive acts during the index treatment,[8] and higher levels of agreeableness.[32] Poor outcomes were predicted by a variety of factors related to greater severity and chronicity of illness, higher degrees of comorbidity, and history of childhood adversity. More specifically, predictors of poor outcome included higher levels of affective instability,[33] chronic dysphoria,[28] younger age at first treatment,[28] longer length of previous hospitalizations,[33] history of antisocial behavior,[27] history of substance abuse,[27] family history of psychiatric illness,[28] history of parental brutality,[32] and having a problematic relationship with one's mother (but not father).[34]

Although important in their scope and using state-of-the-art methods of their time, these studies were nonetheless limited methodologically. For one, length of follow-up was not consistent across participants in each study but was rather an average across participants, thus making conclusions based on timing less precise. Second, patients were diagnosed using retrospective chart review. Third, not all interviewers or raters were blind to diagnosis. Fourth, patients had to provide retrospective reports for at times very long periods of follow-up, which could have led to inaccuracies or biases in reporting. Fifth, only 1 long-term follow-up study used a socioeconomically diverse sample. Finally, in several of these studies, a much smaller pool of patients agreed to participate/complete assessments than the pool initially identified by chart review, perhaps indicating some selection bias in the final samples.

Prospective, Longitudinal Follow-up Studies

In part to address some of these design limitations, beginning in the 1990s, 2 National Institutes of Mental Health (NIMH)-funded prospective longitudinal studies were launched. Methodologically, these studies differed from previous investigations in that identified participants were diagnosed via standardized assessment and then followed at regular intervals for multiple follow-up waves.

The first large-scale prospective follow-up study of BPD was the McLean Study of Adult Development (MSAD),[35] which began in 1992 and is ongoing (currently in its 26th year). In this study, 290 patients with BPD and a comparison group of 72 patients with other personality disorders (OPD) were recruited from inpatient units at McLean Hospital. Patients were diagnosed using structured diagnostic assessments and administered a broad range of psychosocial assessments. Patients were then followed and reassessed every 2 years by raters blind to previous diagnoses. In terms of remission, 99% of borderline patients achieved a symptomatic remission (defined as a period of 2 years in which they did not meet diagnostic criteria for BPD) by 16-year follow-up.[36] That being said, patients with BPD were slower to remit from their primary disorder than patients with OPD. In terms of global outcome, MSAD researchers defined good recovery as a global assessment of functioning (GAF) score of 61, which was further operationalized as concurrent remission of BPD and good psychosocial and good full-time vocational functioning. They found that 50% of borderline patients had achieved this outcome by 10-year follow-up.[37] Sixty percent had achieved this outcome by 16-year follow-up,[32] with the rate remaining the same at 20-year follow-up.[38] Zanarini and colleagues[38] later examined a more stringent outcome of excellent recovery" which was defined as a GAF score of 71 and operationalized as meeting all the criteria of good recovery plus absence of a comorbid disorder that interfered with functioning. It was found that only 39% of borderline patients (compared with 73% of OPD patients) achieved this outcome by 20-year follow-up.

A second large-scale prospective longitudinal study of the naturalistic course of personality disorders, the Collaborative Longitudinal Personality Disorders Study (CLPS[39]), began in 1996. CLPS was a multisite study of individuals with BPD (n = 175), cluster C OPD (n = 312), and major depressive disorder (MDD; n = 95) who were recruited from outpatient clinics, inpatient units, and the community. Like MSAD, patients were initially diagnosed using structured diagnostic interviews and completed a full psychosocial battery at baseline. They were then reassessed annually for 10 years (with a more thorough battery administered every 2 years). Around a quarter of patients experienced a remission (defined as meeting less than 2 symptoms of BPD) lasting at least 2 months by the 2-year follow-up period.[40] By the 10-year follow-up period, 85% of borderline patients achieved a remission lasting 12 months or more, and 91% had at least a 2-month remission.[41] Patients with BPD were slower to remit than patients with MDD. A GAF score of 71 (defined by the GAF scale's narrative description) represented a good global outcome in the CLPS study. It was found that 21% of borderline patients achieved this outcome (compared with 48% of comparison subjects with cluster C OPDs) by the 10-year follow-up period.

PREDICTORS AND CORRELATES OF LONGITUDINAL OUTCOME
Prediction of Remission from Borderline Personality Disorder

As a part of longitudinal investigations, researchers have also been interested in determining the best predictors of outcome. Predictors of remission over long-term follow-up (ie, 10 years) were only examined in MSAD.[42] Predictors of remission were multifactorial and included the following: younger age at baseline, absence of a history of childhood sexual abuse, no family history of substance use disorder, good vocational record prior to index admission, absence of an anxious cluster personality disorder, lower levels of neuroticism, and higher levels of agreeableness.

Prediction of Recovery

Prospective predictors of recovery (ie, concurrent remission of BPD and good psychosocial and good full-time vocational functioning) were examined in the MSAD sample.[43] The best set of predictors included factors related to personal competence, illness chronicity, comorbidity, and temperament. Specifically, predictors of recovery in MSAD included having a higher IQ, history of no prior hospitalizations, absence of a comorbid anxious cluster OPD, good full-time vocational functioning prior to index admission, higher levels of extraversion, and higher levels of agreeableness. Additionally, 1 study using this sample[38] examined the more stringent positive outcome of excellent recovery, defined as concurrent remission of BPD, good psychosocial and full-time vocational functioning, and absence of a comorbid disorder that interfered with functioning. This outcome was predicted by factors related to capacity and competence (ie, higher IQ, good childhood work history, good adult vocational record) and temperament (ie, lower trait neuroticism, higher trait agreeableness).

Differences Between Recovered Versus Nonrecovered Borderline Patients

Borderline patients who achieve a recovery from the disorder also differ from nonrecovered patients on other important outcomes. Findings from MSAD have highlighted that 2 important areas that distinguish these groups of patients are vocational functioning and physical health difficulties. With respect to the former, it has been found that vocational impairment is the leading reason why patients do not achieve or maintain recovery,[37,44] although the reasons for this are likely multifaceted (eg, caused by symptoms of BPD or other comorbid conditions, or caused patient competence or resilience). Recovery status also differentiates patients on other outcomes, notably in the realm of physical health, which may in turn impact vocational and other domains of functioning. Patients who never experience a recovery from the disorder are more likely than recovered patients to experience serious medical problems, engage in poor health behaviors (eg, pack-a-day smoking, lack of regular exercise), utilize costly medical services, and experience poor sleep quality.[45–49] Additionally, those who demonstrate poorer indicators of health over time, such as increased cumulative body mass index (BMI), are more likely to report adverse psychological outcomes (eg, self-mutilation and dissociation) and other functional deficits (eg, lack of life partner or poor work/school functioning) over time. Additionally, nonrecovered patients are more likely to die prematurely (by any cause) than recovered patients.[50]

STABILITY AND FLUIDITY OF GLOBAL AND SYMPTOMATIC OUTCOMES

The designs of the prospective longitudinal follow-up studies with regular follow-up intervals allowed researchers to examine the fluidity of outcomes in more granular ways. One way in which this has been examined is looking at outcomes in terms of stability and relapse.

In terms of remission, as noted previously, remissions were common in both MSAD and CLPS. In MSAD, varying lengths of remission were studied, and all were found to be common.[36] Specifically, 99% of borderline patients had a 2-year remission; 95% had a remission that lasted 4 years, and 90% had a remission that lasted 6 years. Additionally, 78% had a remission that lasted 8 years. The authors similarly looked at the rate of recurrences, and how the rate of recurrence corresponded to the duration of the remissions. In general, the risk of relapse decreased the longer the remission lasted. In particular, 36% of those with only a 2-year remission had a recurrence, but the rate dropped to 25% for 4-year remissions, 19% for 6-year remissions, and 10% for 8-year remissions. In CLPS, the rate of recurrence at 10-year follow-up was 11% for patients who had at least a 12-month remission previously.[41] This relapse rate was lower than that which was observed for other personality disorders and for MDD.

As noted previously, recoveries are rarer than remissions, and longer-lasting recoveries are rarer still among borderline patients.[36] In MSAD, around 60% of borderline patients achieved a good recovery lasting at least 2 years,[36] and 54% had a recovery lasting 4 years. Forty-four percent had a recovery lasting 6 years, and only 40% had a recovery lasting 8 years (compared with 75% of personality-disordered comparison subjects). Thus, recovery of longer duration is rarer for patients with BPD than patients with other personality disorders. Similarly, loss of recovery was more common than loss of remission status in patients with BPD. For those who had a recovery of 2 years, 44% went on to lose their recovery status; however, the rate of loss of recovery decreased the longer the recovery lasted (ie, 32% for 4-year recovery, 26% for 6-year recovery, and 20% for 8-year recovery). In many cases, these losses of recovery status may be a function of the vocational instability and physical health impairments discussed previously.

Symptom-Specific Change

When examining subsyndromal BPD, studies have indicated that patterns of change over time may differ by symptom type. Studies have indicated that acute symptoms of BPD—dramatic, typically behavioral symptoms specific to BPD (eg, self-mutilation)—tend to remit more rapidly than temperamental symptoms of the disorder, which are more chronic, generally internal symptoms that are less specific to BPD (eg, chronic depressed affect[41,51]). Additionally, when symptoms are examined over time, there is a substantial degree of waxing and waning.

In an examination of the course of individual symptoms over 16 years of follow-up in the MSAD study, Zanarini and colleagues[52] found that remissions (lasting at least 2 years) of all symptoms were extremely common (median rate of 93%). These authors also found that recurrences of symptoms were common after only a 2-year remission (median rate of 75%) but less common when remission of the symptom lasted at least 4 years (median rate of 56%). In terms of symptom types, it was found that over 16 years of follow-up, acute symptoms had higher remission rates and lower recurrence rates than temperamental symptoms, whereas the reverse pattern (ie, lower remission rates, higher recurrence rates) was observed for temperamental symptoms. A similar division was found in CLPS,[53] in which certain symptoms representing pathologic variants of normal personality (eg, affective instability or inappropriate intense anger) were found to be most stable, whereas symptoms representing dysfunctional behaviors undertaken to cope with these dysfunctional traits (eg, self-injury) were found to be least stable.

SUMMARY

Overall, findings from longitudinal studies suggest that most patients with BPD will experience a favorable outcome over the course of their lives. Specifically, long-term studies have consistently found that most patients eventually function in the moderate range, and remissions of the disorder are common. The likelihood of having a good outcome (eg, recovery) increases with time, though rates appear to stabilize over the course of long-term follow-up. It is rarer for patients to have an excellent outcome, but this does happen for a sizable portion of them (32%[38]). Research regarding predictors of outcome has identified several positive and negative prognostic factors. In particular, factors related to competence or resilience are consistently prognostic and are also the predictors that may be most amenable to change.

In terms of more guarded outcomes, a sizable portion of patients (ie, 40% in MSAD) never achieve recovery from BPD. Further, recovery status is associated with many other important outcomes, with nonrecovered patients experiencing significantly higher rates of vocational impairment, disability, physical morbidity, and mortality than recovered patients. These findings highlight a complicated interplay between multiple functional domains and suggest that therapy aimed at rehabilitation may be appropriate and necessary for some patients. Findings also highlight that symptoms of BPD wax and wane over time, and that some symptoms (ie, acute symptoms) change more rapidly and more readily than others (ie, temperamental symptoms). Seeing that most existing treatments for BPD focus largely on acute symptoms, developing interventions that target temperamental symptoms may be fruitful.

Taken together, these studies suggest that promising outcomes for patients with BPD are not only possible, but likely. They also highlight the factors that may interfere with recovery in patients with less favorable outcomes, which in turn suggest potential avenues for further treatment refinement and development.

REFERENCES

1. American Psychiatric Association. Committee on nomenclature and statistics: diagnostic and statistical manual of mental disorders. 3rd edition. Washington, DC: American Psychiatric Association; 1980.
2. Grinker RR, Werble B, Drye RC. The borderline syndrome: a behavioral study of ego functions. New York: Basic Books; 1968. p. 126–40.
3. Werble B. Second follow-up study of borderline patients. Arch Gen Psychiatry 1970;23:3–7.
4. Gunderson JG, Carpenter WT, Strauss JS. Borderline and schizophrenic patients: a comparative study. Am J Psychiatry 1975;132:1257–64.
5. Carpenter WT, Gunderson JG. Five year follow-up comparison of borderline and schizophrenic patients. Compr Psychiatry 1977;18:567–71.
6. Zanarini MC. The longitudinal course of borderline personality disorder. In: Gunderson JG, Hoffman PD, editors. Understanding and treating borderline personality disorder: a guide for professionals and families. Washington, DC: American Psychiatric Publishing, Inc; 2005. p. 83–104.
7. Akiskal HS, Chen SE, Davis GC, et al. Borderline: an adjective in search of a noun. J Clin Psychiatry 1985;46:41–8.
8. Barasch A, Frances A, Hurt S, et al. The stability and distinctness of borderline personality disorder. Am J Psychiatry 1985;142:1484–6.
9. Perry J, Cooper S. Psychodynamic symptoms and outcome in borderline and antisocial personality disorders and bipolar II affective disorder, in the borderline: current empirical research. Washington, DC: American Psychiatric Press; 1985.
10. Nace EP, Saxon JJ, Shore N. Borderline personality disorder and alcoholism treatment: a one-year follow-up study. J Stud Alcohol 1986;47:196–200.
11. Tucker L, Bauer SF, Wagner S, et al. Long-term hospital treatment of borderline patients: a descriptive outcome study. Am J Psychiatry 1987;144:1443–8.
12. Modestin J, Villiger C. Follow-up study on borderline versus nonborderline disorders. Compr Psychiatry 1989;30:236–44.

13. Links PS, Mitton JE, Steiner M. Predicting outcome for borderline personality disorder. Compr Psychiatry 1990;31:490–8.
14. Mehlum L, Friis S, Irion T, et al. Personality disorders 2-5 years after treatment: a prospective follow-up study. Acta Psychiatr Scand 1991;84:72–7.
15. Stevenson J, Meares R. An outcome study of psychotherapy for patients with borderline personality disorder. Am J Psychiatry 1992;49:358–62.
16. Linehan MM, Heard HL, Armstrong HF. Naturalistic follow-up of a behavioral treatment for chronically parasuicidal borderline patients. Arch Gen Psychiatry 1993; 50:971–4.
17. Antikainen R, Hintikka J, Lehtonen J, et al. A prospective three-year follow-up study of borderline personality disorder inpatients. Acta Psychiatr Scand 1995; 92:327–35.
18. Najavits LM, Gunderson JG. Better than expected: improvements in borderline personality disorder in a 3-year prospective outcome study. Compr Psychiatry 1995;36:296–302.
19. Pope HG, Jonas JM, Hudson JI, et al. The validity of DSM-III borderline personality disorder. Arch Gen Psychiatry 1983;40:23–30.
20. Sandell R, Alfredsson E, Berg M, et al. Clinical significance of outcome in longterm follow-up of borderline patients at a day hospital. Acta Psychiatr Scand 1993;87:405–13.
21. Senol S, Dereboy C, Yuksel N. Borderline disorder in Turkey: a 2- to 4-year follow-up. Soc Psychiatry Psychiatr Epidemiol 1997;32:109–12.
22. Links PS, Heslegrave RJ, Mitton JE, et al. Borderline psychopathology and recurrences of clinical disorders. J Nerv Ment Dis 1995;183:582–6.
23. Links PS, Heslegrave RJ, Van Reekum R. Prospective follow-up study of borderline personality disorder: prognosis, prediction of outcome, and axis II comorbidity. Can J Psychiatry 1998;42:265–70.
24. McGlashan TH. The Chestnut Lodge follow-up study. III. Long-term outcome of borderline personalities. Arch Gen Psychiatry 1986;43:20–30.
25. Paris J, Brown R, Nowlis D. Long-term follow-up of borderline patients in a general hospital. Compr Psychiatry 1987;28:530–6.
26. Plakun EM, Burkhardt PE, Muller JP. 14-year follow-up of borderline and schizotypal personality disorders. Compr Psychiatry 1985;6:448–55.
27. Stone MH. The fate of borderline patients. New York: Guilford Press; 1990.
28. Paris J, Zweig-Frank H. A 27-year follow-up of patients with borderline personality disorder. Compr Psychiatry 2001;42:482–7.
29. Endicott J, Spitzer RL, Fleiss JL, et al. The global assessment scale: a procedure for measuring overall severity of psychiatric disturbance. Arch Gen Psychiatry 1976;33:766–71.
30. Luborsky L. Clinician's judgements of mental health: a proposed scale. Arch Gen Psychiatry 1962;7:407–17.
31. Plakun EM. Prediction of outcome in borderline personality disorder. J Pers Disord 1991;5:93–101.
32. Stone MH. Borderline patients: 25 to 50 years later: with commentary on outcome factors. Psychodyn Psychiatry 2017;45:259–96.
33. McGlashan TH. The prediction of outcome in borderline personality disorder: part V of the Chestnut Lodge follow-up study. In: McGlashan TH, editor. The borderline: current empirical research. Washington, DC: American Psychiatric Press; 1985. p. 61–98.
34. Paris J, Nowlis D, Brown R. Developmental factors in the outcome of borderline personality disorder. Compr Psychiatry 1988;29:147–50.

35. Zanarini MC, Frankenburg FR, Hennen J, et al. The McLean Study of Adult Development (MSAD): overview and implications of the first six years of prospective follow up. J Pers Disord 2005;19:505–23.
36. Zanarini MC, Frankenburg FR, Reich DB, et al. Attainment and stability of sustained symptomatic remission and recovery among borderline patients and axis II comparison subjects: a 16-year prospective follow-up study. Am J Psychiatry 2012;169:476–83.
37. Zanarini MC, Frankenburg FR, Reich DB, et al. Time-to-attainment of recovery from borderline personality disorder and its stability: a 10-year prospective follow-up study. Am J Psychiatry 2010;167:663–7.
38. Zanarini MC, Temes CM, Frankenburg FR, et al. Description and prediction of time-to-attainment of excellent recovery for borderline patients followed prospectively for 20 years. Psychiatry Res 2018;262:40–5.
39. McGlashan TH, Grilo CM, Skodol AE, et al. The Collaborative Longitudinal Personality Disorders Study: baseline Axis I/II and II/II diagnostic co-occurrence. Acta Psychiatr Scand 2000;102:256–64.
40. Grilo CM, Shea MT, Sanislow CA, et al. Two-year stability and change in schizotypal, borderline, avoidant, and obsessive-compulsive personality disorders. J Consult Clin Psychol 2004;72:767–75.
41. Gunderson JG, Stout RL, McGlashan TH, et al. Ten-year course of borderline personality disorder: psychopathology and function from the Collaborative Longitudinal Personality Disorders Study. Arch Gen Psychiatry 2011;68:827–37.
42. Zanarini MC, Frankenburg FR, Hennen J, et al. Prediction of the 10-year course of borderline personality disorder. Am J Psychiatry 2006;163:827–32.
43. Zanarini MC, Frankenburg FR, Reich DB, et al. Prediction of time-to-attainment of recovery for borderline patients followed prospectively for 16 years. Acta Psychiatr Scand 2014;130:205–13.
44. Zanarini MC, Jacoby RJ, Frankenburg FR, et al. The 10-year course of social security disability income reported by borderline patients and axis II comparison subjects. J Pers Disord 2009;23:346–56.
45. Frankenburg FR, Zanarini MC. Obesity and obesity-related illnesses in borderline patients. J Pers Disord 2006;20:71–80.
46. Frankenburg FR, Zanarini MC. Relationship between cumulative BMI and symptomatic, psychosocial, and medical outcomes in patients with borderline personality disorder. J Pers Disord 2011;25:421–31.
47. Keuroghlian AS, Frankenburg FR, Zanarini MC. The relationship of chronic medical illnesses, poor health-related lifestyle choices, and health care utilization to recovery status in borderline patients over a decade of prospective follow-up. J Psychiatr Res 2013;47:1499–506.
48. Niesten IJM, Karan E, Frankenburg FR, et al. Prevalence and risk factors for irritable bowel syndrome in recovered and non-recovered borderline patients over ten years of prospective follow-up. Personal Ment Health 2014;8:14–23.
49. Plante DT, Frankenburg FR, Fitzmaurice GM, et al. Relationship between maladaptive cognitions about sleep and recovery in patients with borderline personality disorder. Psychiatry Res 2013;30:975–9.
50. Temes CM, Frankenburg FR, Reich DB, et al. Deaths by suicide and other causes among borderline patients and personality-disordered comparison subjects over 24 years of prospective follow-up. J Clin Psychiatry.
51. Zanarini MC, Frankenburg FR, Reich DB, et al. The subsyndromal phenomenology of borderline personality disorder: a 10-year follow-up study. Am J Psychiatry 2007;164:929–35.

52. Zanarini MC, Frankenburg FR, Reich DB, et al. Fluidity of the subsyndromal phenomenology of borderline personality disorder over 16 years of prospective follow-up. Am J Psychiatry 2016;173:688–94.
53. McGlashan TH, Grilo CM, Sanislow CA, et al. Two-year prevalence and stability of individual DSM-IV criteria for schizotypal, borderline, avoidant, and obsessive-compulsive personality disorders: toward a hybrid model of axis II disorders. Am J Psychiatry 2016;162:883–9.

Borderline Personality Disorder

Barriers to Borderline Personality Disorder Treatment and Opportunities for Advocacy

Paula Tusiani-Eng, LMSW, MDiv[a],*, Frank Yeomans, MD, PhD[b]

KEYWORDS

- Borderline personality disorder • Barriers • Advocacy • Evidence-based treatments

KEY POINTS

- Patients experience difficulty in accessing the evidence-based treatments that exist for borderline personality disorder.
- This article identifies barriers to treatment within the structural, economic, and political US landscape, and how different organizations have advocated for change.
- This article explores how the United States has addressed such barriers, in comparison with other countries.
- Finally, the authors offer recommendations for future advocacy to increase access to treatment for borderline personality disorder.

INTRODUCTION: IDENTIFYING THE PROBLEM: ACCESS TO TREATMENT FOR BORDERLINE PERSONALITY DISORDER

Beginning in the early 1990s, a number of treatments have been developed, tested, and shown to have efficacy for treating individuals with borderline personality disorder (BPD).[1,2] These treatments include transference-focused psychotherapy (TFP),[3] dialectical behavior therapy (DBT),[4] schema-focused psychotherapy,[5] mentalization-based therapy (MBT),[6] and good psychiatric management (GPM).[7] In the context of a field where other treatments have been developed, DBT, MBT, TFP, GPM, and schema-focused psychotherapy have emerged as the "big 5."[2]

Each of these treatments represents versions of psychodynamic and cognitive-behavioral treatment approaches that clinician–researchers refined and modified based on their understanding of the underlying developmental psychopathology,

Conflict of Interest: The authors declare that they have no conflict of interest.
[a] Emotions Matter, Inc, PO Box 7642, Garden City, NY 11530, USA; [b] Personality Disorders Institute (PDI), 122 East 42nd Street, Suite 3200, New York, NY 10168, USA
* Corresponding author.
E-mail address: paula@emotionsmatterbpd.org

clinical experience, and mechanisms of change in therapy so as to better help those suffering from BPD. The evidence to date for these treatments suggests their efficacy.[2] Additionally, a number of adjunctive treatments have been developed, including group therapies such as systems training for emotional predictability and problem solving[8] or family therapy modalities like Family Connections.[9]

Although each of the psychotherapies is distinct in its approach to treating core BPD features, they share certain similarities, particularly in structure.[2] Most of these 5 BPD treatments involve intensive individualized or group therapy, or a combination of the two, often involving several sessions per week. On average, BPD interventions last 1 to 3 years.[10]

Because multiple metaanalyses have found that the various psychotherapies produce similar effects and that there are no striking differences in those effects between treatments, some have suggested that patient choice and the goodness of fit between the patient, therapist, and the specific therapeutic approach may be important to the intervention outcome.[11] These studies find that 40% to 60% of those with BPD who are treated with one of these specialized treatments show significant symptom reduction and increased. It seems clear that, with proper treatment, individuals with BPD can stabilize, meaning that their symptoms remit and they no longer meet the criteria for the diagnosis, and, in some cases, can achieve recovery from the condition. The specialized treatments differ in the ambitiousness of their goals.[1] In comparing treatment for BPD with treatment for other psychiatric conditions, research demonstrates this outcome is more hopeful in terms of stabilization than is found in the treatment of many other mental health diagnoses, such as bipolar disorder.[12–14]

Given that effective evidence-based therapies exist to treat BPD, we might ask why is it so difficult for those diagnosed to access these specific treatments.

Statistics point to the prevalence and severity of BPD. Studies suggest that between 1.6% and 6.0% of the US population is diagnosed with BPD.[15,16] The severity of the disorder is evidenced by the statistics on suicidality. Up to 75% of individuals with BPD attempt suicide during the course of their illness and up to 10% of those diagnosed end their lives by suicide or drug overdose.[17] Therefore, both the prevalence and mortality or morbidity data speak to the importance of addressing the need to provide treatment for those with BPD.

Yet, there is a discrepancy between the availability of and access to effective treatments and the clinical need.[18] A gap exists between optimal care available in the form of one of the evidence-based treatments and actual care delivered in health care systems.[11] This article explores the factors that may contribute to treatment barriers in the United States. It then identifies how concerned stakeholders in the United States have addressed these barriers in comparison with other countries. Finally, it assesses opportunities for future treatment advocacy.

Factors that Contribute to Borderline Personality Disorder Treatment Barriers in the United States

Lack of clinical education and diagnostic training in borderline personality disorder

BPD is a complex mental disorder characterized by 9 diagnosed criteria (*Diagnostic and Statistical Manual of Mental Disorders,* fifth edition). This multilayered mix of symptoms requires careful training for clinicians to make an accurate diagnosis, because it can often be confused with other psychiatric disorders. For example, in the current system, clinicians often mistakenly diagnose patients with BPD as having bipolar disorder or major depression.[19] Clinicians frequently treat the surface symptoms of BPD through psychopharmacology, without recognizing the more complex

BPD pathology as the core psychiatric issue and in a context where there is little evidence for the efficacy of psychopharmacology for BPD.

Training and education in psychiatric residency programs about BPD is woefully inadequate.[18] This factor leads to both misdiagnosis and underdiagnosis. Inaccurate diagnosis can lead to years of misguided treatment, with the personal suffering and missed opportunities for improvement that go along with that.[19] Without adequate training in recognizing and understanding BPD, in addition to missing the diagnosis, doctors in the field can quickly become overwhelmed by the patient with BPD's risky behaviors, needs, and complex forms of attachment.[20] For example, when a patient with BPD presents with suicidal ideation and depression, clinicians often react with feelings of anxiety, guilt, or anger because they are afraid to treat complicated and challenging high-risk cases.[21,22] This situation deters them from working with this particular patient population, as well as from obtaining further training in the field of personality disorders.

Compared with other fields in psychiatry or psychology, the number of graduates annually who pursue a high level of training in BPD-specific therapies is relatively minor. Psychiatry residencies and psychology graduate programs do not provide full training in the specialized treatments for BPD. Postgraduate education is necessary and economics may play a factor in how many graduating psychiatrists and psychologists pursue further training. Training in BPD-specific treatment methods is both costly and time intensive.[23] For example, to become a licensed DBT trained clinician through Behavioral Tech, the corporation responsible for DBT training, takes 2 years of intensive training and costs between $8000 and $10,000.[24] Both TFP and MBT training also take significant training and costs, with ongoing intensive supervision required. One of the objectives of GPM is to provide a more basic training that requires less time and expense.[7] Consequently, owing to the challenge of treating patients with BPD and the extensive nature of training for the evidence-based treatments that have been developed for BPD, there are not enough clinicians to meet the demand.[25] In addition, the majority of clinicians and researchers specializing in the condition reside in urban areas, universities, or psychiatric research centers on the East or West Coasts of the United States, where they have access to supervision and ongoing training. This distribution leaves a wide swath of the BPD population in the middle of America underserved, with few evidence-based treatment options.[18]

Culture of stigma toward the patient with borderline personality disorder

Stigma within the clinical community toward treating individuals with BPD is widespread and often rooted in misperceptions and lack of knowledge about BPD. Research shows professionals routinely stigmatize patients with BPD using negative language, labeling them as manipulative, attention seeking, and not worthy of resources[26,27] and describing their experience working with this population as difficult. This stigma has led to discriminatory practices, because some clinicians refuse to treat patients with BPD.

The relative paucity of medical knowledge, research, and clinical education about BPD has created a situation in which many clinicians, lacking the tools needed to effectively treat this patient population, dismiss patients with BPD as difficult, manipulative, or hard to handle,[28] seeming to view the condition more as a moral failing than a valid psychiatric condition. Such negative attitudes toward those with BPD may result from the clinician unconsciously projecting his or her fears and inadequacies onto the patient, blaming them for their mental disorder instead of acknowledging the clinician's own lack of adequate training as a possible source for their insecurity and frustration. This reaction on the part of clinicians compounds the shame and guilt experience by patients with BPD. These prejudices can be internalized by individuals with BPD, who believe they are not worthy of being treated in a way that fuels negative self-talk and stigma in the person.

A further way in which stigma toward the patient with BPD may become a barrier to treatment is that the patient may reject or resist working with a therapist with a negative view of their disorder.[18] Some patients reject treatment altogether, having experienced clinicians as authority figures who can make them feel invalidated.[29] Clinicians who use stigmatizing language can hinder recovery because individuals with BPD may adopt the clinician's negative narrative based on the rhetoric of stigma as opposed to being able to more fully appreciate their own story.[30]

Stigma also hinders fostering a younger generation of clinicians and researchers interested in BPD. Bias in clinicians who teach in the mental health professions can have negative impact on the willingness of their students to specialize in the treatment of BPD. This pattern not only affects patients and families trying to access mental health care, but also affects the atmosphere throughout the mental health field and expands to limiting the public's knowledge about this disorder.

Lack of medical research to understand borderline personality disorder as a legitimate psychiatric disorder with a strong biological basis

Although the concept of BPD has existed in the psychiatric literature since 1938, BPD as a diagnosis was not entered into the *Diagnostic and Statistical Manual for Mental Disorders* until its third edition in 1980.[4,31] Even with its introduction, BPD and other personality disorders were relegated into a special diagnostic group (Axis II). As a result, many in the field of mental health did not consider BPD a serious mental illness (SMI) of equal standing with other disorders such as bipolar disorder, schizophrenia, or major depression.[4,32] In addition, in comparison with other major psychiatric conditions, relatively little medical research exists today to help clinicians and researchers understand the etiology and biology of BPD as a brain disorder.[33] According a report from the National Institute of Mental Health, BPD received the least amount of funding for research grants compared with other major mental health disorders from 2009 to 2013.[34] Despite its prevalence and devastating impact on both individuals and society, BPD continues to be largely unrecognized as a priority and public health crisis by the psychiatric research community and government funding agencies.[35]

The cost of treatments for borderline personality disorder and the organization of insurance guidelines

Although evidence-based treatments have been shown to be effective, the cost of such therapies makes it difficult for the majority of those with BPD to access them.[36] This situation is largely due to the fact that most BPD-specific treatments are not adequately covered by health insurance companies in the United States. Insurers' mental health medical necessity guidelines are generally geared to cover treatment to resolve acute psychiatric symptoms (eg, acute depression, suicidal feelings) with the goal of restoring the patient to his or her baseline condition before symptom onset, even if that condition is a chronically pathologic one. Many health insurance companies in the United States base their coverage of treatments on the somewhat elusive term of medical necessity. Although the term sounds medical, it is rooted more in the writings of the insurance industry[37–39] and is used to justify treating only acute symptoms rather than underlying conditions. The treatment of deeper, more chronic aspects of illness, which create ongoing vulnerability to more acute episodes, is generally not covered.[37] In other words, insurers set up their guidelines to pay for brief acute treatments, but not the long-term continuous treatments addressing the underlying factors of illness required to help patients with BPD in a meaningful way. This approach is akin to reducing a fever without treating its underlying cause[37] and does not allow for treatment of the root of the problem. Currently, not treating the underlying condition may be illegal if insurer's coverage does not respect the law mandating parity in terms of the coverage of psychiatric and medical illnesses.[37] In addition to these concerns, many insurance companies will not accept BPD as a billable diagnosis.[40] Because of these reasons, the evidence-based treatments for BPD are generally not covered by health insurance plans. These treatments, by virtue of being long term, are costly and most patients are required to pay out of pocket to access them,[18,36] creating a situation where, for the most part, access to the evidence-based treatments for BPD is limited to patients and families in the middle and upper classes of society.

Evidence-based therapies are not widely accessible in publicly funded treatment settings either.[38] In many places, it is difficult to find Medicaid or Medicare providers who treat BPD. Therapists in private practice knowledgeable in specialized treatments tend not to accept these forms of reimbursement. Clinics who do accept Medicare and Medicaid may not have therapists trained in the evidence-based treatments, especially outside of urban centers.[18] Receiving the appropriate level of care is also an issue. Although the majority of patients with BPD can be treated as outpatients, many require inpatient hospitalization, long-term residential treatment, or intensive day treatment to stabilize and move on to outpatient treatment. These levels of care are often not covered or only partially covered by health insurance. As a result of all of these factors, many impacted by BPD go without treatment.

Federal and state policies that do not list borderline personality disorder as a serious mental illness

In 1992, the Alcohol Drug Abuse and Mental Health Administration Reorganization Act mandated the Department of Health and Human Services to distinguish SMI from other forms of mental illness for the purpose of distributing grants to states. According to the Alcohol Drug Abuse and Mental Health Administration Reorganization Act, the federal definition of SMI was a condition that impacts an individual who is at least 18 years of age, with a diagnosable mental disorder in the *Diagnostic and Statistical Manual of Mental Disorders,* 3rd edition, resulting in behavioral or emotional disorder of sufficient duration that results in significant impairment which substantially limits one or more of life's major activities, such as maintaining interpersonal relationships, activities of daily functioning, self-care, employment, and recreation.[41] This definition shifted mental health policy in the United States to focus on prioritizing funding based on impairment severity.[42]

According to the Substance Abuse and Mental Health Services Administration, the diagnoses most commonly associated with Serious Mental Illness under this definition are schizophrenia, bipolar disorder, and major depressive disorders[43] Borderline Personality Disorder is not specifically named in this list, although it is stated that "one or more disorders may also fit the definition of SMI if those disorders result in functional impairment."[43] Because BPD is not named as a SMI by SAMHSA, the classification is not universally accepted among the 50 states that have flexibility in identifying specific diagnosis they use to establish eligibility. In many states, the list of SMI diagnoses is limited to schizophrenia, other psychotic disorders, bipolar disorder, mood disorders, and major depression. Some states include personality disorders, but the decision is subject to their understanding of the severity of BPD, the degree of impairment to the individual, and the state's perception of duration of the disorder.[44] States can develop specifications for the number of domains that an individual must be impaired in to receive services, as well as for the duration of impairment. For instance, in some states only those with severe and persistent mental illness that is considered chronic, in contrast with a condition that can respond to treatment, qualify for reimbursement; this excludes many with BPD and keeps treatment out of reach for many people who could improve.[45] Thus, eligibility and access to BPD treatment differs in every state where health care policies are subject to state regulations.

Similarly, SMI definitions can vary among health care delivery reimbursement systems, which interpret state laws and determine eligibility of services. For example, Blue Cross Blue Shield of Illinois specifically categorizes BPD as a Non-Serious Mental Illness under state law in its provider manual.[46] In contrast, anorexia nervosa, bulimia nervosa, and obsessive-compulsive disorder are listed as SMIs. In states like this, individuals with BPD are more likely to qualify for some type of insurance coverage based on a comorbid diagnosis, such as depression, to treat their systems than they are for their actual diagnosis. This circumstance is both unfair and unwise, because it denies patients information and treatment for their actual diagnosis, often providing treatment only for 1 aspect of their total condition.[45] This policy results in bad medicine; research has shown that patients suffering from depression in the context of BPD do not respond to the treatment for depression until the underlying personality disorder is addressed.

Just as BPD is not well-understood in the clinical community and is shrouded by stigma, misperceptions persist through the governmental and for-profit economic health care systems leading to discriminatory health care delivery services. Although research and personal experience with BPD clearly point to BPD fulfilling criteria for SMI classification, the way the US governmental system classifies and understands BPD within the larger framework creates significant barriers to treatment.

Responses to Treatment Barriers: Efforts to Improve Access to Treatment Through Advocacy in the United States

Research and clinical advocacy

Since the 1990s, with the first treatment outcome studies, barriers to BPD treatment in the United States have been addressed through advances in research. More recently, organizations have been created to bring researchers together to communicate across different research sites and help coordinate and focus efforts. In 2012, the North American Society for the Study of Personality Disorders was founded as a professional organization for clinicians and scientists devoted to research in personality disorders. Its mission emphasizes new research pointing to positive treatment outcomes for those with personality disorders, sharing this research with the clinical community and public, and advocating for research funding. Annual North American Society for the Study of Personality Disorders conferences are held to present new research and cultivate a new generation of young researchers.[47] Similar efforts are carried out at the international level by the European Society for the Study of Personality Disorders and the International Society for the Study of Personality Disorders.

As a result of these and other efforts to bring attention to BPD, new research has emerged on how to conceptualize the disorder, on the biological and social/interpersonal aspects of BPD, on the effectiveness of treatment, on diagnostic tools for aid clinicians, on the rates of underdiagnosis, and on the cost effectiveness of treatment versus nontreatment. Research has increased our understanding of the problem of BPD and suicide and the need for more community resources. In recent years, a body of research has focused on the Global Alliance for the Prevention and Early Intervention for Borderline Personality Disorder, advocating for early intervention and prevention.[48] These efforts have called more attention to the problem of BPD and the barriers to treatment.

The National Institute of Mental Health (NIMH) provides much of the funding for mental health research in this country. The amount of funding that has been granted for studies related to BPD is relatively small.[34] Nevertheless, in 2012 NIMH introduced the Research Domain Criteria system to evaluate and fund research. This system organizes levels of research from the basic biological to the social/interpersonal level and has helped researchers to focus their investigations in the appropriate domain of study. In 2016, a privately funded think tank of leading researchers convened to explore novel approaches to understand BPD under the new Research Domain Criteria system. A White Paper coming out of the meeting identified 6 areas for future research to consider new efforts in brain and psychosocial studies.[49] These include emotional dysregulation, interpersonal and social deficits, impulsive aggression, the genetics of BPD, social stressors in BPD, and animal models to study the neurobiology of BPD.[49]

Efforts have also been made by clinicians and private foundations to recruit and support young researchers to study BPD. Clinical research teams in DBT, TFP, GPM, and MBT continue to combine a focus on training with ongoing research, introducing graduate students and residents to evidence-based treatments, and generating interest in studying BPD. Families for Borderline Personality Disorder Research was founded in 2011 at the Brain and Behavior Research Foundation (www.bbrfoundation.org).[50] It has funded 5 BPD researchers through National Alliance for Research in Schizophrenia and Affective Disorders (NARSAD) Young Investigator Grants of $70,000 each from the Brain and Behavior Research Foundation (http://www.familiesforbpdresearch.org).[51]

Role of nonprofit organizations in advocacy

Given the challenges to providing appropriate care to the borderline population delineated, family and peer-run nonprofit organizations developed address treatment barriers through a focus on education, community support, and resources. Valerie Porr was the first to gain the public's attention when her loved one was diagnosed with BPD. She found very little information about BPD and how it could be treated effectively. This energized her to establish the Treatment and Research Advancements National Association for Personality Disorder in New York.[52] Porr developed a treatment for individuals and families called the TARA Method, which is an 8-week class that includes elements of dialectical behavioral therapy, MBT, transference-focused psychotherapy, and education about the neurobiology of BPD.[53] Porr was an early voice advocating for the BPD population, with an emphasis on education and communicating developments in neurobiological social cognition research.

The National Education Association for Borderline Personality Disorder (NEA-BPD), a second national organization founded to meet the needs of family members, was founded by Perry Hoffman, PhD, in 2001.[54] Along with Alan Fruzzettii, Hoffman developed a 12-week course called Family Connections[9] that is administered by trained leaders and covers education and skills training based on DBT for family members with loved ones impacted by BPD. The NEA-BPD received government grants to pursue its mission of sponsoring regional and international conferences on BPD and expanding the Family Connections teaching program. The NEA-BPD introduced a model in which conferences targeted individuals with BPD and their family members as well as clinicians and researchers, sometimes including family and client participation as conference presenters. According to its website, the NEA-BPD has hosted more than 65 professional conferences to date.[54]

Through a partnership with the National Alliance for Mental Illness, the NEA-BPD was instrumental in requesting a Congressional Report on BPD from the Substance Abuse and Mental Health Association. This marked the first time that BPD was entered into the Congressional Record as a SMI.[55] Additionally, NEA-BPD worked with Representative Tom Davis (R-VA-11) to sponsor House Resolution 1005, Supporting the

Goals and Ideals of Borderline Personality Disorder Awareness Month in the 110th Congress in 2008.[56]

The New York-Presbyterian Hospital Borderline Personality Disorder Resource Center (BPDRC) was founded 2003 by the Michael and Beatrice Tusiani, in memory of their daughter Pamela Tusiani, who died as a result of BPD and negligent mental health care.[57] The BPDRC's mission is to provide the public information about BPD and help in seeking appropriate treatment. The BPDRC maintains the largest database in the world of clinicians, facilities and programs specifically trained in BPD, and refers callers to appropriate resources.[58] Since its inception, the BPDRC has received more than 13,000 calls, averaging 130 calls per month.[58] "Back from the Edge", an educational video on the Center's website has been viewed almost 1,800,000 times. A study of the data accumulated by the BPDRC from 2008 to 2015 determined that stigmatization, financial concerns, and comorbid disorders are the most significant obstacles for those seeking care for BPD.[18]

In May of 2015, a new US nonprofit called Emotions Matter, Inc, composed of individuals with BPD, family members, and clinicians, was launched to empower and connect individuals impacted by BPD and to raise awareness and advocate for improved mental health care.[59] Emotions Matter differs from TARA, NEA-BPD, and the BPDRC in that individuals with BPD are central in its leadership and programming, promoting empowerment and recovery in addition to helping the organization understand the experience and needs of individuals with BPD.

Emotions Matter launched grassroots campaigns to address treatment barriers on social media. In April of 2016, it created a petition on Change.org addressed to Dr Bruce Cuthbert, then the Acting Director of NIMH, requesting more funding for BPD research. In 6 weeks, petition received more than 5000 signatures, leading to a meeting at NIMH.[59] The NIMH subsequently updated its webpage on BPD, demonstrating the impact that individuals can have by advocating for BPD in the government agencies. Twenty months later, the NIMH published its first public education brochure on BPD.[60]

In May 2017, Emotions Matter initiated a campaign to encourage members of congress to sign a Congressional Letter sponsored by Representative Barbara Comstock, to recognize BPD as an SMI. This letter addressed the fact the BPD was not listed as such in the 21st Cures Act of 2016, which allocated significant federal mental health funding to states. Emotions Matter succeeded in mobilizing 5 additional members of congress to sign the letter. The outcome from this effort is pending, but communication about BPD has increased with both NIMH and Substance Abuse and Mental Health Services Administration as a result.[59]

LEARNING FROM OTHER COUNTRIES

Efforts to advocate for patients with BPD are often intertwined with a country's system of health care delivery. Countries that have more coordinated health care systems can provide organizational structures that help to move advocacy efforts forward.

For example, in the United Kingdom, the National Institute for Clinical Excellence (NICE) was established in 1999 by the Secretary of State for Health. The original aim of NICE was to ensure that the most clinically and cost effective drugs and treatments were made available widely in the country's National Health Service.[61] The government believed that creating NICE could advance the pace at which good value treatments were used across the National Health Service, in turn promoting successful innovation on the part of clinicians, pharmaceutical companies, and the medical devices industry. NICE has established a worldwide reputation for producing authoritative evidence-based advice and guidelines.

The NICE guidelines for managing BPD were published in 2009.[61] They issued 4 important recommendations with the goal of improving access to treatment. First, people with BPD should not be excluded from any health care or social service because of their diagnosis or self-harm. Second, clinicians working with people with BPD should explore treatment options with hope and optimism, articulating that recovery is possible. Third, drugs should not be prescribed for individuals with BPD. Fourth, mental health clinicians should work with multidisciplinary specialists or services to support those with BPD in the community.[61]

The NICE guidelines represent a significant paradigm shift in clinical thinking about BPD not yet seen in the United States to the same degree. They educate the clinical community about BPD being treated through therapy and multidisciplinary supports, without relying on medication alone. They reduce stigma by encouraging optimism about treatment. The NICE guidelines also establish the vital role that community services play in BPD recovery, promoting multidisciplinary collaboration. The closest equivalent to the NICE guidelines in the United States are the guidelines for treating specific disorders by the American Psychiatric Association (APA), published in 2001,[62] which have less influence than the NICE guidelines because they are issued by a professional organization rather than a government agency. The APA guidelines for BPD also stipulate that psychotherapy is the first line of treatment for BPD, rather than medication. But the guidelines of a professional organization do not have the same weight in determining treatment delivery and reimbursement as those developed with the authority of a government agency in a country with a unified system of health care delivery. Guidelines such as those of the APA can influence clinical and cultural attitudes about BPD, but without as much of an impact as governmental directives.

Australia might provide us with the best example of effective BPD advocacy. Janne McMahon, OAM, has been instrumental in engaging government support, starting a submission to the Australian Parliament, Senate Community Affairs Committee that was supported by a group of service user and family organizations. The initial goal was to establish a task force to look into issues of access to treatment. The initiative was supported by the Australian Medical Association, the Royal Australian and New Zealand College of Psychiatrists, key nonprofit organizations, and key researchers.[63] The next step was the establishment of an Expert Reference Group and the development of the *National Health Medical Research Council – Clinical Practice Guidelines for the Management of Borderline Personality Disorder*.

As in the United States, there was also a successful effort for the federal government to recognize the importance of BPD when the Australian upper house (senate) established the first week in October as BPD Awareness Week starting in October 2014 (in the United States, May is BPD Awareness Month). Advocacy groups in Australia use the official recognition as a marker for a number of advocacy initiatives. Advocacy efforts in the state of South Australia continued, with many submissions and letters to consolidate across benches of the parliament's upper house. A recent success has been receiving funding of $10.25 million over 4 years to establish a BPD Center of Excellence and a statewide BPD service in Southern Australia. These developments demonstrate the potential impact of the cooperation between advocacy groups and clinicians and researchers.

Advocacy efforts in Australia have also included the establishment of the Australian BPD Foundation, a fledgling nonprofit organization established by a group of service users, families, and clinicians on a voluntary basis. The group now organizes 7 annual national conferences around the country with the project of developing a National Training Strategy to provide training and professional development for clinicians and those working in the service area.

Another significant strategy to bring more attention to BPD treatment across Australia involved research. Researchers in Australia showed that BPD is a leading contributor to the burden of disease (BOD) in the community.[64] BOD is a measure used by the World Health Organization to assess qualify of life, disability, loss of health, and mortality related to disease.[65] The BOD is used as essential scientific evidence to influence public health data and policy. Researchers have linked BPD with poor life outcomes, including severe and functional disability,[66] high family and career burden, poor physical health,[67] and premature mortality/suicidality.[68] Andrew Chanen, a leading Australian researcher on BPD, outlines specific recommendations for the Australian health system to manage those with BPD.[64] Chanen places explicit emphasis on access to treatment and clinical training to improve BOD outcomes.

Additionally, research in Australia has also included an important focus on the patient with BPD's experience. In a survey of 153 people diagnosed with BPD, a study by Lawn and McMahon[69] showed that patients continue to experience significant discrimination in Australia in both public and private health services. It was found that patients who disclosed their BPD diagnosis were being systematically denied access to treatment resources by health care providers, especially during emergency room visits, as compared with other mental illnesses. The study documented underdiagnosis of BPD, misdiagnosis, and misinformation about the condition. Lawn and McMahon concluded that better clinical education and attitudes are needed to improve the patient experience. Although research in the United States and Europe has looked into social and economic costs of BPD,[13,66,70] it has fallen behind Australia in developing studies to understand the patient with BPD's experience. By focusing on the patient with BPD, Australian researchers have gathered vital information to understand how the health care system itself may negatively impact patients' symptoms, self-concept, and resistance to treatment.

It is clear that misunderstanding and stigma regarding BPD have been major impediments to providing adequate treatment resources. As these problems are slowly improving, the clinical, research, and government communities have begun to more adequately address the needs of the BPD community. This change involves the need for clinicians, researchers, and government officials to take their share of responsibility for the patient's experience and to continue to adopt more positive attitudes and structures to improve access to treatment. Putting priority on the patient's needs involves, among other things, validating the trauma that individuals may have experienced in a system that has chronically included unfounded stigma of those with BPD. In summary, the different approaches within Australian advocacy efforts have been successful thus far in placing an emphasis on the patient, the disorder's severity, and discrimination in the health care system.

DISCUSSION: FUTURE DIRECTIONS FOR TREATMENT ADVOCACY IN THE UNITED STATES

After reviewing barriers to accessing treatment for BPD and comparing US efforts to address these barriers with some other countries, the following recommendations are made to advance BPD treatment advocacy in the United States:

1. Create centralized standards for categorizing BPD by a government agency to manage BPD in place of a system where 50 states set standards in a decentralized way.
2. Encourage the APA and the government to work more closely together.
3. Increase work by advocacy groups and clinicians to lobby for state legislation to mandate health insurance coverage for evidence-based BPD treatments.

4. Increase the mobilization of government agencies, researchers, clinicians, patients, and family members working together for reform. Even though progress has been made, Zimmerman[35] contends that, compared with other mental disorders, the BPD clinical community lacks an advocacy strategy. Zimmerman[35] attributes this to a lack of an advocacy strategy on the part of clinicians, who have largely ignored BPD and have not done a good job highlighting the public health implications of the disorder.

5. Use laws that exist to advocate for the BPD population. Although the federal parity law requiring insurance companies to cover mental illness at an equal level to other illnesses should, in theory, have established fair insurance reimbursement for the treatment BPD, evidence suggests that the parity law is largely not respected.[38] While these breeches in the application of the parity law are being pursued in court, further economic and social impact studies of BPD will help evidence for the wisdom and need for insurance coverage for the treatments specific to BPD. Class action lawsuits have a role in this effort.

6. Increase the inclusion of the patient experience in advocacy efforts.

7. Better educate the general public on the severity of the disorder and its cost to society. Without treatment, the high cost to society will continue, given that untreated BPD contributes to the suicide rate and other social problems, such as homelessness, children in foster care, incarceration, and unemployment.

8. Increase clinical education. Future efforts for advocacy at the clinical level should include mandating education about BPD in medical and mental health training, developing a comprehensive antistigma campaign specifically geared toward clinicians, advocating for better accounting of prevalence and suicide statistics, advocating for adequate insurance coverage for treatment, and advocating for increased funding for research.

REFERENCES

1. Gunderson J. Borderline personality disorder: ontogeny of a diagnosis. Am J Psychiatry 2009;166:530–9.

2. Sledge W, Plakun E, Bauer S, et al. Psychotherapy for suicidal patients with borderline personality disorder: an expert consensus review of common factors across five therapies. Borderline Personal Disord Emot Dysregul 2014;1:16.

3. Yeomans F, Clarkin J, Kernberg O. Transference-focused psychotherapy for borderline personality disorder: a clinical guide. Washington, DC: American Psychiatric Publishing, Inc; 2015.

4. Linehan M. DBT skills training manual. 1st edition. New York: Guilford Publications Inc; 1993.

5. Kellogg S, Young J. Schema therapy for borderline personality disorder. J Clin Psychol 2006;62(4):445–58.

6. Bateman A, Fonagy P. Mentalization based treatment for borderline personality disorder. World Psychiatry 2010;9(1):11–5.

7. Gunderson JG. Handbook of good psychiatric management for borderline personality disorder. Washington, DC: American Psychiatric Association Publishing; 2011.

8. Choi-Kain LW, Finch E, Masland S, et al. What works in the treatment of borderline personality disorder. Curr Behav Neurosci Rep 2017;4:21–30.

9. Fruzzetti A, Shenk C, Hoffman P. Family interaction and the development of borderline personality disorder: a transactional model. Dev Psychopathol 2005; 17:1007–30.

10. Biskin RS. The lifetime course of borderline personality disorder. Can J Psychiatry 2015;60(7):303–8.
11. Hermens M, van Splunteren P, van den Bosch M, et al. Barriers to implementing the clinical guideline on borderline personality disorder in the Netherlands. Psychiatr Serv 2011;62(11):1381–3.
12. Paris J, Gunderson JG, Weinberg I. The interface between borderline personality disorder and bipolar spectrum disorder. Compr Psychiatry 2007;48:145–54.
13. Zanarini M, Frankenburg F, Hennen J, et al. The longitudinal course of borderline psychopathology: 6-year prospective follow-up of the phenomenology of borderline personality disorder. Am J Psychiatry 2003;160:274–83.
14. Paris J. The outcome of borderline personality disorder: good for most but not all patients. Am J Psychiatry 2012;169(5):445–6.
15. Grant B, Chou S, Goldstein R, et al. Prevalence, correlates, disability, and comorbidity of DSM-IV borderline personality disorder: results from the wave 2 national epidemiologic survey on alcohol and related conditions. J Clin Psychiatry 2008; 69(4):533–45.
16. Lenzenweger MF. Current status of the scientific study of the personality disorders: an overview of epidemiological, longitudinal, experimental psychopathology, and neurobehavioral perspectives. J Am Psychoanal Assoc 2010;58: 741–78.
17. Goodman M, Alvarez Tomas I, Temes C, et al. Suicide attempts and self-injurious behaviours in adolescent and adult patients with borderline personality disorder. Personal Ment Health 2017;11(3):157–63.
18. Lohman M, Whiteman K, Yeomans F, et al. Qualitative analysis of resources and barriers for BPD in the U.S. Psychiatr Serv 2017;68(2):167–72.
19. Paris J. Why psychiatrists are reluctant to diagnose borderline personality disorder. Psychiatry 2007;(1):25–39.
20. Hong V. Borderline personality disorder in the emergency department: good psychiatric management. Harv Rev Psychiatry 2016;24(5):357–66.
21. Hersh R. Confronting myths and stereotypes about borderline personality disorder. Soc Work Ment Health 2008;6(1–2):13–32.
22. Chartonas D, Kyratsous M, Dracass S, et al. Personality disorder: still the patients psychiatrists dislike? BJ Psych Bull 2017;41(1):12–7.
23. Okamura KH, Benjamin Wolk CL, Kang-Yi CD, et al. The price per prospective consumer of providing therapist training and consultation in seven evidence-based treatments within a large public behavioral health system: an example cost-analysis metric. Front Public Health 2018;5:356.
24. Behavioral Tech: a Linehan Institute Training Company. Dialectical behavior therapy intensive training. Available at: https://behavioraltech.org/event/5093-dialectical-behavior-therapy-intensive-training/. Accessed December 15, 2017.
25. Howe E. Five ethical and clinical challenges psychiatrists may face when treating patients with borderline personality disorder who are or may become suicidal. Innov Clin Neurosci 2013;10(1):14–9.
26. Lewis G, Appleby L. Personality disorder: the patients psychiatrists dislike. Br J Psychiatry 1988;153(1):44–9.
27. Fallon PG. Traveling through the system: the lived experience of people with BPD in contact with psychiatric services. J Psychiatr Ment Health Nurs 2003;10(4): 393–401.
28. Sulzer SH. Does "difficult patient" status contribute to de facto demedicalization? The case of borderline personality disorder. Soc Sci Med 2015;142:82–9.

29. Kling R. Borderline personality disorder, language and stigma. Ethical Hum Psychol Psychiatry 2014;16(2):114–9.
30. Errerger S, Foreman A. That's so borderline – language matters when talking about BPD. Harrisburg (PA): Spring The New Social Worker; 2016.
31. Kernberg O. Borderline conditions and pathological narcissism. New York: Jason Aronson; 1975.
32. Tyrer P. Borderline personality disorder: a motley diagnosis in need of reform. Lancet 1999;354:2095–6.
33. Lis E, Greenfield B, Henry M, et al. Neuroimaging and genetics of borderline personality disorder: a review. J Psychiatry Neurosci 2007;32(3):162–73.
34. Insel T. The anatomy of NIMH funding from 2009-2013. Bethesda (MD): National Institute of Mental Health; 2015. Available at: http://nimh.nih.gove/funding/funding-strategy-for-research-grants/the-anatomy-of-nimh-funding.
35. Zimmerman M. Borderline personality disorder: in search of advocacy. J Nerv Ment Dis 2015;203(1):8–12.
36. Maclean JC. Borderline personality disorder: insight from economics. 2013. Available at: http://scattergoodfoundation.org/activity/general/borderline-personality-disorder-insight-economics#.V9hANPorLIU. Accessed September 13, 2016.
37. Lazar S, Bendat M, Gabbard G, et al. Clinical necessity guidelines for psychotherapy, insurance medical necessity and utilization review protocols, and mental health parity. Washington, DC: Coalition for Psychotherapy Parity; 2018. Available at: https://www.coalitionforpsychotherapyparity.org/.
38. Kealy D, Ogrodniczuk J. Marginalization of borderline personality disorder. J Psychiatr Pract 2010;16(3):145–54.
39. Knoepflmacher D. Medical necessity in psychiatry: whose definition is it anyway? New York: Psychiatric Times; 2016. Available at: https://psychnews.psychiatryonline.org/doi/full/10.1176/appi.pn.2016.9b14.
40. Bendat M. The devil is in the details: contracting with managed care. Psychiatric News 2017. Available at: https://psychnews.psychiatryonline.org/doi/full/10.1176/appi.pn.2017.9b14.
41. Insel T. Getting serious about mental illness. Bethesda (MD): National Institute of Mental Health; 2013. Available at: https://www.nimh.nih.gov/about/directors/thomas-insel/blog/2013/getting-serious-about-mental-illnesses.shtml.
42. Goldman H, Grob G. Defining mental illness in mental health policy. Health Aff (Millwood) 2006;25(3):737–49.
43. The way forward: federal action for a system that works for all people living with SMI and SED and their families and caregivers. Interdepartmental Serious Mental Illness Coordinating Committee (ISMICC) Report to Congress. December 13, 2017. Available at: https://www.samhsa.gov/ismicc. Accessed September 4, 2018.
44. U.S. Department of Health and Human Services, Office of the Assistant Secretary for Planning and Evaluation (ASPE). Medicaid and permanent supportive housing for chronically homeless individuals: emerging practices from the field: who qualifies for Medicaid mental health services? 2014.
45. Patients with borderline personality disorder challenge HCH clinicians. Helping Hands: A Publication of the Helping Hands Clinician Network, National Health Care for the Homeless Council 2003;7(4):1–6.
46. Blue cross blue shield of Illinois provider manual. 2018. Available at: https://www.bcbsil.com/provider/standards/serious_vs_non_serious.html. Accessed March 8, 2018.

47. National Association for the Study and Advancement of Personality Disorders (NASSPD). Available at: http://www.nasspd.org. Accessed March 8, 2018.

48. Chanen A, Sharp C, Hoffman P, Global Alliance for Prevention and Early Intervention for Borderline Personality Disorder. Prevention and early intervention for borderline personality disorder: a novel public health priority. World Psychiatry 2017;16(2):215–6.

49. Stanley B, Perez-Rodriquez M, Labouliere C, et al. A neuroscience-oriented approach to borderline personality disorder. J Personal Disord 2018;32:1–39.

50. The Brain and Behavior Research Foundation (BBRF). Available at: https://bbrfoundation.org/. Accessed December 15, 2017.

51. Families for Borderline Personality Disorder Research (FBPDR). Available at: http://www.familiesforbpdresearch.org. Accessed December 15, 2017.

52. Nielsen L. From anger to compassion: resources at US based TARA National Association for Personality Disorder. Here to Help: British Columbia's Mental Health and Addictions Journal 2011;7(1):18. Available at: http://www.heretohelp.bc.ca/visions/borderline-personality-disorder-vol7. Accessed September 4, 2018.

53. Porr V. Overcoming borderline personality disorder: a family guide for healing and change. New York: Oxford University Press; 2010.

54. National education alliance for borderline personality disorder (NEA-BPD). Available at: http://www.borderlinepersonalitydisorder.com. Accessed October 11, 2017.

55. Substance Abuse and Mental Health Services Administration (SAMSHA). Report to congress on borderline personality disorder. Washington, DC: United States Department of Health and Human Services; 2010. HHS Publication No. SMA-11-4644. 2010.

56. 110th Congress (2007-2008). House Resolution 1005: supporting the goals and ideals of Borderline Personality Disorder Awareness Month. Rep. Davis, Tom [R-VA-11], Sponsor. Available at: https://www.congress.gov/bill/110th-congress/house-resolution/1005/text. Accessed October 11, 2017.

57. Tusiani B, Tusiani P, Tusiani-Eng P. Remnants of a life on paper: a mother and daughter's struggle with borderline personality disorder. New York: Baroque Press; 2013.

58. Borderline Personality Disorder Resource Center (BPDRC). Reports. New York: Presbyterian Hospital; 2016. Available at: http://www.nyp.org/bpdresourcecenter.

59. Emotions Matter, Inc. Available at: www.emotionsmatterbpd.org.

60. United States Department of Health and Human Services. National Institute of Health. National Institute of Mental Health. NIH Publication No. QF 17-4928. Borderline Personality Disorder. 2018. Available at: https://www.nimh.nih.gov/health/publications/borderline-personality-disorder/index.shtml. Accessed December 15, 2017.

61. National Institute for Clinical Excellence (NICE). Borderline personality disorder: recognition and management: clinical guideline. 2009. Available at: https://www.nice.org.uk/guidance/CG78. Accessed March 8, 2018.

62. American Psychiatric Association. Practice guideline for the treatment of patients with borderline personality disorder. Washington, DC: American Psychiatric Association; 2001.

63. Australian Government National Health and Medical Research Council. Clinical Practice Guidelines for the Management of Borderline Personality Disorder. Canberra: National Health and Medical Research Council. 2013; 1–6.

64. Chanen A, Thompson K. Proscribing and borderline personality disorder. Aust Prescr 2016;39:49–53.

65. World Health Organization. Health information on burden of disease: 2004 report. Available at: http://www.who.int/healthinfo/global_burden_disease/GBD_report_2004update_part3.pdf. Accessed March 8, 2018.
66. Gunderson J, Stout R, McGlashan T, et al. Ten-year course of borderline personality disorder: psychopathology and function from the collaborative longitudinal personality disorders study. Arch Gen Psychiatry 2001;68(8):827–37.
67. Zanarini M, Frankenburg F, Reich DB, et al. Time to attainment of recovery from borderline personality disorder and stability of recovery: a 10 year prospective follow-up study. Am J Psychiatry 2010;167(6):663–7.
68. El-Gabalway R, Katz L, Sareen J. Comorbidity and associated severity of borderline personality disorder and physical health conditions in a nationally representative sample. Psychosom Med 2010;72(7):641–7.
69. Lawn S, McMahon J. Experiences of care by Australians with a diagnosis of borderline personality disorder. J Psychiatr Ment Health Nurs 2015;22:510–21.
70. Soeteman M, Hakkaart-van Roijen L, Verheul R, et al. The economic burden of personality disorders in mental health care. J Clin Psychiatry 2008;69:259–65.

Treatment of Borderline Personality Disorder

Kenneth N. Levy, PhD[a,b,*], Shelley McMain, PhD[c], Anthony Bateman, MA, FRCPsych[d], Tracy Clouthier, MS[a,e]

KEYWORDS

- Borderline personality disorder • Psychotherapy • Treatment
- Dialectical behavior therapy • Mentalization-based therapy
- Transference-focused psychotherapy

KEY POINTS

- There are several treatments for borderline personality disorder (BPD) that have shown efficacy in one or more randomized controlled trials; these treatments include those based on cognitive behavior theories (eg, dialectical behavior therapy [DBT] and schema-focused psychotherapy) and psychodynamic theories (eg, mentalization-based therapy and transference-focused psychotherapy).
- Regardless of theoretic origin, most treatments for BPD have been modified based on unique problems presented by the disorder and tend to be integrated to some degree, if not explicitly then implicitly.
- Randomized controlled trials and meta-analyses suggest that patients treated with one of these treatments are better off than those on waiting lists and in treatment as usual. Direct comparisons of active treatments, however, are uncommon and show few reliable differences.
- In addition to these specialty treatments, there are several generalist approaches and adjunctive treatments that show promise and could have widespread applicability. These include good psychiatric management, step-down treatment, Systems Training for Emotional Predictability and Problem Solving, and motive-oriented psychotherapy.
- Although DBT has been studied the most, a series of meta-analyses suggest little to no differences between any active specialty treatments for BPD; there are no differences between DBT and non-DBT treatments or between cognitive behavior theory–based and psychodynamic theory–based treatments. Thus, clinicians are justified in using any of these efficacious treatments and might consider developing expertise in more than one approach.

Disclosure: The authors report no relationship or financial interest with any entity that would pose conflict of interest with the subject matter of this article.
[a] Department of Psychology, The Pennsylvania State University, State College, PA 16802, USA; [b] Department of Psychiatry, Joan and Sanford I. Weill Medical College of Cornell University, New York, NY 10065, USA; [c] Department of Psychiatry, Centre for Addiction and Mental Health, University of Toronto, Toronto, Ontario, M5S 2S1, Canada; [d] Mentalization Training Unit, Saint Ann's Hospital, North London, NW3 5SU, UK; [e] Department of Psychiatry, Upstate Medical University, Syracuse, NY 13210, USA
* Corresponding author. Department of Psychology, The Pennsylvania State University, University Park, 362 Bruce V. Moore Building, State College, PA 16802.
E-mail address: klevy@psu.edu

Psychiatr Clin N Am 41 (2018) 711–728
https://doi.org/10.1016/j.psc.2018.07.011
0193-953X/18/© 2018 Elsevier Inc. All rights reserved.

Borderline personality disorder (BPD) is a serious mental health disorder characterized by instability in relationships, emotions, identity, and behavior.[1,2] Approximately 2% to 6% of the general population suffer from BPD,[3] which thus is more common than schizophrenia, bipolar disorder, and autism. Clinical studies have found that 15% to 20% of outpatients[4] and up to 25% of inpatients[5] are diagnosed with BPD. Health care providers should keep in mind that the risk of suicide in BPD is high. An estimated 60% to 85% of individuals with BPD attempt suicide once (mean = 3.3 suicide attempts[6,7]; 8% complete suicide).[8,9] In this article, the authors examine the major treatments developed for BPD. Treatment rationales, techniques, and evidence are described. Special attention is paid to identifying potential mechanisms of change, identifying predictors of long-term outcome, and prescriptive indications for patient-treatment matching. Similarities and differences between treatment approaches and outcome are highlighted. Commonalities across these treatments suggest several important evidence-based guidelines for integrated care.

BPD has historically been viewed as difficult to treat using either psychotherapeutic or psychopharmacologic treatment modalities. Patients with BPD have been noted to frequently not adhere to treatment recommendations, use services chaotically, and repeatedly drop out of treatment. Many clinicians are intimidated by the prospect of treating BPD patients and are pessimistic about the outcome of treatment. Therapists treating patients with BPD have displayed high levels of burnout and have been known to be prone to enactments and even engagement in iatrogenic behaviors. This perspective arose in part due to the publication of case material that tended to be focused on difficult cases and situations within cases. The publication of these cases, although selected and thus not representative of outcome, was important because it helped articulate problem areas for focus and the development of techniques to address these issues. It also contributed, however, to the belief that those diagnosed with BPD were difficult if not impossible to treat. Consistent with this there is little evidence demonstrating for the efficacy of standard forms of cognitive behavior therapy (CBT) and psychoanalytic/psychodynamic therapy (PDT) for treating BPD.[10]

In recent years, however, there has been a burgeoning empirical literature on the treatment of BPD. Beginning with Linehan's[11] seminal randomized controlled trial (RCT) of dialectical behavior therapy (DBT), there is now a range of treatments—deriving from both the cognitive behavior and psychodynamic traditions—that have shown efficacy in RCTs and are now available to clinicians. Some of these treatments were derived from the cognitive behavior tradition. The best known and most widely tested of these is DBT,[11] discussed later. Others include schema-focused therapy (SFT),[12] Systems Training for Emotional Predictability and Problem Solving (STEPPS),[14] emotion regulation group therapy,[15–17] and motive-oriented therapeutic relationship (MOTR).[18] Other BPD-specific psychotherapies were derived from the psychoanalytic/psychodynamic tradition. The best known are mentalization-based therapy (MBT)[19] and transference-focused psychotherapy (TFP),[20–22] both of which are discussed later. Another psychodynamic treatment of BPD, dynamic deconstructive psychotherapy, also has demonstrated efficacy.[23]

The results of these efficacy studies suggest important evidence-based principles. First, BPD is a treatable disorder. Second, because BPD is chronic, its treatment seems to require longer-term efforts (all efficacious approaches conceptualize treatment as a multiyear process) and high levels of intensity; nonetheless, important and significant gains can be made in a relatively short time. Third, therapists have a range of options across several orientations available to them and it is premature to foreclose on any one of the available options that have been tested. Although there have been few direct comparisons, enough data now exist from RCTs and meta-analyses to suggest that no one approach has been consistently found superior to another.

Treatments, such as DBT, schema-focused psychotherapy (SFT), MBT, and TFP, have been described as specialty treatments because they represent modifications of standard CBT and PDT developed specifically for BPD. Kernberg[24] began identifying modifications to standard psychoanalytic therapy during his time at the Menninger Clinic and as part of the Menninger Psychotherapy Research Project. He based these modifications on pragmatic observations and the differing developmental psychopathology of BPDs, as he articulated it, which required changes to the 1-size-fits-all psychoanalytic model at that time. These modifications included a more active stance, explicit setting of the frame, increased emphasis on life outside the therapy (eg, a focus on productive investments and developing a hierarchy for session focus that emphasized events outside session, such as suicidality), the explication and increased efforts to the maintenance of a nonjudgmental stance (called technical neutrality), and, relatedly, a de-emphasis on overt supportive techniques, and finally modifications to the interpretive process. Similarly, Linehan[11] describes developing DBT as a modification of standard CBT, which she believed was not well suited for BPD patients due to a host of different issues that these patients were grappling with. Thus, she developed structures and skill modalities that targeted the difficulties seen in BPD. Young,[12] in developing SFT, also modified the standard CT of Beck[13] for use with BPD patients.

In developing these specialized treatments, these clinical investigators either implicitly or explicitly modified and integrated perspectives outside their home orientations or developed techniques that were consistent with other orientations. Thus, each of these treatments is integrative. For example, in SFT, they explicitly acknowledge the integration of attachment theory and object relational approaches.

In this section, the authors focus on the following 3 treatments for BPD: DBT, MBT, and TFP. Each treatment and evidence for its efficacy in the treatment of BPD is first described and then similarities and differences across these 3 treatments examined.

DIALECTICAL BEHAVIOR THERAPY

DBT is an integrative model that blends elements from traditional CBT with acceptance-based practice drawn from Zen and humanistic approaches. DBT originally developed within the context of treating BPD; however, it has evolved as a treatment of multidisordered, complex client populations. The DBT biosocial theory conceptualizes BPD as a disorder of pervasive emotional dysregulation characterized by high emotional vulnerability and deficits in the ability to modulate emotions.[11] Emotion regulation disturbances develop as a consequence of transaction between biological anomalies resulting in emotional vulnerability and a relational history characterized by invalidating experiences. Borderline symptoms are viewed as a byproduct or consequence of dysregulated emotions. DBT targets all elements of the emotion regulation system, including cognitions, phenomenological experience, expressive–motor behavior, and action tendencies.

The DBT intervention framework dialectically balances a focus on change and acceptance/validation strategies. The overarching goal of all treatment interventions is to enhance emotion regulation. The treatment model balances a structured approach with therapist flexibility and responsivity. The intervention framework is diverse and includes a broad range of change-based interventions, such as exposure-based procedures, problem assessment and solution analysis, exposure, and structural strategies, along with acceptance-based strategies, including validation and a reciprocal communication style. The focus on balancing change and acceptance cuts across DBT's 4 skills modules: mindfulness, distress tolerance, emotion regulation, and interpersonal effectiveness.

Standard DBT has multiple modes that address the following functions:

1. Improving capabilities and skills
2. Enhancing motivation to change
3. Generalizing treatment gains to the client's natural environment
4. Structuring the environment to facilitate and maintain progress
5. Enhancing and maintaining therapist motivation and capabilities

These functions are achieved through the treatments' 4 modes:

1. Weekly individual therapy session to focus on client motivation managing crises and addressing how to help the client develop a life worth living
2. A 2-hour weekly skills training group that emphasizes the acquisition of mindfulness, emotion regulation, interpersonal effectiveness, and distress tolerance skills and is designed to enhance capabilities
3. Access to client-therapist telephone consultation 24 hours a day to ensure
4. Weekly therapist consultation meetings to enhance therapist motivation and improve competence

Among psychotherapies for BPD, DBT has garnered the most robust evidence base. To date, 14 randomized clinical trials (RCTs) have examined the effectiveness of DBT for BPD (including BPD traits). Of these, 7 trials compared DBT with nonspecific controls for BPD.[26–32] The findings indicate that DBT is consistently superior to nonspecific comparators in reducing suicidal and self-harm behavior, health care utilization (eg, inpatient psychiatric hospital admissions and emergency department visits), Clarkin, and improving treatment retention. DBT in comparison to well-defined comparator treatments has also been examined in 8 RCTs.[33–45] DBT has been shown as effective as other well-structured treatments and is associated with improvement across a broad range of outcomes, including suicidal and self-harm behavior, health care utilization, symptoms (depression and anger), and general functioning. Furthermore, the effects of treatment are durable postdischarge.[43] Although general levels of functional impairment show improvement over the course of treatment, they remain remain poor post-treatment.

DIALECTICAL BEHAVIOR THERAPY SKILLS ONLY

DBT skills training offered as adjunctive or stand-alone intervention has become increasingly popular. In the current health care climate of rising costs and limited resources, and with the demand for specialist services exceeding available resources, DBT skills groups are popular because they offer a less resource intensive alternative to standard DBT. DBT skills training groups are increasingly delivered across a variety of contexts, including residential, inpatient, addiction, correctional, forensic, and emergency room services. Skills training groups are easier to disseminate than standard DBT because they require fewer resources and less staff training.

Three RCTs have evaluated DBT skills–only groups for BPD. Soler and colleagues[46] compared 13 weeks of DBT skills training with standard group therapy for individuals diagnosed with BPD. The results indicated that the DBT skills group was superior to the standard group therapy on the following outcomes: BPD symptoms, depression, anxiety, anger, and affect instability. There were no between-group differences on suicidal and self-harm behavior although individuals were not specifically recruited for these behaviors and there was considerable between-subject variance. In another trial, which recruited suicidal and self-injuring BPD clients, Linehan and colleagues[40] randomly assigned participants to a 1 year of standard DBT, DBT skills group plus intensive case management, or DBT individual therapy. Participants enrolled in the arms with skills training—standard DBT or DBT skills training plus intensive care management—had superior outcomes to DBT individual therapy.

In a third trial, McMain and colleagues[47–49] randomized 84 chronically suicidal individuals diagnosed with BPD to 20 weeks of DBT skills training or an active wait-list condition. The DBT group had superior outcomes compared with the active wait-list control on the following outcomes: self-destructive (eg, suicidal and self-harm) behaviors, aggressive behavior (eg, anger), and coping skills (eg, distress tolerance and emotion regulation).

In sum, these trials suggest that DBT skills training as a stand-alone intervention may be especially helpful for high-risk behaviors and symptoms associated with the acute phase of BPD; further research is needed.

MENTALIZATION-BASED THERAPY

MBT is a structured psychodynamic psychotherapy that has been applied in both individual and group formats. In this approach, many of the symptoms of BPD are viewed as resulting from a distortion of, or reduction in, a social cognitive capacity called mentalizing. Mentalizing is defined as the ability to understand the actions of oneself and others in terms of mental states, including both thoughts and feelings. This ability is viewed as critical to everyday interactions and impacts an individual's capacity to experience one's behavior as coherently organized by mental states and to experience oneself as differentiated from others. These capacities may readily be weakened in individuals with a personality disorder, particularly when faced with interpersonal stress, resulting in a loss of cognitive and emotional coherence and differentiation between self and other. In this framework, the symptoms of BPD are understood as resulting from deficits in mentalizing capacities that are particularly pronounced in affectively charged interpersonal situations as well as a pressure to externalize intolerably painful internal states.[19] These deficits are believed to result from disruptions in early attachment relationships.

The core goal of MBT is to improve clients' capacity to mentalize by helping them to regain mentalizing when it is lost, maintain it when it is present, and to increase clients' ability to maintain a mentalizing stance in situations where it otherwise might be lost. Given that clients with BPD are particularly likely to lose mentalizing in interpersonal situations, the relationship between client and therapist is a key area of focus. In this approach, it is thought to be especially important that the client experiences the therapist (or someone else) as keeping the client's mental state in mind.

MBT involves a collaborative and structured approach to working to gently expand mentalizing and helping the client to identify mental states that were previously outside the client's awareness. This approach involves the therapist exhibiting empathy and providing validation of the client's experience, clarifying and exploring the client's narrative, and identifying the affective focus of the session. The therapist then helps broaden the client's perspective on the events presented in the client's narrative by presenting alternative perspectives. The work to expand the client's mentalizing primarily focuses on the here and now of the session and gradually comes to involve relationships with core attachment figures and other key people in the client's life, how these relationships become activated with the therapist, and how they influence mentalizing. The therapist works to encourage mentalizing the therapeutic relationship and takes into account both transference and countertransference reactions, which are specifically defined in terms of technical application. As mentalizing improves, the client becomes increasingly able to alternative representations of important relationships.

The beginning of treatment in MBT involves the establishment of goals with the client. Initial goals are to include commitment to and engagement in treatment as well as an agreement to reduce harmful and self-destructive behaviors. Attachment strategies activated in relationships are mapped out with the client and a joint formulation agreed. A longer-term goal is the improvement of personal and social relationships as well as engagement in constructive activity. MBT was initially developed and tested as an 18-month treatment program that included both group and individual sessions; however, in clinical settings, it has been offered for shorter periods of time and in formats that include only individual or group therapy. Currently, there is no research evidence regarding the optimal format or length of MBT treatment.

To date, 3 RCTs have tested the efficacy of MBT for the treatment of BPD. The first trial of MBT[50] compared it to treatment as usual and found MBT superior in reducing self-harm, suicidality, hospitalization, need for medication, and self-report measures of depression, anxiety, symptom severity, and social adjustment. These results were maintained at an 18-month follow-up[51–57] that also found continued improvement in social and interpersonal functioning. An 8-year follow-up study[58] found that MBT remained superior to treatment as usual in the following outcomes: suicidality, diagnostic status, outpatient service use, need for medication, and social adjustment. Another trial of 134 clients comparing MBT to a structured clinical management (SCM) outpatient program for the treatment of BPD[59] found that MBT was superior with regard to the following outcomes: suicidality, severe self-harm, and client-reported symptom severity, depression, interpersonal problems, and social adjustment. Results also suggested that the rate of change of symptoms differed based on treatment: in MBT, there was more rapid improvement in mood, interpersonal functioning, and social adjustment, whereas the rate of improvement in self-harm was slower in MBT (although the ultimate improvement was greater compared with the SCM group). A follow-up analysis examining clients from this trial with comorbid BPD and antisocial personality disorder found that MBT was also efficacious in reducing anger, hostility, paranoia, self-harm, suicide attempts, negative mood, general psychiatric symptoms, and interpersonal problems and in improving social adjustment in this subgroup of clients.[60] A more recent trial of 85 clients diagnosed with BPD compared MBT to a manualized supportive group therapy[61,62] and found that both treatments were associated with improvements in psychological and interpersonal functioning as well as a decrease in the number of criteria met for BPD; MBT was found to have superior outcomes in clinician-rated functioning. Treatment effects were found sustained 18 months after the trial, with three-quarters of both groups achieving sustained diagnostic remission, and half of the MBT group meeting criteria for functional remission (compared with less than one-fifth of the comparison group). Another relevant study examined MBT in the treatment of self-harming adolescents,[63] 73% of whom met criteria for BPD, and found MBT superior to treatment-as-usual in reducing self-harm, suicidality, and depression. Taken together, these results suggest that MBT is efficacious in treating BPD, including clients with comorbid antisocial personality disorder, and that improvements are sustained long after treatment has ended.

TRANSFERENCE-FOCUSED PSYCHOTHERAPY

TFP is a principle-based manualized individual outpatient psychodynamic psychotherapy tailored specifically for the treatment of severe personality disorders, including BPD. It was developed based on Kernberg's[25] theory of the developmental origins of BPD, in which the symptoms of BPD are understood as arising from unintegrated affectively charged representations of self and others. This lack of integration means that totally negative representations of self and other—and the associated affects—are split off from totally positive representations, leading to instability in affects, identity, and relationships. The goal of

TFP is to integrate these unintegrated representations, leading to a more coherent sense of identity, better affect regulation, a reduction in self-destructive behavior, more balanced and constant relationships, and improved overall functioning.

The primary focus of TFP is on the affect-laden themes that arise in the relationship between client and therapist within sessions; attention is also paid to the client's life outside sessions. Sessions typically take place twice per week. The treatment begins with contract-setting that clarifies the therapeutic frame, the method of treatment, and the responsibilities of both client and therapist. In this contract-setting phase, the therapist is careful to elicit and address any concerns the client may have about the treatment frame. This treatment frame is intended to help contain the client's acting out behaviors. Particularly in the first year of treatment, TFP focuses on a hierarchy of treatment goals: addressing behaviors that pose a risk to self or others (including suicidal and self-destructive behavior), therapy-interfering behaviors, and identifying predominant object relational patterns as they emerge in the here-and-now transference relationship with the therapist.

To date, 3 trials have assessed the efficacy of TFP in the treatment of BPD. Two of thes,[36,64] are discussed previously. In the Clarkin and colleagues[36] trial, although no treatment was found superior in terms of symptom change, TFP was found superior to both DBT and supportive psychodynamic (SPT) in terms of change in attachment patterns and reflective functioning,[65] which is consistent with the mechanisms of change hypothesized by the underlying theory of TFP. In another trial of 104 clients comparing TFP to treatment by an experienced community psychotherapist, TFP was found more efficacious in reducing suicide attempts, inpatient admissions, BPD symptoms, psychosocial functioning, and personality organization.[66,67] In summary, the results of these trials suggest that TFP is efficacious in the treatment of BPD symptoms and overall functioning and may be particularly efficacious in improving attachment patterns and reflective functioning.

In contrast to these specialty treatments, Gunderson and Paris independently have described what they call generalist approaches to psychotherapy and treatment of BPD. Gunderson with Links[68] developed what was originally called general psychiatric management, now named good psychiatric management (GPM). GPM was originally developed as a control condition for an RCT in comparison to DBT[44] and was based on recommendations from the *Guidelines for the Treatment of BPD* published by the American Psychiatric Association in 2001.[69] GPM served as an active and credible control in an RCT examining the efficacy of DBT. In that trial, no between-group differences were found across a broad range of outcomes at end of treatment (12 months) and 24 months postdischarge.[43,44] GPM has evolved since the original trial and what follows is a description of the treatment as it was evaluated.

GPM consists of 3 modes of intervention, including

1. Case management
2. Psychodynamically informed individual psychotherapy
3. Symptom-targeted medication management

Derived from the care promoted in the APA *Guidelines*, emphasizes psychotherapy as the first-line treatment of BPD. GPM's psychotherapeutic approach is well organized and informed by Gunderson's[70] psychodynamic approach treating BPD. The following principles guide the practice of GPM:

1. Clients are viewed and treated as competent adults.
2. Therapists are encouraged to be flexible in terms of the treatment focus.
3. Attention is accorded to client's role functioning.[71,72]

GPM conceptualizes intolerance of aloneness as the core problem underlying BPD. Disturbed attachment relationships contribute to the relational aspects of this disorder. Accordingly, the assessment of problematic patterns in relationships is a focus of treatment.[70] Emotion-processing problems figure centrally in disturbed attachment relationships and consequently GPM has an emotion focus.[71]

In the original trial, GPM was a comprehensive format involving weekly individual therapy sessions (50 minutes), weekly therapist group, and case management. There are a variety of treatment strategies in the model and these include responding to crises, safety monitoring, establishing and monitoring a therapeutic framework and alliance, educating the client and the client's family about the disorder, facilitating adherence to the treatment regimen, coordinating multimodal therapies, and monitoring clinical status and treatment plans. The GPM approach commonly includes medication management and in the original trial this was based on a symptom-targeted approach. Ancillary treatments are tailored to the client's needs and guided by a view that a multimodal and community approach is most effective with suicidal individuals.[73] In the GPM model, therapists are not available outside of working hours and clients are instead encouraged to exercise control over their behavior and seek out emergency services as needed.

With similar intentions, Bateman and Fonagy[59] in the United Kingdom developed a similar manualized approach for BPD that they called SCM, delivered by generalist mental health clinicians without specialist training. SCM was used as a distinct comparison treatment in an RCT comparing MBT for BPD.[59] Focusing less on psychodynamic relational elements in treatment and more on emotional management and impulse control than GPM, the treatment did remarkably well on self-harm and suicide attempts although it was less effective than MBT over time, particularly with the more severe clients.[60,74,75] SCM has been developed further[74] and is currently organized to meet the UK standards for treatment of BPD when delivered by nonspecialists within general mental health services.[76]

Another similar approach is the stepped care rehabilitation model articulated by Paris and colleagues[77–79] as an alternative to extended treatment of BPD. Paris notes that BPD is characterized by both acute and chronic phases. Although BPD presents significant clinical challenges in its acute phase, most patients show steady improvement over time and eventually recover or remit. Despite improvements, those with BPD show residual difficulties, particularly in work and relationships, which can benefit from further treatment. Paris[77] views this residual period as the chronic phase of BPD and suggests that BPD patients have available to them treatments that they can access intermittently on an as-needed basis. In this approach, Paris[77] contends that various empirically supported approaches and derived principles can be applied flexibly. Although no efficacy data from a RCT exist testing this approach, Paris[77] has presented pre–post data on 130 treated individuals. Paris[77] found reductions in somatization, obsessive-compulsive symptoms, interpersonal sensitivity, depression, anxiety, hostility, paranoia, and psychoticism on the Symptom Checklist–90. Additionally, there were reductions in depression, impulsivity, dysfunctional attitudes, and number of emergency department visits and hospital admissions. These findings notwithstanding, this treatment awaits further testing using more rigorous designs that control for issues that pre–post designs cannot account for (eg, regression to the mean).

In addition to the treatments discussed previously, there is preliminary evidence to support other treatments for BPD based on studies using pre–post or quasiexperimental designs or in case studies or in RCTs with ambiguous results. These include the conversational model,[80] cognitive analytical therapy,[81] modified cognitive therapy,[82] clarification-oriented psychotherapy,[83] interpersonal psychotherapy,[84] interpersonal group psychotherapy,[95] and emotion-focused psychotherapy.[86]

DIRECT COMPARISONS

Although most trials of psychotherapies designed specifically for the treatment of BPD have compared these BPD-specific treatments to treatment as usual or a non–BPD-specific treatment, a few trials have directly compared the efficacy of BPD-specific treatments. One trial[64,87] comparing TFP and SFT found that both treatments were efficacious in reducing general and BPD-specific symptoms and improving quality of life but found SFT superior at the 3-year mark with regard to these outcomes, although the TFP cell contained more suicidal patients and showed less adherence.[88,89] Similarly, the therapeutic alliance was rated as higher in SFT compared with TFP,[90] although many of the alliance ratings were made after dropout. Another trial[36] compared TFP, DBT, and an SPT designed for the treatment of BPD (SPT). Results suggested that all 3 treatments (TFP, DBT, and SPT) were generally equivalent in showing statistically significant improvement in multiple symptom domains relevant to BPD, whereas TFP was found superior to both DBT and SPT in terms of change in attachment patterns and reflective functioning.[65] Finally, a year-long trial of 180 clients compared DBT to GPM and found both efficacious in treating suicidal behavior, borderline symptoms, general distress, depression, anger, and health care utilization and in improving interpersonal functioning.[44] A 2-year follow-up study[43] found that these improvements either continued or were sustained over follow-up. Neither treatment was found superior to the other.

META-ANALYSES

As research has been conducted examining the efficacy and effectiveness of psychotherapeutic treatments for BPD, researchers have begun to use systematic reviews and meta-analyses to examine whether any conclusions and recommendations can be drawn from the existing literature. Binks and colleagues[90] initially conducted a systematic review of 7 studies of psychotherapy for BPD, 6 of which were of DBT trails. Although there was evidence of moderate effect sizes (ESs), the confidence intervals were so large as to render the interpretations unreliable. Thus, these investigators concluded that therapy may help treat some problems experienced by BPD clients, including self-harm, hospital admission, depression, and anxiety; however, because of the large confidence intervals, they cautioned that all treatments "remain experimental".[90[p21]] Subsequently, a meta-analysis focused on trials examining the efficacy of DBT[91] found a moderate ES of .39 across 16 studies. Moderator analyses, however, revealed a difference in ES depending on whether the comparison condition was a BPD-specific treatment; the ES was estimated at .51 when DBT was compared with psychotherapies not specifically intended for the treatment of BPD (eg, treatment as usual), but the ES was not significant (estimated at 0.01) when DBT was compared with other BPD-specific treatments, such as TFP or GPM. A later review and meta-analysis of treatments for BPD[92] found there were indications of beneficial effects for comprehensive psychotherapies (defined as treatments where individual psychotherapy was a substantial part of the treatment). Additionally, noncomprehensive psychotherapeutic interventions (treatments where individual psychotherapy was not a substantial part of the treatment, such as psychoeducation and skills training) were also helpful although they were evaluated in only a few trials. The investigators noted that although DBT has been studied most intensely, followed by MBT, TFP, SFT, and STEPPS, they did not consider any of the treatments to have a robust base of evidence and raised concerns about the quality of individual studies. The investigators concluded that psychotherapy is critical to the treatment of BPD; however, replication studies are needed.

More recently, Cristea and colleagues[93,94] conducted a meta-analysis of 33 trials and more than 2000 clients. They found small-to-moderate ESs—ranging between .32 and .44—across types of psychotherapies and outcome variables. No difference was found between DBT and psychodynamic approaches. The investigators concluded that psychotherapy is effective for treating BPD symptoms but cautioned that effects were small, may be inflated by risk of bias and publication bias, and may not be stable at follow-up.

Levy and colleagues[95,96] have also recently completed a comprehensive meta-analysis and metaregression examining treatment of BPD. Levy and colleagues[95] undertook a different approach in that they gathered all studies of psychotherapy for BPD regardless of randomization. In total, they identified 73 unique studies that included more than 1700 patients. By including a wide range of studies with diverse methods, Levy and colleagues[95] were able to examine methodological moderators in addition to study and patient moderators. Although the within-group effects were large (ES = .86), the between-group effects were more moderate. Across all controlled studies, the ES = .36, translating into an effect of number needed to treat (NNT) of 8. Compared with TAU, however, the ES increased to 498 and the NNT became a more robust 5. Compared with wait-list controls, the ES = .646, and the NNT was 4. There were no differences between PDT and CBT treatments or between DBT and other treatments. There was no difference in independently and reliability-rated quality of studies between PDT and CBT. The only consistent moderators were methodological ones: in addition to control condition reported earlier, higher study quality led to weaker effects, dichotomous outcomes had larger effects, observer-rated outcomes had larger effects than self-report, nonblind raters had larger effects, and completer analyses showed larger effects.

TREATMENT GUIDELINES

There are several treatment guidelines and reviews, including the Society of Clinical Psychology Committee[97] on Science and Practice, the United Kingdom National Institute for Health and Care Excellence guidelines,[75] the Cochrane Collaboration reviews,[54] and the Netherlands Multidisciplinary Directive for Personality Disorders,[98] the National Health and Medical Research Council of the Australian Government Clinical Practice Guideline[99] for the Management of Borderline Personality Disorder. These guidelines tend to be consistent in recommending the big five psychotherapies (DBT, MBT, TFP, SFT, and GPM) for treating BPD.

EVIDENCE-BASED CONCLUSIONS

There are several treatment implications of this review. First, there are multiple treatments available to patients with BPD and the clinicians who treat them. Although these treatments derive out of different theoretic orientations and do have some differences, they all tend to be integrative, either explicitly or implicitly. Despite the use of different terms and jargon, there are more similarities across these treatments than is often recognized. This may be in large part given that these treatments are derived from similar clinical experiences in adapting to the challenge of treating clients with BPD, and treatments have been developed and refined in part based on knowledge derived from the broader literature on psychotherapy for BPD. All these treatments tend to be long term, with clinical trials lasting 12 months to 18 months and naturalistic treatment often lasting longer. All 3 include the provision of supervision and consultation for therapists (or intervision for more experienced therapists), with the explicit goal of protecting against therapist burnout, enactments, passivity, iatrogenic behaviors, and colluding with clients' pathology. Similarly, to avoid splitting across providers, each treatment emphasizes integration of different services received by clients and communication among providers. Each treatment is based on a coherent and principle-based theoretic model that guides interventions and is presented to the client so that it makes sense to both the therapist and the client. Additionally, each of these treatments pays a great deal of attention to the structure and frame of therapy: the roles and responsibilities of both client and therapist are clearly established, a great deal of time is dedicated to discussing the treatment frame and addressing treatment-interfering behaviors, and there is a clear focus and set of priorities in treatment to guide the focus of individual sessions. In particular, all treatments involve a commitment to reduce self-destructive behaviors. In both TFP and DBT, there is an explicit focus on prioritizing, respectively, self-destructive behaviors, therapy-interfering behaviors, and behaviors that interfere with quality of life, including a detailed analysis of events when the client does engage in these behaviors. Further, although the reduction of self-destructive behavior is a top priority in each of these treatments, so too is comprehensive change above and beyond symptom reduction. MBT focuses on developing the capacity to mentalize that contributes to intraperseonal and interpersonal functioning, DBT builds toward a "life worth living," whereas TFP aims for clients to develop the capacity "to love and to work." Additionally, each of these treatments places a great deal of emphasis on the therapeutic relationship. Another commonality across these treatments is facilitating the client integrating disparate views, particularly in the context of intense affect, whether via dialectical thinking (DBT) or the exploration of possible alternative perspectives (TFP and MBT).

In these treatments, therapists to take an active role in treatment, adopt a nonjudgmental and flexible stance and to empathize with the client without reinforcing distortions in the perception of self or others. Many treatments for BPD use group therapy in addition to individual therapy: DBT includes skills groups, MBT has traditionally included group therapy, and STEPPS and emotion regulation group therapy are group psychotherapies for BPD. Other forms of treatment, such as dynamic deconstructive psychotherapy, may encourage but not require involvement in group psychotherapy. Additionally, there is a common focus on emotion regulation, views of self and other, and on addressing unintegrated or polarized mental states. The specific form this takes may differ by treatment; for instance, DBT focuses on dialectical thinking, TFP focuses on vacillations in object-relations dyads (affectively charged representations of self and other in relationship) and in integrating self and other representations, whereas SFT focuses on abrupt shifts between schema modes (thoughts, behaviors, and emotions that reflect the emotional/behavioral state of the person at any given moment). MBT emphasizes shifts in mentalizing from effective mentalizing process to nonmentalizing modes. Furthermore, there is a common focus on helping clients to link and integrate their emotions, thoughts, and behaviors. Finally, treatments for BPD generally include a focus on self-observation as well as considering alternative perspectives. Despite this evidence, at this point there are few prescriptive indicators suggested in the literature.

Second, there seem few reliable differences between these treatments when well delivered. In the absence of evidence supporting the superiority of one psychotherapy approach over another, an effective system of care for BPD should include multiple treatment options. Some clients have preferences for specific therapeutic models and this issue warrants consideration. Research on client preference indicates that preferences may have an impact on treatment engagement and the development of a positive therapeutic alliance[100–104] and, therefore, client preferences for specific approaches may be relevant to treatment planning.

Additionally, BPD, like many other disorders, is heterogeneous. As such, it would be shortsighted to think that one treatment approach is best for all presentations. It is likely that some patients might do better in an MBT approach, others DBT, and still others in TFP. At this point, little is known about which type of borderline patients will do best in which specific treatments. Brief treatments and nonspecialty treatments, such as GPM, SCM, and step-down care, are an important part of a broader continuum of care and an alternative to evidence-based lengthy structured treatments. There is growing evidence for the efficacy of abbreviated and adjunctive treatments, such as DBT skills training, STEPPS, emotion regulation groups, and MOTR. Access to comprehensive, lengthy treatments is a global problem due to limited resources, a shortage of well-trained clinicians, and wait-lists. Because evidence-based comprehensive structured treatments for BPD can be costly and complex to deliver to all clients who need it, brief skills-based treatment models may play an important role. Brief interventions are more feasible to implement and disseminate, especially within poorly resourced health care contexts. Furthermore, brief treatments may be suitable for some clients, especially those with less severity and chronicity.

Nonetheless, many patients may desire or require more lengthy and intensive treatments. Given the relative equivalence of the various treatments, patient preferences, limited resources, and patient heterogeneity, it is important for communities to have more than one type of treatment available, most likely from different perspectives (eg, CBT vs PDT). Additionally, individual therapists and their patients may benefit from treaters knowing and having been trained in more than one type of treatment. Increasingly, training institutions and therapists are learning more than one modality. This allows them to integrate various aspects of the treatments, to sequence treatments, and to be responsive to patient needs.

In sum, there are several treatments available to the practicing clinician. The big five psychotherapies for treating BPD are

1. DBT
2. MBT
3. TFP
4. SFT
5. GPM (with PDT)

Outcome data, direct comparisons, and meta-analyses all suggest few reliable differences between these treatments and that no one treatment is more effective than the other. In addition, there are several adjunctive treatments (DBT skills group, STEPPS, and MOTR) that may be useful. Finally, there are several other treatments that show promise and warrant additional study.

Despite these conclusions, treatment research for BPD is relatively impoverished compared with other conditions. This relative lack of research has impeded the field. What is needed are large-scale, multisite studies that compare 2 active treatments with enhanced treatment as usual that allow making inferences about noninferiority and examine moderators.[105–107] Studies selecting patients based on prescriptive indicators would be useful too and allow answering Gordon Paul's[78] iconic question, What treatment, by whom, is most effective for this individual, with that specific problem, and under which set of circumstances?

REFERENCES

1. American Psychiatric Association. Practice guideline for the treatment of patients with borderline personality disorder. Am J Psychiatry 2001;158:1–52.

2. American Psychiatric Association. Diagnostic and statistical manual of mental disorders. 5th edition. Washington, DC: American Psychiatric Association; 2013.

3. Grant BF, Chou SP, Goldstein RB, et al. Prevalence, correlates, disability, and comorbidity of DSM-IV borderline personality disorder: results from the wave 2 national epidemiologic survey on alcohol and related conditions. J Clin Psychiatry 2008;69(4):533–45.

4. Zimmerman M, Rothschild L, Chelminski I. The prevalence of DSM-IV personality disorders in psychiatric outpatients. Am J Psychiatry 2005;162(10):1911–8.

5. Zanarini MC, Frankenburg FR, Hennen J, et al. Mental health service utilization of borderline patients and Axis II comparison subjects followed prospectively for six years. J Clin Psychiatry 2004;65(1):28–36.

6. Black DW, Blum N, Pfohl B, et al. Suicidal behavior in borderline personality disorder: prevalence, risk factors, prediction and prevention. J Pers Disord 2004; 18(3):226–39.

7. Soloff PH, Lynch KG, Kelly TM. Childhood abuse as a risk factor for suicidal behavior in borderline personality disorder. J Pers Disord 2002;16(3):201–14.

8. Pompili M, Girardi P, Ruberto A, et al. Suicide in borderline personality disorder: a meta-analysis. Nord J Psychiatry 2005;59(5):319–24.

9. Pos AE, Greenberg LS. Emotion-focused therapy: the transforming power of affect. J Contemp Psychother 2007;37(1):25–31.

10. Yeomans FE, John FC, Levy KN. Psychodynamic psychotherapies. In: Oldham JM, Skodol AE, Bender DS, editors. Textbook of personality disorders. Arlington (VA): American Psychiatric Publishing; 2005. p. 275–88.

11. Linehan MM. Cognitive behavioural treatment of borderline personality disorder. New York: Guilford Press; 1993.

12. Young JE, Klosko J, Weishaar ME. Schema therapy: a practitioner's guide. New York: Guilford Press; 2003.

13. Beck AT, Freeman A. Associates. Cognitive therapy of personality disorders. New York: Guilford Press; 1990.

14. Blum N, Pfohl B, John DS, et al. STEPPS: a cognitive-behavioral systems-based group treatment for outpatients with borderline personality disorder–a preliminary report. Compr Psychiatry 2002;43(4):301–10.

15. Gratz KL, Gunderson. Extending research on the utility of an adjunctive emotion regulation group therapy for deliberate self-harm among women with borderline personality pathology. Personal Disord 2006;2(4):316–26.

16. Gregory RJ, Chlebowski S, Kang D, et al. A controlled trial of psychodynamic psychotherapy for co-occurring borderline personality disorder and alcohol use disorder. Psychotherapy (Chic) 2008;45(1):28–41.

17. Gross R, Olfson M, Gameroff M, et al. Borderline personality disorder in primary care. Arch Intern Med 2002;162(1):53–60.

18. Kramer AD, Guillory JE, Hancock JT. Experimental evidence of massive-scale emotion contagion through social networks. Proc Natl Acad Sci U S A 2014; 111(24):8788–90.

19. Bateman AW, Fonagy P. Mentalization-based treatment of BPD. J Pers Disord 2004;18(1):36–51.

20. Clarkin JF, Yeomans FE, Kernberg OF. Psychotherapy for borderline personality: focusing on object relations. Washington, DC: American Psychiatric Press; 2006.

21. Comtois KA, Elwood L, Holdcraft LC, et al. Effectiveness of dialectical behaviour therapy in a community mental health center. Cogn Behav Pract 2007;14(4): 406–14.

22. Comtois KA, Russo J, Snowden M, et al. Factors associated with high use of public mental health services by persons with borderline personality disorder. Psychiatr Serv 2003;54(8):1149–54.

23. Gregory RJ, Remen AL. A manual-based psychodynamic therapy for treatment-resistant borderline personality disorder. Psychotherapy 2008;45:15–27.

24. Kernberg OF. Severe personality disorders: psychotherapeutic strategies. New Haven, CT: Yale University Press; 1984.

25. Kernberg OF. Summary and conclusions of psychotherapy and psychoanalysis: final report of the Menninger Foundation's psychotherapy research project. Int J Psychiatry 1973;11(1):62–77.

26. Carter GL, Willcox CH, Lewin TJ, et al. Hunter DBT project: Randomized controlled trial of dialectical behaviour therapy in women with borderline personality disorder. Aust N Z J Psychiatry 2010;44(2):162–73.

27. Koons CR, Robin CJ, Tweed LJ, et al. Efficacy of dialectical behavior therapy in women veterans with borderline personality disorder. Behav Ther 2001;32(2):371–90.

28. Linehan MM. Cognitive-behavioral treatment of chronically parasuicidal borderline patients. Arch Gen Psychiatry 1991;48(12):1060.

29. Linehan MM, Schmidt H, Dimeff LA, et al. Dialectical behavior therapy for patients with borderline personality disorder and drug-dependence. Am J Addict 1999;8(4):279–92.

30. Priebe S, Bhatti N, Bremner K, et al. Effectiveness and cost-effectiveness of dialectical behaviour therapy for self-harming patients with personality disorder: a pragmatic randomised controlled trial. Psychother Psychosom 2012;81(6):356–65.

31. Verheul R, Van Den Bosch LM, Koeter MW, et al. Dialectical behaviour therapy for women with borderline personality disorder: 12-month, randomised clinical trial in The Netherlands. Br J Psychiatry 2003;182(2):135–40.

32. Sachse S, Keville S, Feigenbaum J. A feasibility study of mindfulness-based cognitive therapy for individuals with borderline personality disorder. Psychol Psychother 2011;84(2):184–200.

33. Andreasson K, Krogh J, Wenneberg C, et al. Effectiveness of dialectical behavior therapy versus collaborative assessment and management of suicidality treatment for reduction of self-harm in adults with borderline personality traits and disorder: a randomized observer-blinded clinical trial. Depress Anxiety 2016;33(6):520–30.

34. Andrews HE, Hulbert C, Cotton SM, et al. Relationships between the frequency and severity of non-suicidal self-injury and suicide attempts in youth with borderline personality disorder. Early Interv Psychiatry 2017;1–8. https://doi.org/10.1111/eip.12461.

35. Ansell EB, Sanislow CA, McGlashan TH, et al. Psychosocial impairment and treatment utilization by patients with borderline personality disorder, other personality disorders, mood and anxiety disorders, and a healthy comparison group. Compr Psychiatry 2007;48(4):329–36.

36. Clarkin JF, Levy KN, Lenzenweger MF, et al. Evaluating three treatments for borderline personality disorder: a multiwave study. Am J Psychiatry 2007;164(6):922–8.

37. Clarkin JF, Levy KN, Lenzenweger MF, et al. The personality disorders institute/borderline personality disorder research foundation randomized control trial for borderline personality disorder: rationale, methods, and patient characteristics. J Pers Disord 2004;18(1):52–72.

38. Harned MS, Korslund KE, Linehan MM. A pilot randomized controlled trial of dialectical behavior therapy with and without the dialectical behavior therapy prolonged exposure protocol for suicidal and self-injuring women with borderline personality disorder and PTSD. Behav Res Ther 2014;55:7–17.
39. Linehan MM, Comtois KA, Murray AM, et al. Two-year randomized controlled trial and follow-up of dialectical behavior therapy vs therapy by experts for suicidal behaviors and borderline personality disorder. Arch Gen Psychiatry 2006; 63(7):757–66.
40. Linehan MM, Korslund KE, Harned MS, et al. Dialectical behavior therapy for high suicide risk in individuals with borderline personality disorder: a randomized clinical trial and component analysis. JAMA Psychiatry 2015;72(5):475.
41. Linehan MM, Korslund KE, Harned MS, et al. Faculty of 1000 evaluation for dialectical behavior therapy for high suicide risk in individuals with borderline personality disorder: a randomized clinical trial and component analysis. JAMA Psychiatry 2015;72(5):475.
42. Linehan MM, Dimeff LA, Reynolds SK, et al. Dialectical behavior therapy versus comprehensive validation therapy plus 12-step for the treatment of opioid dependent women meeting criteria for borderline personality disorder. Drug Alcohol Depend 2002;67(1):13–26.
43. McMain SF, Guimond T, Streiner DL, et al. Dialectical behavior therapy compared with general psychiatric management for borderline personality disorder: clinical outcomes and functioning over a 2-year follow-up. Am J Psychiatry 2012;169(6):650–61.
44. McMain SF, Links PS, Gnam WH, et al. A randomized trial of dialectical behavior therapy versus general psychiatric management for borderline personality disorder. Am J Psychiatry 2009;166(12):1365–74.
45. Turner RM. Naturalistic evaluation of dialectical behavior therapy-oriented treatment for borderline personality disorder. Cogn Behav Pract 2000;7(4):413–9.
46. Soler J, Pascual JC, Tiana T, et al. Dialectical behaviour therapy skills training compared to standard group therapy in borderline personality disorder: a 3-month randomised controlled clinical trial. Behav Res Ther 2009;47(5):353–8.
47. McMain SF, Guimond T, Barnhart R, et al. A randomized trial of brief dialectical behaviour therapy skills training in suicidal patients suffering from borderline disorder. Acta Psychiatri Scand 2017;135(2):138–48.
48. National Health and Medical Research Council. Clinical practice guideline for the management of borderline personality disorder. Melbourne (Australia): National Health and Medical Research Council; 2012.
49. National Institute for Health and Care Excellence. Personality disorders: borderline and antisocial. England (United Kingdom): Quality Standard QS88; 2015. Available at: https://wwwniceorguk/guidance/qs88.
50. Bateman AW, Fonagy P. Effectiveness of partial hospitalization in the treatment of borderline personality disorder: a randomized controlled trial. Am J Psychiatry 1999;156(10):1563–9.
51. Bateman AW, Fonagy P. Treatment of borderline personality disorder with psychoanalytically oriented partial hospitalization: an 18-month follow-up. Am J Psychiatry 2001;158(1):36–42.
52. Bateman AW, Fonagy P. Health service utilization costs for borderline personality disorder patients treated with psychoanalytically oriented partial hospitalization versus general psychiatric care. Am J Psychiatry 2003;160(1):169–71.
53. Bateman AW, Fonagy P. Mentalization based treatment for borderline personality disorder. World Psychiatry 2010;9(1):11–5.

54. Bateman AW, Krawitz R. Borderline personality disorder: an evidence-based guide for generalist mental health professionals. Oxford (United Kingdom): Oxford University Press; 2013.
55. Bender DS, Dolan RT, Skodol AE, et al. Treatment utilization by patients with personality disorders. Am J Psychiatry 2001;158(2):295–302.
56. Binks C, Fenton M, McCarthy L, et al. Psychological therapies for people with borderline personality disorder (Review). Cochrane Database Syst Rev 2006;(8):CD005652.
57. Binks C, Fenton M, McCarthy L, et al. Psychological therapies for people with borderline personality disorder (Review). Cochrane Database of Systematic Reviews. Chichester, UK: John Wiley & Sons. 2006. https://doi.org/10.1002/14651858.CD005652.
58. Bateman AW, Fonagy P. 8-year follow-up of patients treated for borderline personality disorder: Mentalization-based treatment versus treatment as usual. Am J Psychiatry 2008;165(5):631–8.
59. Bateman A, Fonagy P. Randomized controlled trial of outpatient mentalization-based treatment versus structured clinical management for borderline personality disorder. Am J Psychiatry 2009;166(12):1355–64.
60. Bateman AW, Fonagy P. Mentalization based treatment for personality disorders: a practical guide. Oxford (United Kingdom): Oxford University Press; 2016.
61. Jorgensen CR, Freund C, Boye R, et al. Outcome of mentalization based and supportive psychotherapy in patients with borderline personality disorder: a randomised controlled trial. Acta Psychiatr Scand 2013;127(4):305–17.
62. Jorgensen CR, Kjolbye M, Freund C, et al. Level of functioning in patients with borderline personality disorder. The Risskov-I study. Nord Psychol 2009;61(1):42–60.
63. Rossouw T, Fonagy P. Mentalization-based treatment for self-harm in adolescents: a randomized controlled trial. J Am Acad Child Adolesc Psychiatry 2012;51:1304–13.
64. Giesen-Bloo J, van Dyck R, Spinhoven P, et al. Outpatient psychotherapy for borderline personality disorder: randomized trial of schema-focused therapy vs transference-focused psychotherapy. Arch Gen Psychiatry 2006;63(6):649–58.
65. Levy KN, Meehan KB, Kelly KM, et al. Change in attachment patterns and reflective function in a randomized control trial of transference-focused psychotherapy for borderline personality disorder. J Consult Clin Psychol 2006;74:1027–40.
66. Doering S, Hörz S, Rentrop M, et al. Transference-focused psychotherapy v. treatment by community psychotherapists for borderline personality disorder: Randomised controlled trial. Br J Psychiatry 2010;196(5):389–95.
67. Feigenbaum JD, Fonagy P, Pilling S, et al. A real-world study of the effectiveness of DBT in the UK National Health Service. Br J Clin Psychol 2012;51(2):121–41.
68. Gunderson JG, Links PS. Borderline personality disorder: a clinical guide. Washington, DC: American Psychiatric Publishing; 2008.
69. Oldham et al. 2001.
70. Gunderson JG. Borderline personality disorder: a clinical guide. Washington, DC: American Psychiatric Publishing Inc; 2001.
71. Links PS. Introduction. In: Links PS, editor. Clinical assessment and management of severe personality disorders. Washington, DC: American Psychiatric Press; 1996.

72. Markowitz JC, Weissman MM. Interpersonal psychotherapy: Past, present and future. Clin Psychol Psychother 2012;19(2):99–105.
73. Leenaars AA. Psychotherapy with suicidal people: the commonalities. Arch Suicide Res 2006;10:305–10.
74. Bateman AW, Fonagy P. Impact of clinical severity on outcomes of mentalisation-based treatment for borderline personality disorder. Br J Psychiatry 2013;203(3):221–7.
75. Bateman AW, Fonagy P. Randomized controlled trial of out-patient mentalization based treatment versus structured clinical management for borderline personality disorder. Am J Psychiatry 2009;166(12):1355–64.
76. National Institute for Health and Care Excellence. Personality disorders: borderline and antisocial. National Institute for Health and Care Excellence website. https://www.nice.org.uk/guidance/qs88. Updated June 2015. Accessed October 16, 2017.
77. Paris J. Stepped care for borderline personality disorder: making treatment brief, effective, and accessible. London: Academic Press; 2017.
78. Paul GL. Strategy of outcome research in psychotherapy. J Consult Psychol 1967;31:109–18.
79. Perry JC, Herman JL, Van der Kolk BA, et al. Psychotherapy and psychological trauma in borderline personality disorder. Psychiatr Ann 1990;20:33–43.
80. Meares R. The conversational model: An outline. Am J Psychother 2004;58(1): 51–66.
81. Ryle A, Leighton T, Pollock P. Cognitive analytic therapy and borderline personality disorder: The model and the method. Chichester: Wiley; 1997.
82. Brown GK, Newman CF, Charlesworth SE, et al. An open clinical trial of cognitive therapy for borderline personality disorder. J Pers Disord 2004;18(3):257–71.
83. Sachse R. Klärungsorientierte psychotherapie [Clarification-oriented psychotherapy]. Göttingen: Hogrefe; 2003.
84. Markowitz JC, Skodol AE, Bleiberg K. Interpersonal psychotherapy for borderline personality disorder: Possible mechanisms of change. J Clin Psychol 2006;62(4):431–44.
85. Marziali E, Munroe-Blum H. Interpersonal group psychotherapy for borderline personality disorder. New York: Basic Books; 1994.
86. Pos AE, Greenberg LS. Organizing awareness and increasing emotion regulation: Revising chair work in emotion-focused therapy for borderline personality disorder. J Pers Disord 2012;26(1):84–107.
87. Zanarini MC, Frankenburg FR, Hennen J, et al. Mental health service utilization by borderline personality disorder patients and Axis II comparison subjects followed prospectively for 6 years. J Clin Psychiatry 2004;65(1):28–36.
88. Levy KN, Meehan KB, Yeomans FE. An update and overview of the empirical evidence for transference-focused psychotherapy and other psychotherapies for borderline personality disorder. In: Levy KN, Ablon JS, Kachele H, editors. Psychodynamic psychotherapy research. New York: Springer; 2012. p. 139–67.
89. Yeomans FE. Questions concerning the randomized trial of schema-focused therapy vs. transference-focused therapy. Arch Gen Psychiatry 2007;58: 590–610.
90. Spinhoven P, Giesen-Bloo J, van Dyck R, et al. The therapeutic alliance in schema-focused therapy and transference-focused psychotherapy for borderline personality disorder. J Consult Clin Psychol 2007;75(1):104–15.

91. Kliem S, Kroger C, Kosfelder J. Dialectical behavior therapy for borderline personality disorder: a meta-analysis using mixed-effects modeling. J Consult Clin Psychol 2010;78(6):936–51.
92. Stoffers JM, Vollm BA, Rucker G, et al. Psychological therapies for people with borderline personality disorder. Cochrane Database Syst Rev 2012;(8):CD005652.
93. Cristea IA, Gentili C, Cotet CD, et al. Efficacy of psychotherapies for borderline personality disorder: a systematic review and meta-analysis. JAMA Psychiatry 2017;74(4):319–28.
94. de Groot ER, Verheul R, Trijsburg RW. An integrative perspective on psychotherapeutic treatments for borderline personality disorder. J Pers Disord 2008;22(4): 332–52.
95. Levy K, Ellison W, Temes C, Khalsa S. The outcome of psychotherapy for borderline personality disorder: A meta-analysis. Paper presented at: the 1st Annual Meeting of the North American Society for the Study of Personality Disorders; 2013 Apr 20-21; Boston, MA.
96. Lieb K, Zanarini MC, Schmahl C, et al. Borderline personality disorder. Lancet 2004;364(9432):453–61.
97. Society of Clinical Psychology Committee on Science and Practice. Diagnosis: borderline personality disorder. Society of Clinical Psychology website. https://www.div12.org/diagnosis/borderline-personality-disorder/. Updated 2015. Accessed October 16, 2018.
98. Landelijke Stuurgroep Multidisciplinaire Richtlijnontwikkeling in de GGZ [National Steering Committee on Multidisciplinary Guideline Development in Mental Health]. Multidisciplinaire richtlign persoonlikheidsstoornissen: richtlijn voor de diagnostiek en behandeling van volwassen patiënten met een persoonlijkheidstoornis [Multidisciplinary directive personality disorders: Guideline for the diagnosis and treatment of adult patients with personality disorders]. Utrecht: Trimbos Instituut; 2008.
99. National Health and Medical Research Council. Clinical practice guideline for the management of borderline personality disorder. Melbourne: National Health and Medical Research Council; 2012.
100. Iacoviello BM, McCarthy KS, Barrett MS, et al. Treatment preferences affect the therapeutic alliance: implications for randomized controlled trials. J Consult Clin Psychol 2007;75(1):194–8.
101. Lindhiem O, Bennett CB, Trentacosta CJ, et al. Client preferences affect treatment satisfaction, completion, and clinical outcome: A meta-analysis. Clin Psychol Rev 2014;34(6):506–17.
102. Swift JK, Callahan JL. The impact of client treatment preferences on outcome: a meta-analysis. J Clin Psychol 2009;65(4):368–81.
103. Turner RM. Understanding dialectical behavior therapy. Clin Psychol: Science and Practice 2006;7(1):95–8.
104. Warwar SH, Links PS, Greenberg L, et al. Emotion focused principles for working with borderline personality disorder. J Psychiatr Pract 2008;14:94–104.
105. Levy KN. Treating borderline personality disorder. In: Koocher GP, Norcross JC, Greene BA, editors. The psychologist's desk reference. 3rd edition. Boston: Oxford University Press; 2013. p. 193–6.
106. Levy KN, Yeomans FE, Denning F, et al. Commentary on the UK NICE guidelines for the treatment of borderline personality disorder. Personal Ment Health 2010; 4:54–8.
107. Levy KN, Scala JW. Integrated treatment for personality disorders: a commentary. J Psychothor Integr 2015;25(1):49–57.

Psychotherapy for Borderline Personality Disorder in Adolescents

Alan S. Weiner, PhD[a],*, Karin Ensink, PhD[b], Lina Normandin, PhD[b]

KEYWORDS

- Psychotherapy • Borderline personality disorder • Adolescents • Diagnosis

KEY POINTS

- The rapid proliferation of research on borderline personality disorder (BPD) in adolescence has helped to clarify the characteristics of BPD in young people, distinguished it from the vicissitudes of normal adolescence, and has made comparisons with adult manifestations of the disorder.
- The considerable emotional and economic cost to individuals, families, and society associated with adolescent BPD supports calls for early intervention and requires that the assessment of personality functioning be an essential component in the psychological evaluation of adolescents.
- Adult treatment models with demonstrated efficacy have been adapted for adolescents, including dialectical behavior therapy, mentalization-based therapy, transference focused psychotherapy, and cognitive-analytical therapy.
- The implementation in adolescence of these empirically supported treatment approaches are described after first reviewing factors that frequently complicate the recognition and diagnosis of BPD in young people, followed by an overview of research on BPD in adolescents that delineates its clinically relevant features.

The rapid proliferation of research on borderline personality disorder (BPD) in adolescence has helped to clarify the characteristics of BPD in young people, described its course, distinguished it from the vicissitudes of normal adolescence, and has made comparisons with adult manifestations of the disorder.[1–7] The considerable emotional and economic cost to individuals, families, and society associated with adolescent BPD[8] supports calls for early intervention[9] and requires that the assessment of personality functioning be an essential component in the psychological evaluation of adolescents. As a result, adult treatment models with demonstrated efficacy have been adapted for adolescents, including dialectical behavior therapy (DBT),[10] mentalization-based therapy (MBT)[11] transference-focused psychotherapy

a Weill Cornell Medical College, Personality Disorders Institute, 21 Bloomingdale Road, White Plains, NY 10605, USA; b Université Laval, École de psychologie, 2325 rue des Bibliothèques, Québec, Québec G1V 0A6, Canada
* Corresponding author. 2600 Netherland Avenue, Suite 107, Riverdale, NY 10463.
E-mail address: aweiner.phd@gmail.com

Psychiatr Clin N Am 41 (2018) 729–746
https://doi.org/10.1016/j.psc.2018.07.005
0193-953X/18/© 2018 Elsevier Inc. All rights reserved.

(TFP),[12-14] and cognitive-analytical therapy (CAT).[15] The implementation in adolescence of these empirically supported treatment approaches are described after first reviewing factors that frequently complicate the recognition and diagnosis of BPD in young people, followed by an overview of research on BPD in adolescents that delineates its clinically relevant features. Increasing the accurate identification of BPD in this population is necessary for facilitating appropriate targeted psychotherapeutic intervention.

OBSTACLES TO RECOGNIZING AND DIAGNOSING BORDERLINE PERSONALITY DISORDER IN ADOLESCENTS

The 5-fold increase in research on BPD in young people in the last decade[16] has generated a wealth of findings[6,17,18] that should dispel any hesitancy about diagnosing BPD in young people.[19] However, recent surveys indicate that many clinicians remain reluctant to do so and doubt the validity of this diagnosis for this age group[20,21] despite diagnostic guidelines that recognize its presence and the need to diagnose BPD in adolescents (Diagnostic and Statistical Manual of Mental Disorders [DSM]-5, 2013).[22]

BPD has a prevalence rate of 3.27% in young people[23] and it has been shown to affect as many as 22% of adolescent outpatients[24] and 33% of adolescent inpatients.[25] Therefore, it is likely that clinicians who see teenagers have had contact with adolescents who have this disorder, but only half or fewer of those surveyed think it is a valid diagnosis, 25% or less indicate that they have made this diagnosis, and less than 10% indicate that they have treated youngsters with this diagnosis.[20,21] They consider that these types of problems are transient in this age group (41%), that the DSM-IV Text Revision does not allow personality disorder diagnoses in adolescents (26%), or are concerned that it would be stigmatizing (9%).[21] However, because most psychotherapeutic approaches with demonstrated efficacy with adults with BPD advocate discussing the diagnosis with the patient,[26] it is important that clinicians become familiar and comfortable with making and discussing the diagnosis of BPD with adolescents and parents.

BPD in adolescence also may be under-recognized by clinicians, not just reluctantly underdiagnosed. Shared risk factors commonly underlie mental disorder in young people[27] and the diagnostic process can be confounded by the high rate of comorbidity associated with BPD. For example, BPD features such as impulsivity, emotional instability, and dysregulation are not unique to BPD, are likely contributors to the comorbidity of BPD and mood/internalizing and externalizing disorders, and are mediated by the prefrontal cortex, which may be involved in a variety of mental disorders and which undergoes significant development during adolescence.[28] Inpatient adolescents with BPD have higher rates of mood disorders, anxiety disorders, and externalizing difficulties than adolescents with no personality disorder.[25] Prospective studies show that impulsivity and affective and behavioral dysregulation in childhood, and symptoms of oppositional defiant disorder and attention-deficit/hyperactivity disorder in children and adolescents, predict BPD symptoms in early adolescence[29] and young adulthood, respectively.[30] Therefore, it is likely that the clinician's interview of adolescents and parents is dominated by descriptions of long-standing depressed mood, anxiety, or conduct problems, including impulsivity, that offer a satisfying diagnostic understanding and serve as impressive targets for behavioral and pharmacologic intervention. However, although the internalizing and externalizing qualities seen in childhood precede personality disorder and then remain comorbid with it,[31] the symptoms that characterize BPD and cluster B disorders are more stable than internalizing and externalizing difficulties, and BPD goes beyond issues of mood, anxiety, or behavioral problems in understanding the adolescent's functioning.[6] Kernberg and colleagues[19] (2000) suggested that clinicians might be more alert to the presence of BPD if they were sensitive to a behavior's multiple meanings and, as an example, noted that items from the Achenbach System of Empirically Based Assessment Child Behavior Checklist,[32,33] such as "complains of loneliness; cruelty to others; deliberately harms self or attempts suicide; impulsive; sudden changes in mood; complains that no one loves him/her," which happen to load on both internalizing and externalizing factors, are features that can signal the presence of BPD.[34]

DIAGNOSTIC FEATURES

The range of behaviors that characterize BPD, providing both diagnostic features and treatment goals, can be placed in categories such as affective instability/dysregulation, impulsivity/behavioral dysregulation, and disturbed relatedness/interpersonal dysfunction.[29] For example, emotional dysregulation[35] subsumes BPD features such as poor distress tolerance, lack of persistence, prolonged anger, poor inhibition of negative emotions, increased impulsivity associated with negative moods, shifting mood states, and difficulty identifying emotions associated with distress. Social dysfunction includes symptoms that indicate fearful or preoccupied attachment, expectations of social rejection, difficulty tolerating aloneness, hypervigilance to others' hostility, and mistrust of others. In addition, individuals with BPD show more frequent dissociation, disturbed sense of identity, potential for exaggerated inner pain, intense experience of shame, impulsivity (eg, suicidality), and breakdowns in mentalization when faced with stress.[35] They show poorer problem solving when upset, and have difficulty self-soothing.[29] Categorizations such as these map well onto interventions that attempt to enhance self-regulatory strategies and reflect goals that are consistent with the changes in cognitive control and planning mechanisms that occur during the course of adolescent neurodevelopment. It is also evident that this broad range of BPD symptoms allows for considerable observable differences to exist among the young people with this diagnosis.

An alternative conceptualization emphasizes identity integration, the quality of object relations,[36] and mentalization about the self and others,[37] perspectives that are consistent with[16] the suggestion that 5 key BPD symptoms (abandonment fears, unstable relationships that alternate between idealization and devaluation, identity disturbance, paranoid ideation, and chronic feelings of emptiness) arise from an individual's dysfunctional internal images of self and others. The other DSM-5 BPD symptoms (intense anger and its controllability, affective instability, recurrent suicidal behavior, impulsivity) are displayed in interpersonal contexts and have a significant impact on relationships. By emphasizing self and interpersonal functioning, this framework is consistent with the DSM-5 alternative model for personality disorders (DSM-5, 2013), as well as with those treatment models that highlight the individual's representational world, including the individual's identity and the integration or coherence of internal images and their impact in daily life and relationships. These organizational schemes capture the classification framework of behavioral and psychodynamic approaches to psychotherapy that have been used with adults with BPD.[38]

PSYCHOTHERAPY FOR BORDERLINE PERSONALITY DISORDER IN YOUNG PEOPLE

The effectiveness of psychotherapy for young people with BPD can be viewed in the context of:

1. The developmental course of BPD in adolescence
2. The general effectiveness of psychotherapy for children and adolescents

Evidence indicates that BPD begins in childhood and is clearly diagnosable in adolescence; its symptoms increase in early adolescence, tend to reach a peak in midadolescence, and then begin to decline in frequency in most, but not all, adolescents as they move toward young adulthood.[39] A similar pattern is observed with personality traits. In general, maladaptive childhood personality traits such as disagreeableness and emotional instability decline in young adolescents but less so in those who had obtained more extreme trait scores.[40] Although there is a general trend for positive traits (eg, affiliation, conscientiousness) to increase and negative traits (eg, neuroticism) to decrease as personality disorder symptoms decline, this is not the case in adolescents who develop personality disorders.[8] Identity status also matures across adolescence[41] but, with a clinical sample, level of identity integration is not associated with age but is associated with the presence or absence of mental disorder.[4] These findings, using different indices of growth and disorder, suggest that there is a subset of adolescents with more severe mental disorder (ie, symptom severity, higher trait scores) who do not manifest the developmental trend toward more mature, less pathologic personality functioning. They include those who meet full criteria for a formal BPD diagnosis and are the most resistant to change following psychotherapy.

A recent meta-analysis[42] of 50 years of psychotherapy research with children who ranged in age from 4 to 18 years suggests that modest expectations about psychotherapy outcome with adolescents with BPD would be understandable. Positive results were most often found in patients with anxiety disorders for which there is a well-developed and tested model, but effect size was much smaller with mood and behavioral disorders. Interventions with multiproblem youngsters, which typify those with BPD,[25] showed the smallest, nonsignificant effect size.

These patterns suggest that:

1. It will be necessary to consider how to distinguish treatment effects from normative developmental changes, and not just from control group effects
2. A major challenge will be to develop an understanding of how best to identify those adolescents who are least likely to show normative improvement in functioning and to develop treatment approaches for them
3. The task ahead may be difficult because young people with complex disorders historically have been resistant to improvement following psychotherapeutic intervention

Thus far, several interventions have been developed that apply adult models to adolescent dysfunction.

Dialectical Behavior Therapy

Miller, Rathus, and others[43–47] have developed and applied extensive adaptations of the adult DBT treatment model[10] to adolescents (DBT-A) who are typically diagnosed with 2 to 4 DSM-5 disorders and have difficulty coping with emotional dysregulation. They show a range of behavior problems that include suicidal behavior, nonsuicidal self-injury, risky sexual behaviors, eating disorders, substance use disorder, anger problems, school avoidance, difficulty sustaining relationships, and poor awareness of emotions and motives.[47]

The construct of dysregulation is broadly used in the DBT model[47] and includes emotion dysregulation (eg, emotional vulnerability, angry outbursts, shame, anxiety, guilt), interpersonal dysregulation (eg, conflicts with others, attempts to avoid abandonment, difficulty getting needs met in relationships), cognitive dysregulation and family conflict (eg, black-or-white thinking and acting, poor perspective taking, invalidation of self and others), and self-dysregulation (eg, impulsivity, poor awareness of emotions, poor attentional control, identity confusion, and sense of emptiness). Thus, features of BPD that are described by others as indications of identity diffusion, problems in attachment, deficits in mentalization, defenses such as splitting, or other personality features such as pathologic narcissism are described in the DBT model as byproducts of various forms of dysregulation to be treated by learning skills modules that have been developed for each type of dysregulation. For example, cognitive dys-regulation and family conflict is treated with the module of Walking the Middle Path, developed specifically for working with adolescents and their families.[48] This module tries to teach how to reduce extreme, all-or-nothing thinking and move toward a dia-lectical style that incorporates both/and rather than either/or thinking. Multifamily groups and individual therapy may be used to teach how to overcome an invalidating parental style.[47] Mindfulness is a module that may be taught in multifamily groups and used to target dysregulation of sense of self (eg, unawareness of feelings and goals), of cognition (eg, dissociation and depersonalization), of emotions, relationship prob-lems, and regulating impulsivity.[47]

LENGTH OF TREATMENT

There is an initial 16-week program and the adolescents may choose to recontract for another 16 weeks and may reenroll as needed. A graduate group provides an addi-tional 4 months of treatment of those adolescents with multiple problems and depres-sion. This format potentially allows for the reduction of serious presenting problems followed by the pursuit of other treatment goals, and provides adolescents a sense of mastery over their treatment.[44] Included is a 4-week specialized parent-adolescent skills module.

ASSESSMENT

Five areas associated with adolescent BPD are assessed: confusion about self, impul-sivity, emotional dysregulation, interpersonal problems, and adolescent family prob-lems. Measures can include semistructured interview (K-SADS),[49] a personality measure, or a brief self-report (Life Problems Inventory).[47] These results determine the skills modules selected for each individual's intervention.

CONTRACTING

A variety of interactive strategies attempt to ensure commitment to the treatment. A quick agreement to participate is not accepted; instead, the adolescents are chal-lenged to think about and justify their decisions and consider alternatives, including pros and cons about participating, before a final acceptance is offered.[47]

TREATMENT PROCESS

Modes of DBT intervention for treating disorders of dysregulation include individual psychotherapy, group skills training, telephone coaching between sessions for adolescent and parent as needed, and meetings of the therapist consultation team for planning and support. There are well-defined treatment goals that include:

1. Create a life worth living by motivating a wish to change and replace maladaptive behaviors with adaptive ones
2. Promote growth in the adolescent's skills and abilities

3. Promote the generalization of new skills from the treatment modality to everyday life
4. Modify the adolescent's environment when needed to support the new skills
5. Support the therapist's motivation and ability to perform the treatment model

The adolescents are taught to self-monitor their dysfunctional behaviors and their times of occurrence, which are recorded on a diary card. Factors that cause and maintain sequences of maladaptive behaviors are identified so that a particular skill can be selected to replace a problem behavior to produce a more adaptive outcome.

Evaluation

There have been several attempts to evaluate DBT-A effectiveness, typically targeting adolescent suicidal and self-harming behaviors.[43] Mehlum and colleagues[50,51] (2014) conducted a single-blind randomized controlled trial (RCT) comparing DBT-A with enhanced usual care (EUC) over the course of 19 weeks with a follow-up evaluation 1 year after treatment. The DBT-A condition included 39 subjects who received 1 weekly individual session, 1 weekly multifamily skills training session (120 minutes), family therapy, and telephone coaching with the individual therapist, as needed. Fifteen naive therapists received extensive DBT training and supervision for 12 months. The 8 who were most adherent during training were selected to be DBT-A study therapists. The EUC, which was not manualized or monitored for adherence, used 30 therapists with varied professional backgrounds to treat 38 adolescents for 19 weeks with psychodynamically oriented or cognitive behavior therapy treatment plus medication when appropriate. The enhancement was that the subjects received at least 1 weekly treatment session. The subjects displayed at least 2 self-harming episodes within the previous 4 months and met at least 2 DSM-IV BPD criteria. Self-reports were obtained at 9, 15, and 19 weeks and interviewing was also done at 19 weeks.

Taking the treatment and follow-up studies together, the frequency of self-harming behavior declined from weeks 9 to 15 with DBT-A but not EUC, and a significant difference between groups was maintained at the 1-year follow-up. The difference seen on measures of suicidal ideation, hopelessness, depression, and borderline symptoms after the initial treatment phase were no longer significant at 1-year follow-up. Thus, DBT-A was associated with more notable long-term reduction in self-harm and more rapid reduction in suicidal ideation, depression, and BPD symptoms, but EUC patients showed continued improvement such that group differences only remained for self-harm.

Unambiguous interpretation of RCT findings are often elusive and, because these are carefully planned studies, they are instructive for thinking about intervention more generally. It is not known whether the greater number of group sessions experienced by individuals with DBT-A, the additional sessions sought by some of them, or continued therapy experienced by many EUC patients affected outcome. Although DBT-A therapists received intensive, manualized, structured training that was carefully observed and supervised, EUC consisted of many therapist who were not trained to use a common procedure and who used either psychodynamic approaches that have been found to have some positive effect with BPD or cognitive approaches that have not.[38] Therefore, there is the risk that the patients with DBT-A received the kind of special attention that can enhance treatment effects.[38] The results on follow-up are consistent with meta-analyses that reported that control conditions, other than nonactive options such as wait-list controls, are often associated with improvement or as effective as treatment conditions.[12]

Mentalization-Based Therapy

MBT was originally developed as a day-hospital treatment program for adults with BPD[52,53] and was adapted for adolescents who self-harm, have BPD, and manifest suicidality.[37,54–57] The aim of MBT for adolescents (MBT-A) is to help adolescents more accurately represent theirs and others' feelings in the moment, particularly when they are emotionally aroused or dealing with interpersonal stressors.

Mentalizing is thought to develop within early attachment relationships when the caretaker, by engaging in marked affect mirroring,[58] reflects back the emotion that the infant is experiencing for the infant, and so provides them with a representation of how the infant's own affect looks and thereby facilitates the development of an early sense of self. By helping infants to develop a representation of their own minds, the parents facilitate their communication with others' minds. However, when the response to the infant's affect experience is inaccurate or inappropriate, such as can occur with abuse or neglect, the hostile or inaccurate representations of affect lead to the development of an alien self that can be particularly persecutory as the capacity to mentalize collapses. Relief from the destabilization and primitive fears of abandonment associated with the alien self is obtained via externalization in the form of self-harm or suicidality. The impact of MBT in reducing self-harm seems to be mediated by a reduction in avoidant attachment and an improvement in the capacity to mentalize.[37]

FOUR PHASES OF MENTALIZATION-BASED THERAPY FOR ADOLESCENTS
Assessment

A 2-week assessment involves 1 or 2 sessions with the individual and the family therapist (MBT-F). Diagnostic, cognitive, and mentalizing measures are also administered.

Initial Phase

A collaborative written formulation is developed and discussed in both the individual and family treatment components. It includes a detailed crisis plan that suggests how to reinstate mentalization when disrupted by emotional dysregulation and impulsive behavior. A contract incorporates an agreement about the treatment plan (eg, duration of treatment, required commitments). Psychoeducation introduces the ideas underpinning MBT.

Middle Phase

Nine to 10 months are devoted to improving adolescent and family mentalizing skills and focus on the mental states evoked by current or recent interpersonal experiences. Specific interventions are used to manage a variety of impulsive behaviors, including suicidality, substance use, or bingeing and purging.

Final Phase

This 2-month phase develops independence by building relational stability and supporting the patients' sense of agency and autonomy within their relational networks. A coping plan is formulated of what to do when difficulties recur.

INTERVENTIONS AND STRATEGIES

A variety of strategies have been developed to help adolescents enhance or redeploy their mentalizing function and identify when certain intense emotions or aspects in a relationship became excessive and lead to a suspension of a mentalizing attitude. These strategies include the mentalizing stance of the therapist, which uses an empathic attitude that respects the adolescents' agency and promotes their understanding of their feelings in the moment; a series of techniques such as a mentalizing functional analysis to identify when suicidality or self-harm took on a compulsive quality so that this cycle can be intercepted to prevent future collapses in mentalization; and affect clarification and elaboration by which intense distress is clarified and then seen as emotional rather than overwhelming reality, especially in the context of attacks from the alien self when the individual may feel hopeless, unlovable, angry, and ashamed.

MENTALIZATION-BASED TREATMENT OF FAMILIES

Family therapy is a key modality of MBT-A. Its goal is to reduce impulsive enactments, coercion, affect storms, and nonmentalizing interactions by helping families develop an awareness of each person's state of mind and how these mental states affect one another, including how the breakdown in mentalizing undermines the ability of the family members to respond resiliently and supportively to each other's needs.

The concept of the mentalizing loop[59] works toward family members becoming more inclined to focus on thinking about feelings before planning any action. The therapist works with the family to identify, highlight, and name a nonmentalizing moment and uses this to systematically mentalize and make sense of what each family member experienced, including the inner and external representations of the family in the mind of each family member.

The pause-and-review technique uses the sequence of (1) action, (2) pause, and (3) reflection to restore balance to mentalizing. Successful rebalancing is reflected in relevant commentary that implies:

1. Curiosity
2. Respect for the opacity of other minds
3. Awareness of the impact of affects on the self and others
4. Perspective taking
5. Narrative continuity
6. A sense of agency and trust

Evaluation

In an RCT of MBT-A,[37] 80 adolescents presenting to mental health services with self-harm during the preceding month were randomized to MBT or treatment as usual (TAU); 97% received a diagnosis of depression and 73% met the criteria for borderline personality disorder. At the end of 12 months of treatment, MBT-A was found to be superior to TAU in reducing self-harm and depression. The recovery rate was 44% for MBT-A versus 17% for TAU based on self-report, and 57%versus 32% based on interviews. A larger reduction in depressive symptoms and BPD diagnoses and traits was also found in the MBT-A group. After 12 months, self-harm remained significantly lower in the MBT-A group,[37] although 69% of the sample were still self-harming at 12 months.

Transference-Focused Psychotherapy for Adolescents

TFP for adolescents (TFP-A[36,60]) is an adaptation of TFP for adults with personality disorders,[12–14,61–63] a contemporary psychoanalytic object relations model that has found support in evidence-based and neurobiological research with adult subjects.[64–67] TFP-A was inspired by Paulina Kernberg, who long advocated that personality disorder symptoms and structure were observable in children and adolescents and were unlikely to resolve without specific intervention.[19]

The adolescent's observable behaviors, dysfunctions, and subjective disturbances are seen as being derived from their level of personality organization, which can range from normal to neurotic, borderline, and psychotic levels. The level is a function of their degree of identity integration and it provides the framework for treatment recommendations and planning. Improvement is achieved as integrated representations of self and others develop, use of primitive defenses is reduced, and self-esteem and confidence in others are enhanced. Specific aims of TFP-A include (1) improve self-regulation; (2) develop the capacity for gratifying relationships with family, friends, and possibly a romantic partner; and (3) invest in school or work, develop interests and future goals, and move on to a healthy developmental trajectory by mastering these tasks of adolescence.

Basic elements of TFP-A include (1) evaluating the adolescent's identity development to differentiate identity diffusion, which underlies personality disorders, from identity confusion (or crisis), seen more commonly in normal adolescence; (2) engaging the adolescent in a contract that helps contain self-destructive behaviors and creates a reflective mental space to facilitate the exploration of conflicts and intense affects; and (3) a consistent analysis and interpretation of transference and countertransference reactions activated in the here-and-now interactions with the therapist, which provides access to the dominant pathologic object relations and manifestations of the internal split, dissociated psychological structure underlying identity diffusion, acting out, and interpersonal difficulties.

Assessment

The assessment maintains an awareness of the different physical and emotional changes and developmental tasks that adolescents have to engage with while integrating a coherent sense of identity. This assessment requires that the clinician have firm knowledge of the adolescent's developmental history and current functioning with family, peers, school, or work. The procedure attempts to identify the adolescent's habitual ways of responding to anxiety; meeting developmental challenges; and integrating new body-sensual, cognitive-affective, and social experiences.

Integrated identity

Self-integration is reflected in the adolescent's capacity to describe an internal state of turmoil from the perspective of an implicit integrated view of self and of the most important members of the family despite turmoil and conflict in their relations; the presence of a well-integrated system of moral values; the commitment to ideals beyond self-serving objectives; the capacity for friendships, including romantic feelings; and good functioning at school. Findings here indicate whether they have attained a level of self-reflection (or mentalization) that supports self-examination.

Personality assessment interview

The personality assessment interview (PAI)[68] focuses specifically on the moment-to-moment interaction between the therapist and the adolescent to gather information about the quality of object relations and the dominant affect. The PAI technique consists of systematically asking questions that tap into self and others: representation, mentalization capacities, affect, and cognitions (eg, "Tell me about yourself and your understanding of why we are meeting." "Now that we have met for a while, what have you learned, about me, yourself?" "Was it like what you expected?"). The PAI contributes to the differentiation between normal identity confusion and identity diffusion as well as the capacity of the adolescent to engage in psychotherapy and sustain a working alliance when affect is activated.[19]

Contract

The contract is undertaken before psychotherapy begins. Its purpose is to clarify and delineate expectations and responsibilities of the adolescent, the caretaker, and the therapist in order to minimize interruptions or threats to the treatment from acting out or self-destructive behaviors so that exploration of the adolescent's mind is possible. The contract also identifies specific ways of engaging with parents to help the adolescent develop autonomy and assume responsibility for the difficulties.

In formulating the contract, the parties:

1. Hear the clinician's assessment and come to agree on a shared understanding of the adolescent's problems with regard to personality disorders and identity diffusion
2. Establish the frame of the treatment, as clarified by the clinician, in which management plans for attendance and possible dangerous behaviors, such as drug abuse and antisocial behaviors, are agreed on so as to reduce threats to the viability of the treatment while still maintaining confidentiality
3. Anticipate and prevent forms of resistance that could threaten the continuation of the treatment
4. Begin reworking maladaptive functioning such as lack of motivation, avoidance of productive activities (school, work), regression to states of dependency, frantic quest for pleasure and liberty to avoid anxiety reflective of maladaptive object relations dyads that are best explored through behavioral activation[69]
5. Agree to engage with developmental tasks
6. Establish the basis of collaboration with parents

The relationship with parents in all phases of the treatment process is complex. TFP-A considers 3 options:

1. When family dynamics are unproblematic, foster a mental space for the adolescent to develop autonomy and assume responsibility for the difficulties, with parents becoming collaborators, not patients. Parental involvement is sought during episodes when the adolescent is putting themselves, others, or the treatment, at risk.
2. Using family therapy to reduce high-conflict interactions.
3. In cases in which there is severe family dysfunction, including parental mental illness, substance abuse, and minimal parental involvement, the focus becomes helping the adolescent avoid assuming parental responsibilities in family contexts that are abusive, that undermine their self-organization and movement toward autonomy, and are a threat to their mental health.

Individual psychotherapy

To facilitate identity integration, the TFP-A therapist uses the strategies of TFP-A to integrate part-self and part-object representations and mark underlying representations and characteristic patterns of experiencing and interpersonal relations that disrupt development. TFP-A's 5 basic techniques are:

1. Interpretative process, including clarification, confrontation, and interpretation
2. Analysis of transference
3. Analysis of countertransference reactions
4. Technical neutrality
5. Leveling of developmental challenges

These techniques are described more fully in Ref.[60] As an example, a very intelligent 16-year-old boy with narcissistic and borderline features told the therapist he viewed him as a "brick wall" and therefore was impervious to the therapist and what he thought or felt or said did not matter to this adolescent. Confrontation, clarification, and interpretation of the transference while using the metaphor of the brick wall, over time, elucidated for him a defensive structure that contributed to a decline in a paranoid quality with the therapist and peers.

Evaluation

Krischer and colleagues[70] analyzed the effectiveness of a day clinic treatment program based on TFP-A, focusing on improving core symptoms such as affective problems, aggressive behavior against self and others, and interpersonal problems. It consisted of 32 female and male adolescent patients who had undergone at least 12 weeks of partial inpatient TFP-A therapy. Despite the small sample size, both the self-injurious behavior and the self-directed aggression decreased significantly, suggesting that TFP-A can contribute toward an increase in behavioral control and affect regulation in adolescents in an inpatient setting.

Cognitive-Analytical Therapy

Chanen and colleagues[9,15] have adapted CAT[71] to treat adolescents with BPD. Noting that stable signs and symptoms of BPD can be identified in childhood and early adolescence, they advocate early intervention before a more complex, integrated form of BPD develops, with the goal of fostering a return to adaptive developmental pathways. Their Helping Young People Early (HYPE) intervention, for individuals 15 to 25 years of age, is a 16-session program that can be extended to 24 sessions if needed, with follow-up meetings to monitor progress. Individual practitioners provide psychotherapy and case management, and psychoeducation is offered for patients, families, schools, or others in the patients' lives. Patients are chosen for HYPE who show 3 or more DSM-IV BPD features and they do not have to meet the full criterion for the BPD diagnosis.

Consistent with its object relations roots, the CAT model views mental disorder as reflecting maladaptive or distorted reciprocal roles, with the more impaired adolescents having a much less integrated self, poorer reflective capacity, and executive functioning; an absence of a coherent identity; and possible dissociation derived from abusive and traumatic experiences.[9] In a clinical example, the patient and therapist established treatment goals; identified maladaptive reciprocal roles; formulated an understanding of the patient's difficulties, including problems with relationships as seen in therapy and in daily life; and explored relationship patterns and more effective ways of coping with problems. To do this they jointly constructed diagrams that concretely depicted causal connection among relationships, feelings, and events, and the therapist provided a written summary at the end of the opening phase to provide a "route map" that guided the therapy's attempt to revise the representational roles and the affects, thoughts, and perceptions associated with them.[9] A written understanding of the patient was also provided at the end of treatment. Improved mood and reduced risk taking were achieved.

Evaluation

An RCT[15] examined adolescents who ranged in age from 15 to 18 years and displayed 2 to 9 DSM-IV BPD criteria along with other features in childhood that have been found to be predictive of personality disorder in young adults. The therapists received 9 months of training and supervised practice by the originators of CAT and did not begin psychotherapy until adherence was attained. CAT was compared with good clinical care (GCC), a standardized problem-solving model that included modules devoted to problems such as depression and anxiety. Both groups significantly improved over 2 years with the CAT intervention associated with a faster rate of improvement than GCC in externalizing and internalizing behaviors, whereas GCC showed faster improvement in general functioning. Importantly, there was no difference between groups in the rate of change for BPD total scores and frequency of parasuicidal behavior.

SUMMARY

More than a decade of expanding research supports the necessity to assess personality functioning when evaluating an adolescent's mental health and to treat personality disorders and their features as early as possible because untreated BPD is likely to undermine adolescents' current functioning and subsequent development, affecting functioning and relationships into adulthood.[8] Because symptoms and risk factors for BPD overlap with those of both internalizing and externalizing disorders,[72–74] it is important to develop a clinical mindset in which personality and personality disorders are actively considered.

Current interventions with adolescents have most often focused on reducing suicidal and self-harming behaviors, an understandable and worthy goal, leaving unanswered how these interventions will fare with other maladaptive features of BPD. More generally, it was noted that normatively, by late adolescence a decline in borderline symptoms, an increase in positive and a decline in negative personality traits, and an increase in identity status consolidation are seen. Treatment effects need to be judged in relation to these developmental trends as well as in comparison with study control conditions. Regarding study control conditions, current favored treatments seem to produce more rapid improvement but it remains to be seen whether these will stabilize as more enduring effects. Over time, treatment and especially well-executed control condition outcomes seem to be less distinct, notably with adult as well as adolescent patients.

It was noted that some treatment models focused on overt behavioral symptoms and deployed interventions that emphasized the learning of skills to reduce dysregulation and enhance behavioral and emotional control. Others emphasized the adolescents' mental lives and sought to enhance an awareness of theirs or others' internal worlds and to promote identity integration, believing that this would promote greater emotional control. Independent of the type of effort, it seems clear that there is a subset of adolescents who do not show a normative decline in maladaptive personality functioning nor does it respond well to treatment, even when the treatment is intense and the clinicians are attentive to identity status.[4] Thus, there seems to be a group of borderline patients who are more resistant to change, both in adolescence and adulthood, especially with regard to their functional (work, school) and interpersonal behavior, perhaps reflecting more severe mental disorder. One goal of future research might be to attain better understanding of these young people and identify their defining characteristics to guide the development of more effective treatment.

Recent work on the structure of mental disorder has identified in adults and adolescents a general factor (termed p) that includes several borderline features as well as thought problems, but a separate borderline factor does not emerge in these analyses.[75–78] It has been suggested that p may reflect severity or vulnerability[75,76] and a general liability for mental disorder. If developmental approaches to personality disorder and its treatment in young people incorporate severity and vulnerability concepts, it is evident that interventions will have to be further tailored to address these issues and so new applications may be expected,[79,80] perhaps including a reexamination of the role of resiliency in the presence of vulnerability. The psychotherapy research on BPD in adolescents, thus far, consists of just a few studies, and the absence of severity indices contributes to the difficulty in assessing their relative effectiveness.

There are some important common features in the psychotherapy programs reviewed in this article, although they are implemented differently, depending on the model's theory of change:

1. Contract with parents and teenagers. There are many challenges to maintaining treatment with this high-risk population. All approaches show empathy and support for adolescents and their families and try to motivate regular participation but also recognize that adolescents and their parents may have difficulty maintaining commitment to treatment, attend irregularly, or engage in acting out that undermines treatment. The treatment contract/agreement tries to prevent such events from intruding into or undermining the therapy process but also provides a frame for intervention when it occurs. The contracting is often the first window into individualizing the treatment and establishing the alliance with both the adolescent and the caretaker.

2. Parental involvement. This involvement is often seen as an essential component in treating youth BPD, although there may be mixed evidence about the impact of caregiver or family involvement more generally.[42,81] Maladaptive parenting, including abuse, can contribute to the development and maintenance of BPD and so it is often essential to carefully consider how to involve caretakers. Efforts may include trying to reduce negative affect and improve self-regulation in all parties, promoting the development of autonomy in these young people and guiding parents to either less restrictive or more appropriate involvement that is experienced as nurturant rather than critical and controlling, and clarifying and reducing role reversal. TFP involves parents in formulating and carrying out the treatment contract, whereas other approaches may be more likely to involve parents in groups that include psychoeducation and instruction or techniques that help parents identify maladaptive interactive styles to be replaced by patterns that are thought to be more effective or at least less hurtful to the adolescents or harmful to their relationships.

3. Alertness to factors that may undermine psychotherapy. A variety of strategies have been described for dealing with adolescent resistance.[81] Adolescents are likely to manifest behaviors that can interfere with psychotherapy and all approaches try to deal with that. These behaviors include their ambivalence about change, demands for autonomy, aversion to dependency, avoidance of asking for help and rejection of it when offered; and often resistance to accepting or acknowledging praise and reward.

4. All acknowledge that the therapist must actively engage with the adolescent, rather than having a passive interactive style, and that it is important to have clear plans for dealing with crisis and safety issues should they arise.

5. Coherence, consistency, and continuity are critical features of effective, specialized psychotherapies used with adults, arguably because they provide external cognitive structuring for these patients who have poor metacognitive organization.[54,82] This point is likely to be even more critical for adolescents considering their developmental immaturities.

REFERENCES

1. Bornovalova MA, Hicks BM, Iacono WG, et al. Stability, change, and heritability of borderline personality disorder traits from adolescence to adulthood: a longitudinal twin study. Development Psychopathology 2009;21(4):1335–53.
2. Casey BJ, Duhoux S, Cohen MM. Adolescence: what do transmission, transition, and translation have to do with it? Neuron 2010;67:749–60.
3. DeFife JA, Malone JC, DiLallo J, et al. Assessing adolescent personality disorders with the Shedler-Westen Assessment Procedure for Adolescents. Clinical Psychology: Science and Practice 2013;20(4):393–407.
4. Feenstra DJ, Hutsebaut J, Verheul R, et al. Identity: empirical contribution: changes in the identity integration of adolescents in treatment for personality disorders. J Personal Disord 2014;28(1):101–12.
5. Hutsebaut J, Feenstra DJ, Luyten P. Personality disorders in adolescence: label or opportunity? Clinical Psychology: Science and Practice 2013;20(4):445–51.
6. Sharp C, Fonagy P. Practitioner review: borderline personality disorder in adolescence – recent conceptualization, intervention, and implications for clinical practice. J Child Psychol Psychiatry 2015;56(12):1266–88.
7. Westen D, Waller NG, Shedler J, et al. Dimensions of personality and personality pathology: factor structure of the Shedler-Westen Assessment Procedure-II (SWAP-II). J Personal Disord 2014;28(2):281–318.
8. Wright A, Zalewski M, Hallquist M, et al. Developmental trajectories of borderline personality disorder symptoms and psychosocial functioning in adolescence. J Personal Disord 2016;30(3):351–72.
9. Chanen A, McCutcheon L, Kerr I. HYPE: a cognitive analytic therapy-based prevention and early intervention program for borderline personality disorder. In: Sharp C, Tackett J, editors. Handbook of borderline personality disorder in children and adolescents. New York: Springer; 2014. p. 361–83.
10. Linehan MM. DBT® skills training manual. 2nd edition. New York: Guilford Press; 1993/2015.
11. Bateman A, Fonagy P. Mentalization-based treatment for borderline personality disorder: a practical guide. Oxford (United Kingdom): Oxford University Press; 2006.
12. Clarkin JF, Yeomans FE, Kernberg OF. Psychotherapy for borderline personality: focusing on object relations. Arlington (VA): American Psychiatric Publishing, Inc; 2006.
13. Kernberg OF, Selzer MA, Koenigsberg HW, et al. Psychodynamic psychotherapy of borderline patients. New York: Basic Books; 1989.
14. Yeomans FE, Clarkin JF, Kernberg OF. Transference-focused psychotherapy for borderline personality disorder: a clinical guide. Washington, DC: American Psychiatric Publishing; 2015.
15. Chanen AM, Jackson HJ, McCutcheon LK, et al. Early intervention for adolescents with borderline personality disorder using cognitive analytic therapy: randomised controlled trial. Br J Psychiatry 2008;193(6):477–84.
16. Sharp C. Current trends in BPD research as indicative of a broader sea-change in psychiatric nosology. Personal Disord 2016;7(4):334–43.
17. De Fruyt F, De Clercq B. Personality and psychopathology: a field in transition. Eur J Pers 2014;28(4):388–9.
18. Shiner RI, Allen TA. Assessing personality disorders in adolescents: seven guiding principles. Clinical Psychology: Science and Practice 2013;20(4):361–77.

19. Kernberg PF, Weiner AS, Bardenstein KK. Personality disorders in children and adolescents. New York: Basic Books; 2000.
20. Griffiths M. Validity, utility and acceptability of borderline personality disorder diagnosis in childhood and adolescence: survey of psychiatrists. Psychiatrist 2011;35(1):19–22.
21. Laurenssen EMP, Hutsebaut J, Feenstra DJ, et al. Diagnosis of personality disorders in adolescents: a study among psychologists. Child Adolesc Psychiatry Ment Health 2013;7(1):3.
22. National Institute for Health and Clinical Excellence (NICE). Borderline personality disorder: treatment and management: clinical guideline. London: National Institute of Health and Clinical Excellence; 2009.
23. Zanarini MC, Horwood J, Wolke D, et al. Prevalence of DSM-IV borderline personality disorder in two community samples: 6,300 English 11-year-olds and 34,653 American adults. J Personal Disord 2011;25(5):607–19.
24. Chanen, McCutcheon. 2015.
25. Ha C, Balderas JC, Zanarini MC, et al. Psychiatric comorbidity in hospitalized adolescents with borderline personality disorder. J Clin Psychiatry 2014;75(5): e457–64.
26. Fonagy P, Allison E, Ryan A. Therapy outcomes: what works for whom?. In: Midgley N, Cooper M, Hayes J, editors. Essential research findings in child and adolescent counselling and psychotherapy. London: Sage; 2017. p. 79–118.
27. Hayden EP, Mash EJ. Child psychopathology: a developmental-systems perspective. In: Mash EJ, Barkley RA, editors. Child psychopathology. New York: Guilford Press; 2014. p. 3–72.
28. MacDonald, et al. 2016.
29. Belsky DW, Caspi A, Arseneault L, et al. Etiological features of borderline personality related characteristics in a birth cohort of 12-year-old children. Development Psychopathology 2012;24(1):251–65.
30. Burke JD, Stepp SD. Adolescent disruptive behavior and borderline personality disorder symptoms in young adult men. J Abnorm Child Psychol 2012;40(1): 35–44.
31. Sharp, Wall. 2018.
32. Achenbach TM. The Achenbach System of Empirically Based Assessment (ASEBA): development, findings, theory, and applications. Burlington (VT): University of Vermont Research Center for Children, Youth, & Families; 2009.
33. Achenbach TM, Rescorla LA. Manual for the ASEBA school-age forms & profiles. Burlington (VT): University of Vermont, Research Center for Children, Youth, & Families; 2001.
34. American Psychiatric Association. DSM-V: diagnostic and statistical manual of mental disorders. 5th edition. Washington, DC. 2013.
35. Fonagy P, Luyten P. A multilevel perspective on the development of borderline personality disorder. Dev Psychopathol 2016;3(17):1–67.
36. Normandin L, Ensink K, Kernberg OF. Transference-focused psychotherapy for borderline adolescents: a neurobiologically informed psychodynamic psychotherapy. J Infant Child Adolesc Psychother 2015;14(1):98–110.
37. Rossouw TI, Fonagy P. Mentalization-based treatment for self-harm in adolescents: a randomized controlled trial. J Am Acad Child Adolesc Psychiatry 2012;51(12):1304–13.
38. Cristea IA, Gentili C, Cotet CD, et al. Efficacy of psychotherapies for borderline personality disorder: a systematic review and meta-analysis. JAMA Psychiatry 2017;74(4):319–28.

39. Courtney-Siedler E, Klein D, Miller A. Borderline personality disorder in adolescents. Clinical Psychology Science and Practice 2013;20:425–44.
40. Klimstra T. Adolescent personality development and identity formation. Child Dev Perspect 2013;7(2):80–4.
41. Meeus, 2016
42. Weisz JR, Kuppens S, Ng MY, et al. What five decades of research tells us about the effects of youth psychological therapy: a multilevel meta-analysis and implications for science and practice. Am Psychol 2017;72(2):79–117.
43. Miller AL, Carnesale MT, Courtney EA. Dialectical behavior therapy. In: Sharp C, Tackett JL, editors. Handbook of borderline personality disorder in children and adolescents. New York: Springer Science + Business Media; 2014. p. 385–401.
44. Miller AL, Rathus JH, DuBose AP, et al. Dialectical behavior therapy for adolescents. In: Dimeff LA, Koerner K, editors. Dialectical behavior therapy in clinical practice: applications across disorders and settings. New York: Guilford Press; 2007. p. 245–63.
45. Miller AL, Rathus JH, Linehan MM. Dialectical behavior therapy with suicidal adolescents. New York: Guilford Press; 2007.
46. Mulder R, Chanen AM. Effectiveness of cognitive analytic therapy for personality disorders. Br J Psychiatry 2013;202(2):89–90.
47. Rathus JH, Miller AL. DBT®skills manual for adolescents. New York: Guilford Press; 2015.
48. Rathus J, Campbell B, Miller A, et al. Treatment acceptability study of walking the middle path, a new DBT skills module for adolescents and their families. Am J Psychother 2015;69(2):163–78.
49. Kaufman J, Birmaher B, Brent D, et al. Schedule for affective disorders and schizophrenia for school-age children-present and lifetime version (K-SADS-PL): initial reliability and validity data. J Am Acad Child Adolesc Psychiatry 1997;36(7):980–8.
50. Mehlum L, Ramberg M, Tørmoen AJ, et al. Dialectical behavior therapy compared with enhanced usual care for adolescents with repeated suicidal and self-harming behavior: outcomes over a one-year follow-up. J Am Acad Child Adolesc Psychiatry 2016;55(4):295–300.
51. Mehlum L, Tørmoen AJ, Ramberg M, et al. Dialectical behavior therapy for adolescents with repeated suicidal and self-harming behavior: a randomized trial. J Am Acad Child Adolesc Psychiatry 2014;53(10):1082–91.
52. Bateman A, Fonagy P. Treatment of borderline personality disorder with psychoanalytically oriented partial hospitalization: an 18-month follow-up. Am J Psychiatry 2001;158(1):36–42.
53. Bateman A, Fonagy P. Effectiveness of partial hospitalization in the treatment of borderline personality disorder: a, randomized controlled trial. Am J Psychiatry 1999;156(10):1563–9.
54. Fonagy P, Rossouw T, Sharp C, et al. Mentalization-based treatment for adolescents with borderline traits. In: Sharp C, Tackett J, editors. Handbook of borderline personality disorder in children and adolescents. New York: Springer Science + Business Media; 2014. p. 313–32.
55. Hutsebaut J, Bales DL, Busschbach JJV, et al. The implementation of mentalization-based treatment for adolescents: a case study from an organizational, team and therapist perspective. Int J Ment Health Syst 2012;6(1):10.
56. Laurenssen E, Hutsebaut J, Feenstra DJ, et al. Feasibility of mentalization-based treatment for adolescents with borderline symptoms: a pilot study. Psychotherapy 2014;51(1):159–66.

57. Laurenssen EMP, Smits ML, Bales DL, et al. Day hospital mentalization-based treatment versus intensive outpatient mentalization-based treatment for patients with severe borderline personality disorder: Protocol of a multicentre randomized clinical trial. BMC Psychiatry 2014;14:301.

58. Gergely G. The social construction of the subjective self: the role of affect-mirroring, markedness, and ostensive communication in self-development. In: Mayes L, Fonagy P, Target M, editors. Developments in psychoanalysis. Developmental science and psychoanalysis: integration and innovation. London: Karnac Books; 2007. p. 45–88.

59. Asen E, Fonagy P. Mentalization-based family therapy. In: Bateman AW, Fonagy P, editors. Handbook of mentalizing in mental health practice. Arlington (VA): American Psychiatric Publishing; 2012. p. 107–28.

60. Normandin L, Ensink K, Yeomans FE, et al. Transference-focused psychotherapy for personality disorders in adolescence. In: Sharp C, Tackett C, editors. Handbook of borderline personality disorder in children and adolescents. New York: Springer Science & Business Media; 2014. p. 333–59.

61. Kernberg OF. Severe personality disorders: psychotherapeutic strategies. New Haven (CT): Yale University Press; 1984.

62. Kernberg OF. Borderline conditions and pathological narcissism. New York: Aronson; 1975.

63. Kernberg OF, Yeomans FE, Clarkin JF, et al. Transference focused psychotherapy: overview and update. Int J Psychoanal 2008;89(3):601–20.

64. Clarkin JF, Posner M. Defining the mechanisms of borderline personality disorder. Psychopathology 2005;38(2):56–63.

65. Clarkin JF, Levy KN, Lenzenweger MF, et al. Evaluating three treatments for borderline personality disorder: a multiwave study. Am J Psychiatry 2007;164: 922–8.

66. Doering S, Hörz S, Rentrop M, et al. Transference-focused psychotherapy v. treatment by community psychotherapists for borderline personality disorder: randomised controlled trial. Br J Psychiatry 2010;196:389–95.

67. Levy KN, Meehan KB, Clouthier TL, et al. In: Fishman DB, Messer SB, Edwards DJA, et al, editors. Case studies within psychotherapy trials: integrating qualitative and quantitative methods. New York: Oxford University Press; 2017. p. 190–245.

68. Selzer MA, Kernberg P, Fibel B, et al. The personality assessment interview: preliminary report. Psychiatry 1987;50(2):142–53.

69. Yeomans FE, Delaney JC, Levy KN. Behavioral activation in TFP: the role of the treatment contract in transference-focused psychotherapy. Psychotherapy (Chic) 2017;54(3):260–6.

70. Krischer M, Ponton-Rodriguez T, Gooran GR, et al. Übertragungsfokussierte Psychotherapie von Borderline-Jugendlichen im tagesklinischen Setting. [[Transference focused psychotherapy for borderline-adolescents in a day clinic treatment program]]. Prax Kinderpsychol Kinderpsychiatr 2017;66(6):445–63 [in German].

71. Ryle A, Fawkes L. Multiplicity of selves and others: cognitive analytic therapy. J Clin Psychol 2007;63(2):165–74.

72. Stepp SD, Lazarus SA, Byrd AL. A systematic review of risk factors prospectively associated with borderline personality disorder: taking stock and moving forward. Personal Disord 2016;7(4):316–23.

73. Venta A, Sharp C, Patriquin M, et al. Amygdala-frontal connectivity predicts internalizing symptom recovery among inpatient adolescents. J Affect Disord 2018; 225:453–9.

74. Weisz JR, Krumholz LS, Santucci L, et al. Shrinking the gap between research and practice: tailoring and testing youth psychotherapies in clinical care contexts. Annu Rev Clin Psychol 2015;11:139–63.
75. Caspi A, Houts RM, Belsky DW, et al. The p factor: one general psychopathology factor in the structure of psychiatric disorders? Clin Psychol Sci 2014;2(2): 119–37.
76. Laceulle OM, Vollebergh WAM, Ormel J. The structure of psychopathology in adolescence: replication of a general psychopathology factor in the trails study. Clin Psychol Sci 2015;3(6):850–60.
77. Patalay P, Belsky J, Fonagy P, et al. The extent and specificity of relative age effects on mental health and functioning in early adolescence. J Adolesc Health 2015;57(5):475–81.
78. Sharp C, Wright AGC, Fowler JC, et al. The structure of personality pathology: Both general ('g') and specific ('s') factors? J Abnorm Psychol 2015;124(2): 387–98.
79. Bjureberg J, Sahlin H, Hellner C, et al. BioMedical Central Open Access Psychiatry 2017;17(411):1–13.
80. Gratz KL, Weiss NH, McDermott MJ, et al. Emotion dysregulation mediates the relation between borderline personality disorder symptoms and later physical health symptoms. J Personal Disord 2017;31(4):433–48.
81. McCutcheon L, Chanen a, Fraser R, et al. Tips and techniques for engaging and managing the reluctant, resistant or hostile young person. Med J Aust 2007; 187(7):S64–7.
82. Fonagy P, Luyten P, Bateman A. Treating borderline personality disorder with psychotherapy: where do we go from here? JAMA Psychiatry 2017;74(4):316–7.

UNITED STATES POSTAL SERVICE® Statement of Ownership, Management, and Circulation
(All Periodicals Publications Except Requester Publications)

1. Publication Title	2. Publication Number	3. Filing Date
PSYCHIATRIC CLINICS OF NORTH AMERICA	000 – 703	9/18/2018

4. Issue Frequency	5. Number of Issues Published Annually	6. Annual Subscription Price
MAR, JUN, SEP, DEC	4	$321.00

7. Complete Mailing Address of Known Office of Publication (Not printer) (Street, city, county, state, and ZIP+4®)

ELSEVIER INC.
230 Park Avenue, Suite 800
New York, NY 10169

Contact Person
STEPHEN R. BUSHING

Telephone (Include area code)
215-239-3688

8. Complete Mailing Address of Headquarters or General Business Office of Publisher (Not printer)

ELSEVIER INC.
230 Park Avenue, Suite 800
New York, NY 10169

9. Full Names and Complete Mailing Addresses of Publisher, Editor, and Managing Editor (Do not leave blank)

Publisher (Name and complete mailing address)

TAYLOR E BALL, ELSEVIER INC.
1600 JOHN F KENNEDY BLVD. SUITE 1800
PHILADELPHIA, PA 19103-2899

Editor (Name and complete mailing address)

LAUREN BOYLE, ELSEVIER INC.
1600 JOHN F KENNEDY BLVD. SUITE 1800
PHILADELPHIA, PA 19103-2899

Managing Editor (Name and complete mailing address)

PATRICK MANLEY, ELSEVIER INC.
1600 JOHN F KENNEDY BLVD. SUITE 1800
PHILADELPHIA, PA 19103-2899

10. Owner (Do not leave blank. If the publication is owned by a corporation, give the name and address of the corporation immediately followed by the names and addresses of all stockholders owning or holding 1 percent or more of the total amount of stock. If not owned by a corporation, give the names and addresses of the individual owners. If owned by a partnership or other unincorporated firm, give its name and address as well as those of each individual owner. If the publication is published by a nonprofit organization, give its name and address.)

Full Name	Complete Mailing Address
WHOLLY OWNED SUBSIDIARY OF REED/ELSEVIER, US HOLDINGS	1600 JOHN F KENNEDY BLVD. SUITE 1800 PHILADELPHIA, PA 19103-2899

11. Known Bondholders, Mortgagees, and Other Security Holders Owning or Holding 1 Percent or More of Total Amount of Bonds, Mortgages, or Other Securities. If none, check box → ☐ None

Full Name	Complete Mailing Address
N/A	

12. Tax Status (For completion by nonprofit organizations authorized to mail at nonprofit rates) (Check one)
The purpose, function, and nonprofit status of this organization and the exempt status for federal income tax purposes:
☒ Has Not Changed During Preceding 12 Months
☐ Has Changed During Preceding 12 Months (Publisher must submit explanation of change with this statement)

PS Form **3526**, July 2014 [Page 1 of 4 (see instructions page 4)]   PSN: 7530-01-000-9931   PRIVACY NOTICE: See our privacy policy on www.usps.com.

---

13. Publication Title		14. Issue Date for Circulation Data Below
PSYCHIATRIC CLINICS OF NORTH AMERICA		JUNE 2018

15. Extent and Nature of Circulation		Average No. Copies Each Issue During Preceding 12 Months	No. Copies of Single Issue Published Nearest to Filing Date
a. Total Number of Copies (Net press run)		234	296
b. Paid Circulation (By Mail and Outside the Mail)	(1) Mailed Outside-County Paid Subscriptions Stated on PS Form 3541 (Include paid distribution above nominal rate, advertiser's proof copies, and exchange copies)	104	125
	(2) Mailed In-County Paid Subscriptions Stated on PS Form 3541 (Include paid distribution above nominal rate, advertiser's proof copies, and exchange copies)	0	0
	(3) Paid Distribution Outside the Mails Including Sales Through Dealers and Carriers, Street Vendors, Counter Sales, and Other Paid Distribution Outside USPS®	73	78
	(4) Paid Distribution by Other Classes of Mail Through the USPS (e.g., First-Class Mail®)	0	0
c. Total Paid Distribution (Sum of 15b (1), (2), (3), and (4))		177	203
d. Free or Nominal Rate Distribution (By Mail and Outside the Mail)	(1) Free or Nominal Rate Outside-County Copies included on PS Form 3541	46	74
	(2) Free or Nominal Rate In-County Copies Included on PS Form 3541	0	0
	(3) Free or Nominal Rate Copies Mailed at Other Classes Through the USPS (e.g., First-Class Mail)	0	0
	(4) Free or Nominal Rate Distribution Outside the Mail (Carriers or other means)	0	0
e. Total Free or Nominal Rate Distribution (Sum of 15d (1), (2), (3) and (4))		46	74
f. Total Distribution (Sum of 15c and 15e)		223	277
g. Copies not Distributed (See Instructions to Publishers #4 (page #3))		11	19
h. Total (Sum of 15f and g)		234	296
i. Percent Paid (15c divided by 15f times 100)		79.37%	73.29%

* If you are claiming electronic copies, go to line 16 on page 3. If you are not claiming electronic copies, skip to line 17 on page 3.

16. Electronic Copy Circulation	Average No. Copies Each Issue During Preceding 12 Months	No. Copies of Single Issue Published Nearest to Filing Date
a. Paid Electronic Copies	0	0
b. Total Paid Print Copies (Line 15c) + Paid Electronic Copies (Line 16a)	177	203
c. Total Print Distribution (Line 15f) + Paid Electronic Copies (Line 16a)	223	277
d. Percent Paid (Both Print & Electronic Copies) (16b divided by 16c × 100)	79.37%	73.29%

☒ I certify that 50% of all my distributed copies (electronic and print) are paid above a nominal price.

17. Publication of Statement of Ownership

☒ If the publication is a general publication, publication of this statement is required. Will be printed in the DECEMBER 2018 issue of this publication.   ☐ Publication not required.

18. Signature and Title of Editor, Publisher, Business Manager, or Owner

STEPHEN R. BUSHING - INVENTORY DISTRIBUTION CONTROL MANAGER

Stephen R. Bushing   Date 9/18/2018

I certify that all information furnished on this form is true and complete. I understand that anyone who furnishes false or misleading information on this form or who omits material or information requested on the form may be subject to criminal sanctions (including fines and imprisonment) and/or civil sanctions (including civil penalties).

PS Form **3526**, July 2014 (Page 3 of 4)   PRIVACY NOTICE: See our privacy policy on www.usps.com

Moving?

Make sure your subscription moves with you!

To notify us of your new address, find your **Clinics Account Number** (located on your mailing label above your name), and contact customer service at:

Email: journalscustomerservice-usa@elsevier.com

800-654-2452 (subscribers in the U.S. & Canada)
314-447-8871 (subscribers outside of the U.S. & Canada)

Fax number: 314-447-8029

Elsevier Health Sciences Division
Subscription Customer Service
3251 Riverport Lane
Maryland Heights, MO 63043

*To ensure uninterrupted delivery of your subscription, please notify us at least 4 weeks in advance of move.